Official health statistics

AN UNOFFICIAL GUIDE

D0589573

Official health statistics

AN UNOFFICIAL GUIDE

Radical Statistics Health Group

Edited by

Susan Kerrison and Alison Macfarlane

A member of the Hodder Headline Group
LONDON

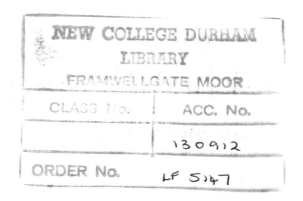
First published in Great Britain in 2000 by
Arnold, a member of the Hodder Headline Group,
338 Euston Road, London NW1 3BH

http://www.arnoldpublishers.com

British Library Cataloguing in Publication Data
A catalogue record for this book is available from the British Library

ISBN 0 340 73132 X (pb)

1 2 3 4 5 6 7 8 9 10

Commissioning Editor: Clare Parker
Project Manager: Paula O'Connell
Production Editor: Wendy Rooke
Production Controller: Iain McWilliams
Cover Design: Terry Griffiths

Typeset in 10pt Palatino by J&L Composition Ltd, Filey, North Yorkshire
Printed and bound in Great Britain by Redwood Books, Trowbridge, Wiltshire

What do you think about this book? Or any other Arnold title?
Please send your comments to feedback.arnold@hodder.co.uk

Contents

Contributors and acknowledgements

Radical Statistics was formed in 1975 by statisticians and other people who shared a common concern about the political implications of statistical work and an awareness of the actual and potential misuse of statistics. The group as a whole publishes *Radical statistics* three times a year and has an annual conference, an email list and a web site. In 1999, it produced a book, *Statistics in society: the arithmetic of politics*, edited by Daniel Dorling and Stephen Simpson and also published by Arnold. Apart from these, most of its activities take place in its subgroups, of which the Radical Statistics Health Group, drawing its membership from people working in health services and medical research and in the National Health Service, has been the most prolific.

Starting in the late 1970s, we published three pamphlets *Whose priorities? Priorities for health and personal social services in England, RAW(P) deals: sharing resources for health in England* and *In defence of the NHS*, which looked critically at the ways in which statistics were used in relation to health service policy under a Labour government. This led us to a critique of the data available and we published the first edition of *The unofficial guide to official health statistics* in 1980 as a 64-page pamphlet, of which we sold 4000 copies.

After a quiet period, the group was very active in the late 1980s and early 1990s in exposing fallacies in the ways in which the Conservative government used statistics to justify its health and health care policies. We did this in a variety of ways, ranging from *Unsafe in their hands,* an 11-page typescript which we invited people to photocopy and pass on, through articles in magazines and peer reviewed journals, including the *Nursing times, Health service journal* and the *British medical journal* to a full length book, *Facing the figures: what really is happening to the National Health Service?* This book, published in 1987, had a considerable impact on government statistics when it was used as source material for a Channel four documentary, *Cooking the books*.

The need for a new edition of the *Unofficial guide* had been apparent for some time and we started work on one, but growing pressures of work gave us less and less 'spare time' in which to organise, research and write it. Had it not been for the generosity of the Lord Ashdown trust, which provided some funding for one of us to work on it, this book would never have come to fruition. We should like to thank the trust for its generosity. In these changed times we looked, for the first time, for a commercial publisher and were delighted that Arnold decided to publish it. We should like to thank Clare Parker, who commissioned it, her successors Cathy Peck and Aileen Parlane, the production editor Wendy Rooke, copy-editor Jane Smith and everyone else at Arnold involved in the publication.

The work of the named contributors to this book would not have been possible without help from the many people who provided information and checked the text for accuracy. As in the past, they include members of the Government Statistical Service. We are glad that, as a consequence of greater openness, we can now thank them publicly, while acknowledging that the views we express are not necessarily shared by the Government Statistical Service. We should like to thank Paul Abberley, Penny Babb, Patsy Bailey, Vera Carstairs, Nish Chaturvedi, Norman Champ, Jim Connelly, Nirupa Dattani, Sue Dodd, Bob Ehrens, Naomi Fulop, Stephanie Goubet, Douglas Harding, Hilary Heine, Gwenda Hughes, Sylvia Kingaby, Lesz Lancucki, Wincen Lowe, Miranda Mugford, Anna McCormack, Corinne McDonald, Helen Maguire, Anna Molesworth, Janet Mortimer, Carol Orchard, Naomi Pfeffer, Ruth Pinder, Allyson Pollock, Steve Price, Vera Ruddock, Melanie Smith, Jim Stokoe, Mark Svenson, Grant Whiting and Richard Willmer.

The people who wrote this book are listed in the table of contents in the order in which their contribution appears, rather than in a way which reflects any hierarchy of authorship. They are also listed in alphabetical order.

Ben Armstrong currently works in the Environmental Epidemiology Unit at the London School of Hygiene and Tropical Medicine. He has been undertaking research on statistics of occupational health risks in England and Quebec since 1978. Ben wrote the section on occupational ill-health statistics in Chapter 6.

Phil Atkinson is a senior scientist working in the London regional office of the Communicable Disease Surveillance Centre, part of the Public Health Laboratory Service. He has been working with communicable disease data for over 6 years, with a particular interest in the geographical aspects of infections. Phil wrote the section on communicable diseases in Chapter 3 in conjunction with John Watson.

Mel Bartley works in the Department of Epidemiology and Public Health at University College London, on the Whitehall Study and other studies of health inequality and social factors in health and disease. She has been a member of the Radical Statistics Group since 1987 and participated in the production of *Facing the figures*. Mel contributed to the section on measuring the health effects of affluence and disadvantage in Chapter 4 in conjunction with Alison Macfarlane.

Yoav Ben-Shlomo is a Senior Lecturer in Clinical Epidemiology at the Department of Social Medicine, University of Bristol. Yoav contributed to the section on housing statistics in Chapter 6 in conjunction with Rebekah Widdowfield.

Annette Boaz is a Senior Research Fellow in the Local Government Centre, University of Warwick and is currently working on the evaluation of Better Government for Older People programme. Annette contributed to the section on diet in Chapter 6 in conjunction with Eric Brunner.

Eric Brunner is Senior Lecturer in Epidemiology at University College London and a member of the International Centre for Health and Society. The role of nutrition and social inequalities in health is a key interest. Eric contributed the section on diet in Chapter 6 in conjunction with Annette Boaz.

Robin Darton is a Research Fellow at the Personal Social Services Research Unit, University of Kent at Canterbury. He has a background in psychology and statistics, and research interests in health and social services provision for elderly people and in methodological issues relating to the design and analysis of studies of health and social care. Robin wrote the section on residential and nursing home statistics in Chapter 9.

Adrian Davis is a Bristol-based consultant specialising in the relationship between transport and health. He is author of the 1997 BMA report Road Transport and Health, and wrote the main transport paper for the Acheson Inquiry on Inequalities in Health. Adrian contributed to the section on transport in Chapter 7 in conjunction with Ben Lane and Stephen Potter.

Danny Dorling is Professor of Human Geography at the University of Leeds. Previously he was a Reader in Human Geography at the School of Geographical Sciences at the University of Bristol. Danny wrote Chapter 2 in conjunction with Mary Shaw and Jenny Grundy.

Declan Gaffney is a research fellow at the Health Policy and Health Services Research Unit at the School of Public Policy, University College London, working on NHS planning, public expenditure and the use of private finance in the public sector. Declan wrote the section on government expenditure on the NHS and financial information in Chapter 8.

Sylvia Godden is a research fellow at the Health Services Policy Research Unit at University College London and also works in the Public Health Department at Merton, Sutton and Wandsworth Health Authority. She is currently undertaking research on the financing of primary care. Sylvia contributed to the section on community and primary care statistics in Chapter 8.

Jenny Grundy teaches geography and sociology at Durham Johnston Comprehensive school, County Durham. Previously she was a research associate at the Department of Geography, Newcastle University. Jenny contributed to Chapter 2 in conjunction with Danny Dorling and Mary Shaw.

Sue Hare is an information co-ordinator at Aric, a research and information centre for Atmosphere, Climate and Environment based at Manchester Metropolitan University. Sue contributed the section on atmospheric pollution in Chapter 7.

Jenny Head is a statistician with an interest in health surveys and official health statistics. She works in the Department of Epidemiology and Public Health at University College London. Jenny wrote the section on ethnic minorities and migrant groups in Chapter 4.

Paul Johnson is currently senior economist at the Financial Services Agency. Previously he was deputy director of the Institute for Fiscal Studies. He is a member of the Pension Provision Group and of the Commission on taxation and citizenship. He is author of many articles and books on pensions, social security, inequality and taxation, including the book *Inequality in the UK* published by Oxford University Press. Paul wrote the section on poverty statistics in Chapter 5.

Susan Kerrison is Rubin Research Fellow in the Health and Health Services Research Unit at the School of Public Policy, University College London. She is currently undertaking research on the regulation of UK health care providers and services. Susan wrote the introduction in conjunction with Alison Macfarlane and contributed the section on disability statistics in Chapter 4 and to Chapter 8.

Ben Lane is a transport consultant based at Ecolane, Bristol, UK. He has conducted work on behalf of the EC-funded Utopia and Strategic Niche Management projects. These European projects investigate the socio-technical issues which can affect the introduction of new transport fuels and vehicle technologies. Ben wrote the section on transport in Chapter 7 in conjunction with Adrian Davis and Stephen Potter.

Alison Macfarlane has been involved with the Radical Statistics Health Group since it first got under way in the 1970s and has contributed to many of its publications. She is a statistician specialising in the interpretation and secondary analysis of official health statistics and works in research on maternity care at the National Perinatal Epidemiology Unit. Alison wrote Chapter 1 and Chapter 8 in conjunction with Susan Kerrison. She wrote the section on registration and notification of vital events, births, congenital anomalies and abortions in Chapter 3 and the section on affluence and disadvantage in Chapter 4 in conjunction with Mel Bartley.

Azeem Majeed is senior lecturer in general practice at the School of Public Policy, University College London. His academic interests include the use of routinely collected health-related information for health services research. Azeem contributed to the section on mortality statistics in Chapter 3.

Nick Miller is Research and Information Manager for a Social Services Department in a large English county. He is involved with health colleagues in developing means of sharing information covering health and social services. He is a member of the national Social Services Research Group. Nick wrote the section on social services statistics in Chapter 8.

Stephen Potter is a senior research fellow in the Technology Faculty at the Open University. He has worked on a variety of research projects covering transport, energy and environmental issues, urban studies and design management, as well as contributing to a number of the Open University's courses, including the new Technology Foundation Course. Stephen wrote the section on transport statistics in Chapter 7 in conjunction with Adrian Davis and Ben Lane.

Mary Shaw is an ESRC research fellow at the School of Geographical Sciences at the University of Bristol and teaches and researches medical geography and sociology. Mary wrote Chapter 2 in conjunction with Danny Dorling and Jenny Grundy.

Sarah Tanner is Programme Co-ordinator of research into pensions, savings and retirement at the Institute for Fiscal Studies. She is the author of a number of publications on savings and pensions, including the recent IFS report *Household saving in the UK*. She is also a participant in the National Bureau of Economic Research International Social Security Project. Sarah wrote the section on wealth statistics in Chapter 5.

Mary Taylor is a senior research officer at Friends of the Earth and has been involved in pollution issues for several years. She is currently working on international legislation on access to information and the development of public participation in environmental decision-making. Mary wrote the section on industrial pollution for Chapter 7.

Ray Thomas is a research fellow at the Open University and an active member of the Radical Statistics Group and the Royal Statistical Society. Ray wrote the section on unemployment statistics for Chapter 5.

Neil Vickers is a literary scholar who was formerly Researcher in Public Health Sciences at St George's Hospital Medical School. He is now Fellow and College Lecturer in English at Corpus Christi College, Cambridge. Neil wrote the section on cancer statistics for Chapter 3.

John Watson is a consultant infectious disease epidemiologist based at the Public Health Laboratory Service, Communicable Disease Surveillance Centre in London. John wrote the section on communicable diseases in Chapter 3 in conjunction with Phil Atkinson.

Rebekah Widdowfield is a research fellow in the Department of City and Regional Planning at the University of Wales, Cardiff. Her research is predominantly concerned with housing, homelessness and related issues. Rebekah wrote the section on housing in Chapter 6 in conjunction with Yoav Ben Shlomo.

Setting the scene

THE GOVERNMENT STATISTICAL SERVICE AND THE COLLECTION OF OFFICIAL HEALTH STATISTICS

Susan Kerrison and Alison Macfarlane

The Government Statistical Service
General guides and collections of data
An overview of official health statistics

Official health statistics: an unofficial guide has been written as a second edition of *The unofficial guide to official health statistics*, which was first published by Radical Statistics Health Group in 1980. The term 'health statistics' is a loose one. It includes the statistics collected about health services and the people who use them and statistics which are collected about the population as a whole. Thus, most relate to illness, death and the use of health services and very few relate to health in a positive sense.

The first edition covered the range of statistics usually acknowledged as being related to health, notably those derived from registration and notification of births and deaths, cancer and communicable disease and statistics about the National Health Service (NHS). In planning this second edition, we took a wider view, as well as covering the original ground more fully. We therefore extended the scope of the publication to describe statistics about known causes of ill-health, such as poverty, unemployment, adverse effects of environmental hazards, air pollution, housing, diet and transport.

The census and official surveys specifically focusing on health, or with a health component, are described in Chapter 2; data collected as by-products of vital events, notably birth, death, diagnosis of a communicable disease or cancer, are described in Chapter 3. Chapters 4 to 7 describe how both surveys and administrative statistics are used in combination to give a picture of health inequalities and the factors associated with poor health, such as poverty, work, housing, diet and the environment. Chapter 8 describes the administrative statistics collected by the NHS, and Chapter 9 those collected by local authority social service departments.

The book concentrates on statistics collected in England, but we have also attempted to describe statistics relating to Wales, Scotland and Northern Ireland. In some cases there is very little difference between data collected in the four countries of the UK, while in others they differ considerably. In particular, Scotland devotes proportionately more resources to data collection and analysis than the other countries and collects more detailed information about the NHS and about residential care. Differences in the datasets and publications may widen as a consequence of devolution, although the pressure to produce 'national statistics' for the UK as a whole might lead to greater consultation and harmonisation.

An important subject, which we have covered only briefly, is the extent to which data are available for local areas. This is important for local planning and resource distribution, particularly in relation to the establishment of primary care groups. Many datasets, especially those designed to produce aggregated totals and those based on samples of areas, cannot be disaggregated to produce data for areas as small as electoral wards, and some data are available only at regional and national level. A further omission is data on health care and the legal system. Medical negligence claims, claims against health authorities about the provision of services and cases before tribunals are playing an increasingly important role in health policy.

We asked contributors to this new and expanded edition to answer four questions about their particular subject areas. They were asked to outline which data are collected, how they are they collected, where they are published and the strengths and limitations of each dataset and the main publications associated with it.

To set the scene for these more detailed accounts, this introduction starts by outlining the development of official data collection and then goes on to give a broad overview of the scope and range of official statistics relevant to health. This raises the question of what we mean by official statistics.

Until relatively recently, 'official statistics' could be defined as statistics collected, processed, analysed and usually published by the government, primarily for its own use. This definition fits less well as the government increasingly contracts out the collection of statistics to other agencies, while also selling data from the Government Statistical Service to health authorities, local authorities, private companies, researchers and others. It also sells services, such as the use of the National Health Service Central Register, for research and other purposes. For the purposes of this guide, 'official statistics' is taken to mean statistics collected, commissioned or published by the central government departments and agencies, local government and the NHS. In addition, we have occasionally included data collected or published by other bodies where they are of major importance and arise from research funded by the government.

The Government Statistical Service

A very brief history

Many of the present systems for collecting routine statistics about the health of the population date back to the mid-nineteenth century, although earlier systems of data collection had been in operation for several centuries. The civil registration of births, marriages and deaths began in 1837, and the General Register Office for England and Wales was set up to co-ordinate the work of local registrars of births, marriages and deaths.[1] The office also took over responsibility for the census, which had been undertaken since 1801. With William Farr as its 'compiler of abstracts', the office began to develop methods for analysing birth and death statistics.[2] An important aspect of this was assessing the impact of social and environmental factors. Data from the General Register Office were influential in arguing for improvements in public health through measures such as sanitation and clean water supplies. General register offices were set up in Scotland and Northern Ireland later in the century.

The Board of Trade set up a statistical department in the 1830s and the army and the poor law commissioners were all collecting data at this period. The Home Office began collecting crime statistics in the mid-nineteenth-century.[2] This was a period when people interested in using statistics to argue for social reform founded statistical societies in major cities. The Statistical Society of London, later to become the Royal Statistical Society, was founded in 1834.

There was considerable interest in hospital statistics at this period and the Statistical Society of London set up a committee on the subject in 1840. As hospitals were not run or funded by the state, they could not be required to collect data for it. The Statistical Society encouraged them to collect data in a comparable way, and Florence Nightingale proposed a 'uniform plan' in a paper written for the International Statistical Congress in London in 1860.[3] This was not adopted and most hospitals continued to compile statistics in their own way. National data collection did not start until some elements of health care began to be funded by the state in the 1920s and 1930s. The wide-ranging collection of data about health care developed under the NHS from 1948 onwards. This association between data collection and the running of services by the state is a major reason for the lack of data about the private sector, a problem which became much more serious as the role of the private sector expanded from the mid-1990s onwards.[4]

Social surveys undertaken by and for the government have a much shorter history. In 1941, stimulated by a wide range of problems which arose in wartime, the government set up a separate agency, the Wartime Social Survey, to carry out questionnaire surveys on a wide range of specific topics for government departments and semi-official organisations.[1] The work continued after the war. As well as doing work for almost all government departments, royal commissions and special inquiries, the agency also developed a programme of continuous surveys.

The Family Expenditure Survey started in 1957 and an annual Food Survey was conducted for the Ministry of Agriculture every year from 1950 onwards. The General Household Survey, which began in 1970, collects more general information about housing and social conditions. This was the year when the General Register Office merged with the Government Social Survey to form the Office of Population Censuses and Surveys (OPCS). The office was accountable to the Department of Health and Social Security and later to the Department of Health.

The other specialised statistical office within government was the Business

Statistics Office, whose role was to collect economic statistics. Many other statisticians worked in individual government departments. The role of government statistics was expanded in the 1960s by Harold Wilson, a prime minister who had started his working life as a government statistician. He gave the director of the Central Statistical Office the additional role of the head of the decentralised Government Statistical Service (GSS). During the 1960s, the collection of social statistics expanded and developed and the annual publication *Social trends* started.

The late 1980s and early 1990s was a period marked by moves towards increasing centralisation in government statistics and by mounting controversy about the quality and credibility of official statistics. After a review by Sir Derek Rayner in 1980, major cuts were made in the Government Statistical Service in the early 1980s.[5] Rayner proposed what became known as the 'Rayner doctrine', that government should collect only the statistics it needs for its own purposes. The contraction led to widespread concern about the quality of government statistics and, in the late 1980s, errors appeared in key economic series. After another review,[6] further changes were made. The Central Statistical Office was moved from the Cabinet Office to the Treasury. It also took over responsibility for statistics in the Department of Trade and Industry, including the Business Statistics Office.

The concern about integrity and quality continued. A Channel Four documentary, *Cooking the books,* based heavily on information from Radical Statistics publications, and Radical Statistics Health Group's book, *Facing the figures,* published in 1987,[7] in particular raised the alarm and articles appeared in the national press. The Royal Statistical Society responded by setting up a committee on official statistics. Its report, *Official statistics: counting with confidence,*[8] recommended an Official Statistics Act which would safeguard the autonomy and constitutional position of official statistics and an independent National Statistics Commission to oversee official statistics.

Despite moves towards greater independence and openness, there is still widespread concern about the integrity of the Government Statistical Service. In 1998, the government published a green paper, *Statistics: a matter of trust,* in which it set out four models for an independent National Statistical Service.[9] Disturbingly, the consultation on the green paper was followed by a long silence. During this there was a review of the Office for National Statistics (ONS) by management consultants KPMG, who suggested privatising many of ONS' activities. Concerns about the reliability of the average earnings index led to an enquiry, whose report was published in March 1999, and the announcement of the early retirement of the head of the Government Statistical Service.

The white paper *Building trust in statistics* eventually emerged in October 1999.[10] It set out arrangements for a Statistics Commission, as an independent, non-executive body with seven members and a small permanent staff. No legislation was proposed to underpin its work on the grounds that 'Demands on legislative time are considerable and likely to remain so.'[10] Instead, the Statistics Commission will be asked to review the need for legislation once it has been in existence for 2 years. The scope of 'national statistics' was defined narrowly as 'too ambitious a programme could pose considerable practical diffi-culties.'[10] Initially, at least, 'national statistics' will include 'all ONS publica-tions and public access databases and, with the agreement of Ministers, other statistics published by Departments'.[10]

The changing structure

In 1995, when the Department of Employment merged with the Department of Education, the Central Statistical Office took over its Labour Market Statis-tics Group. A year later, on 1 April 1996, the Central Statistical Office and the OPCS merged to become a 'next steps' agency, the ONS. The ONS has respon-sibility for the census, the registration of births, marriages and deaths in England and Wales, and the collection of social and economics statistics. The director of the ONS is also head of the Government Statistical Service, but this is a co-ordinating role. Each government department continues its own pro-gramme of data collection, analysis and publication.

The changes set out in *Building trust in statistics* have not altered this greatly. A new Head of National Statistics or National Statistician has taken over the roles of the director of the ONS and has overall professional respon-sibility for 'national statistics'. This includes working closely with the heads of profession for statistics in other departments and taking account of the views of users.

The ONS and the statisticians and related staff who work in individual government departments form the Government Statistical Service. Its struc-ture and activities are described in its *Annual report*.[11] As of 1 April 1998, 4560 full-time equivalent staff worked in the Government Statistical Service. Of the 604 in the Statistician Group, 170 worked in the ONS.[11] The director of the ONS is directly accountable to the Chancellor of the Exchequer, and their rela-tionship is set out in a framework document. The director of ONS is also Reg-istrar General for England and Wales and has a coordinating role as head of the Government Statistical Service. ONS has, in theory at least, a certain amount of managerial and financial freedom from the civil service. It compiles birth and death statistics and collects data about the health of the population in England and Wales, but data about health and social care are collected by the Department of Health and by the National Assembly for Wales, formerly known as the Welsh Office.

The Northern Ireland Statistics and Research Agency (NISRA) was also established as a 'next steps' agency in April 1996. Its responsibilities broadly correspond with those of the ONS. It is an executive agency responsible for registrations, the census in Northern Ireland and statistical research. Some of its statisticians are outposted to other Northern Ireland departments, agencies and non-departmental public bodies. In particular, some work in the Depart-ment of Health, Social Services and Public Safety, whose Regional Information Branch collects data about health and social care. The Northern Ireland Statis-tics and Research Agency is not part of the Government Statistical Service, but has close links with it.

In Scotland, the General Register Office for Scotland is responsible for registration data, the census in Scotland and demographic statistics. The Information and Statistics Division of the Common Services Agency of the NHS in Scotland is responsible for the collection and publication of most data about health care. Data about social care are collected by the Scottish Executive's Community Care and Children's Social Work statistics groups.

In addition to appearing in statistical publications, data from each department appear in its own annual report, in which the government also sets out the expenditure plans for the department concerned. The Department of Health's expenditure plans are described in Chapter 8.

As well as the ONS and the Department of Health, there are a number of executive bodies and regulatory authorities whose functions are related to health and include collecting data. They include the new Care Standards Commission, the National Blood Authority, the Human Fertilisation and Embryology Authority, and the Prescription Pricing Authority. The annual reports of these bodies can be important sources of statistical information. For example, the annual report of the Prescription Pricing Authority contains statistics on prescribing, tabulated by health authority and region. Information about these bodies, including details of the organisation's annual report and where it can be obtained, are published annually by the Cabinet Office in *Public bodies*.

General guides and collections of data

Some guides to official data and publications containing official statistics on a range of subjects, including health and health services, are now published in both print and electronic form. The main guide in print form is the *Guide to official statistics*, the most recent edition of which was published in 2000.[12] This lists sources of government statistics in England, Wales, Scotland and Northern Ireland by topic area. Since this was published, the ONS has been developing a web site, *Statbase*, which includes information about data sources. In addition, the ONS publishes a free catalogue of key Government Statistical Service publications. In 1999 this was called *The source.*

Three main annual compendia are the *Annual abstract of statistics, Regional trends* and *Social trends*. The *Annual abstract* contains tables for the UK and its constituent countries, with trends over the past 10 years or so. These include a useful set of summary tables giving trends in NHS spending and activity. Data for Northern Ireland, Scotland and Wales are published in *Northern Ireland annual abstract of statistics, The Scottish abstract of statistics* and *The digest of Welsh statistics. Regional trends* contains the most recent data available on a variety of subjects for the 'standard' regions of England and for Wales, Scotland and Northern Ireland. *Social trends* draws data together from a wide range of sources and includes sections on health, education, housing and other socioeconomic factors. Each edition includes special coverage of particular issues. The ONS has developed a series of short publications called *Social focus*, containing a range of information on geographical areas and social groups. These include, for example, *Social focus on London, Social focus on*

Northern Ireland, *Social focus on children*, *Social focus on women* and *Social focus on ethnic minorities*. These publications are useful introductions, but their coverage is superficial and their prices are relatively high.

Health and personal social services statistics for England includes a range of data on the subject for England. Data for Wales are divided between *Health statistics Wales* and *Social services statistics Wales*, published by the National Assembly for Wales, formerly the Welsh Office. *Scottish health statistics*, published by the Information and Statistics Division of the NHS in Scotland, contains data about health care. Health and social service data for Northern Ireland are divided between *Hospital statistics* and *Community statistics*. These publications are described more fully in Chapters 8 and 9. General overviews of changes in the health of the population and of key issues in health care can be found in the annual reports of the four chief medical officers. *On the state of the public health* is published annually by the Department of Health and similar reports are published by the other three countries.

This book concentrates on sources available in print, but datasets are becoming increasingly available in electronic form. The *Guide to official statistics* and *Regional trends* are both available on the internet. Every edition of *Social trends* is now available on CD-ROM. Data from the 1991 and 1981 censuses have been made available in computer-readable formats. Many of the ONS's population and vital statistics are available on diskette or CD-ROM. Many data from the General Register Office for Scotland are now available on its web site.

In 1998, the ONS launched a web site called *Statbase*. This consists of a free electronic catalogue of Government Statistical Service publications and a limited database of key economic and social statistics, drawn from *Regional trends* and *Social trends*. *Statbase* is at an early stage in its development at the time of writing and its descriptions of datasets are still very limited.

The Economic and Social Research Council's data archive at the University of Essex is the principal repository for social science and humanities datasets in the UK. Its emphasis is on survey data. The Bibliographical Information Retrieval Online (BIRON) service contains descriptions of what is available. It is mainly geared towards academic users. By 1999, it held approximately 5000 datasets, mostly but not exclusively relating to the second half of the twentieth century. They include the census, the General Household Survey and many of the other surveys mentioned in this guide. The Public Record Office has commissioned the University of London Computer Centre to establish a similar archive of electronic data from government departments. A commercial depository, SPSS MR, formerly Quantime Ltd, in London offers services which include the provision of Labour Force Survey data going back to 1979. A non-commercial depository, the National Online Manpower Information Service (NOMIS), has a wide range of statistics from sources which relate mainly to employment and unemployment as well as online facilities to access data from the Labour Force Survey.

An overview of official health statistics

Most data produced by government or the NHS are collected either through surveys of the population or as a by-product of administrative processes in which data collection is triggered by a particular event such as a birth, seeing a doctor or claiming unemployment benefit.

Each of these two methods of data collection has different strengths and limitations. Surveys are expensive to undertake and the size of the sample is a large element in their cost. For example, the 1991 census in England and Wales, where the whole population of those two countries, some 49 million people, was surveyed, cost £135 million. If surveys are too small, they cannot be used to produce reliable estimates for subgroups within the community. This applies to the problems of deriving data for ethnic minority groups, which are described in Chapter 4. Moreover, unless a survey is very large, the data cannot be disaggregated to produce reliable estimates for health or local authority areas, yet such data are crucial for planning and resource allocation.

The problems associated with administrative statistics are different. They are cheaper to collect, but there can be problems with completeness and accuracy of the data. The event which triggers data recording needs to come to the attention of the person responsible for reporting it. This is seldom a problem with birth and death registration (described in Chapter 3), as there is a statutory requirement to report these and the resulting documents are needed for legal and other purposes. Many factors can impede the reporting of other events, such as communicable diseases (also described in Chapter 3), even though notification is required by law. The staff of the NHS or social services who are required to collect data may be disinterested if data collection is perceived as a burden and irrelevant to their main work and they are not able to use the data to inform their own work. Considerable training and reinforcement are required to ensure the completeness and accuracy of datasets, and feedback of data to people collecting them is crucial to this. In other cases, there may be disincentives to reporting the event to the authorities. For example, as described in Chapter 5, there are considerable disincentives for employers to report incidents of occupational injuries and diseases.

A final problem affecting administrative statistics linked to entitlements to benefits is that when criteria for receiving the benefits are tightened or broadened, this changes the groups of people who should be counted. An extreme example is the data series based on entitlement to benefits under the Industrial Injury Scheme, described in Chapter 6. A legal ruling accepting workers' claims that a particular disease is occupationally caused can result in a large increase in the numbers of people recorded in the statistics for that type of occupational disease. Other well-known examples are the unemployment benefit series (described in Chapter 5), where there have been many changes in entitlement from year to year, or the count of the number of homeless families (described in Chapter 6), where the definition of homelessness changed in the early 1990s. Clearly, tightening the rules for entitlement to benefit not only saves money but also disguises the full extent of social problems and prevents the figures from becoming the focus of unwelcome debate.

One way of illustrating undercounting is to compare data from different sources. The survey data about occupational health (described in Chapter 6), show a markedly higher incidence of occupational disease than administrative statistics, suggesting that these are subject to considerable under-reporting. Where both administrative data and survey data are presented in combination (as with the two unemployment series in Chapter 5), the relationship between the two data series can illuminate the strengths and weaknesses of each.

Who is left out of official health statistics?

During the 1990s, the number of surveys which focus specifically on health expanded considerably. In particular, the programme of health surveys for each of the countries of the UK got under way and the Health Education Monitoring Survey started in 1995. These surveys are described in Chapter 2, along with other surveys which have a general health component, such as the decennial census and the General Household Survey. Many of the new surveys focus specifically on health-related behaviour. As a result, much is now known about the public's attitudes to health and health-related behaviour, but other areas are badly neglected.

A particular problem is the dearth of information about people with disabilities, as no comprehensive survey has been undertaken since the mid-1980s. There is concern that the numbers of children with disabilities may be rising as a result of the increasing survival of very immature babies, but little information is available about the numbers of such children or about their needs. There are also many methodological problems associated with designing surveys of people with disabilities, and these are discussed in Chapter 4.

People who live in institutions form another neglected group with many needs. Many of these are elderly people living in residential care homes. All the nine continuous surveys described in Chapter 2 exclude this group, as they use households as their sampling frame, as do the majority of ad hoc surveys. Apart from the decennial census, which includes people in institutions, the only official survey undertaken in the 1990s which included people in institutions was the survey of diet and health carried out in 1997. This formed part of the series of National Diet and Nutrition Surveys, which is described in Chapter 6. At the time of writing, however, plans are being developed for including people in care homes in the Health Survey for England in 2000.

The administrative data collected about care homes (described in Chapter 9) also suffer from considerable neglect. The care home sector received an estimated £8.3 billion of public funding in 1995,[13] and this sum is likely to have increased since then. Despite this, the only official data collected were the capacity of the homes and the numbers of residents. There is no basic information about the utilisation of care homes, let alone information which could be used to assess residents' health needs or monitor the quality of services provided by homes.

Government priorities tend to focus on highly visible subjects like heart disease, smoking or drugs. Considerable investment in methodology is needed to undertake surveys of disabled people and elderly people. When these factors are coupled with a reluctance to find information that exposes unmet needs, the result is that low priority is given to collecting information about people in these groups.

Keeping pace with policies in a changing world

Organisations responsible for official data have the almost impossible task of keeping up with changing social phenomena and rapidly evolving policies while at the same time maintaining the continuity of particular series. While there is great interest in comparing groups of people with common character-istics, such as people with disabilities or people from ethnic minority groups, defining such groups is far from simple. People may be asked to assign them-selves to a particular group, for example to a category of people with disabil-ities or to an ethnic minority group, but finding categories which are valid, reliable and acceptable to the people concerned is not easy.

In addition, the way people perceive their identities can change over time. There has been a long-running debate with organisations of people with dis-abilities about the definitions that should be used in surveys. It is claimed that the most commonly used definitions, based on the concept of impairment, disability and handicap, ignore the effects of environment on disability. Like-wise, the categories introduced in the 1991 census for classifying people in minority ethnic groups (described in Chapter 4) are considered to be mislead-ing for describing the ethnic diversity of the population of the UK. New cate-gories have been added for the 2001 census, but they too are likely to be hotly debated.

Migration is a dynamic phenomenon and it is difficult to capture data on the subject between censuses, as the description of the statistics on migration in Chapter 4 shows. Another evolving area is the labour market, where work patterns and entitlements to benefits can change rapidly, making interpreta-tion of the statistics extremely difficult, as Chapter 5 shows. The acknowl-edgement that road traffic is the major source of air pollution and a major health hazard (described in Chapter 7), has called into question the relevance of current transport statistics. These were set up primarily to monitor the demand for transport.

Similarly, frequent changes during the 1990s to the NHS and local author-ity social services make it difficult to maintain the relevance of datasets. Both NHS and social services policies increased the amount of care provided by independent, mainly private, providers. Despite this, there has been a reluc-tance to collect data from the private sector, even when care is being publicly funded. The introduction of primary care groups and their counterparts in Wales, Scotland and Northern Ireland means a shift in the focus of care from hospitals to primary and community care services where data collection sys-tems are much less developed than in hospitals. In particular, data about care given by different organisations to the same person are not linked, making it difficult to monitor care received or the health outcomes of that care.

The many changes in health and social care during the 1990s resulted in care being fragmented between many different types of providers. This has increased the difficulties in co-ordinating data collection and in ensuring completeness. At the same time, the government is attempting to monitor and compare the performance of public providers in different areas. As described in Chapter 9, such comparisons are often misleading, because data on the contribution of non-statutory providers are not available and NHS and local authority social services do not share common definitions. Indeed, definitions can even differ between local authority departments.

Finally, the role of central and local government itself is changing from that of directly providing services to commissioning and regulating services provided by private and voluntary agencies. Despite this, the government still has an important role in data collection. It should ensure that data are collected and also has a role in standardising definitions and establishing public access to datasets. If central government fails to undertake these tasks, the data are extremely difficult to obtain and use. For example, Chapter 7 describes a situation where the data on industrial pollution are collected using unstandardised definitions and held locally. This makes it impossible to obtain a comparative or overall picture of industrial pollution. As described earlier, lack of central government direction has also reduced the usefulness of local authority social services statistics.

Since the first edition of this *Unofficial guide* was published in 1980, there have been enormous developments in information technology. This has the potential to make considerable amounts of data available electronically, on diskettes or CD-ROM or via the worldwide web. Indeed, the raw data on air pollution from local monitoring sites (described in Chapter 7) are updated hourly and are available free of charge on the internet. Nevertheless, the significance of these data is difficult to understand without knowledge of the air pollution standards and the rationale for setting them.

This dataset on air pollution is unusual in being made available in an electronic version free of charge. Sizeable charges are made for access to the majority of datasets available in electronic form. At the same time, the cost of printed versions appears to be escalating, while their content becomes slimmer. For example, since 1997, *Health and personal social services statistics for England* has contained fewer data than earlier volumes.

As work on this book has progressed, we have found publications increasingly difficult to find, as cost-conscious academic and public libraries have become less able to maintain series of official publications. As a result, there is a danger that the only people using official data will be specialists. Other people, ranging from health service managers, voluntary agencies and organisations representing users to the general public, will be excluded by cost and by difficulties in accessing data. Further development of the ONS's *Statbase* web site may improve access, but at present it does not give enough background information about each data source to place the data in an overall context.

Accessing data at second hand, when it may be unclear how they were collected and analysed, makes it very difficult to interpret what the data mean.

In describing data about the NHS and social services, we sought to highlight the impact of privatisation on the extent to which official statistics can be used to monitor the delivery of care. At the time of writing, there are plans to privatise parts of the ONS, as recommended by management consultants KPMG. Although this does not include data collection and analysis, it does include the publication and dissemination of statistics. As the main aim is to reduce cost, we have little confidence that this will improve either the public access to these publicly funded statistics or the quality of the product. The government may devolve its responsibility for the publication and dissemination of official statistics to private companies, but it must not abdicate its responsibility to ensure that the public has access to statistics for which it has already paid through taxation.

Key publications

Office for National Statistics: *Annual abstract of statistics*. London: TSO, published annually.
Office for National Statistics: *Regional trends*. London: TSO, published annually.
Office for National Statistics: *Social trends*. London: TSO, published annually.
Office for National Statistics: *Guide to official statistics 2000*. London: TSO, 2000.

Contact addresses and web sites

Office for National Statistics (ONS)
1 Drummond Gate
London SW1V 2QQ
Economic statistics
Telephone: 020 7533 6363/6464
Social statistics
Telephone: 020 7533 6262
Website: http://www.ons.gov.uk/
Statbase: http://www.statistics.gov.uk

The National Assembly for Wales
(formerly the Welsh Office)
General contact for publications:
Publications Unit
Statistical Directorate 5
National Assembly for Wales
Cathays Park
Cardiff CF10 3NQ
Telephone: 02920 825044 or 02920 825054
Fax: 02920 825350
Email: statswales@gtnet.gov.uk

The Scottish Executive Central Statistics Unit
1B-West, 10 Victoria Quay
Edinburgh EH6 6QQ
Telephone: 0131 244 0443
Website: http://www.scotland.gov.uk

Northern Ireland Statistics and Research Agency
McAuley House
2–14 Castle Street
Belfast BT1 1SA
Telephone: 028 9034 8100
Website: http://www.nisra.gov.uk/

The Data Archive
University of Essex Wivenhoe Park
Colchester CO4 3SQ
Telephone: 01206 872322
Email: Essex-archive-all@mailbase.ac.uk
(Information Link)
Website: http://dawww.essex.ac.uk/ or http://biron.essex.ac.uk/

References

1. Nissel M. *People count: a history of the General Register Office.* London: HMSO, 1987.
2. Eyler JM. *Victorian social medicine: the ideas and methods of William Farr.* London and Baltimore: Johns Hopkins University Press, 1979.
3. Nightingale F. Proposal for an uniform plan of hospital statistics. In *programme of the fourth session of the International Statistical Congress.* London: HMSO, 1860.
4. Macfarlane AJ, Pollock AM. Statistics and the privatisation of the National Health Service and social services. In: Dorling D, Simpson S, eds. *Statistics in society: the arithmetic of politics.* London: Arnold, 1998.
5. Rayner D. *Review of the government statistical services: report to the Prime Minister.* London: Central Statistical Office, 1980.
6. Pickford S, Cunningham J, Lynch R, Radice J, White G. *Government economic statistics: a scrutiny report.* London: HMSO, 1989.
7. Radical Statistics Health Group. *Facing the figures: what really is happening to the National Health Service?* London: Radical Statistics, 1987.
8. Royal Statistical Society. Official statistics: counting with confidence. *Journal of the Royal Statistical Society* Series A, 154 Part 1: 23–44, 1990.
9. Office for National Statistics. *Statistics: a matter of trust. A consultation document.* Cm 3882. London: The Stationery Office, 1998.
10. *Building trust in statistics.* Cm 4412. London: TSO, 1999.
11. Government Statistical Service. *Annual report, 1997–98.* London: ONS, 1998.
12. Office for National Statistics. *Guide to official statistics, 2000.* London: TSO, 2000.
13. Laing W, ed. *Laing's review of private healthcare and directory of independent hospitals, nursing and residential homes and related services.* London: Laing and Buisson, 1996.

2 Surveying the population

HEALTH TOPICS IN THE CENSUS OF POPULATION AND OTHER SURVEYS

Mary Shaw, Danny Dorling and Jenny Grundy

The census

Health topics in other general surveys

Population surveys focusing specifically on health and illness

This chapter describes the health information available from the census of population and other official surveys. Surveys which collect such information are of two types: general surveys, where health questions are included among many other different topics, and surveys which focus specifically on health issues. In addition to the census, nine general surveys are regularly undertaken by the Office for National Statistics (ONS): the General Household Survey, the Family Expenditure Survey, the Family Resources Survey, the Survey of English Housing, the Labour Force Survey, the International Passenger Survey, the National Travel Survey, the Omnibus Survey and the National Food Survey. These are often described as continuous surveys, meaning that they have been undertaken regularly, annually or more frequently, for many years and therefore provide information on time trends. The amount of health information in these surveys varies from one or two single questions in the census to the considerable health component in the General Household Survey, which includes questions on the use of health services as well as self-reported illness.

Surveys which focus exclusively on health-related topics may also be part of long-running series. The survey of Infant Feeding has been undertaken every 5 years since 1975, and the Adult Dental Health survey every 10 years since 1968. With the recent introduction of the National Diet and Nutrition Surveys, the Health Surveys for England and Scotland and the Health Education Monitoring Survey, the number of continuous surveys focusing exclusively on health-related topics has increased. From time to time, important occasional, large-scale surveys are undertaken, for example the Office of Population Censuses and Surveys (OPCS) Surveys of Disability (described in Chapter 4) and the OPCS Psychiatric Morbidity Survey. The introduction of market testing means that some surveys originally undertaken by OPCS and its successor the ONS, such as the Health Survey for England, are now contracted out. They are usually contracted to consortia of market research companies and academic institutions.

The census

Counting the population

The census is a count of the number of people normally resident in the UK on a particular night. Using the household as its basic unit of enumeration, the census asks questions about the social and economic condition of the population. It also collects information on the number of houses in the country, family structure and employment. In 1991, questions on ethnicity and health were added, except in Northern Ireland where questions about religion and fertility were included but not the question on ethnic group. It is, thus, a 'snapshot' of the population on one night of the year. In order to gain as complete as possible a set of results, the census was made compulsory through an Act of Parliament, with an assurance to the public that the information collected is both confidential and anonymous. The 1920 Census Act gave the Registrars General for England and Wales and for Scotland a general authority and duty to conduct censuses at intervals no shorter than 5 years. Despite this, each census requires secondary legislation, an Order in Council which determines the date, the broad topics on which questions will be asked and by whom, and to whom returns should be made.

The 2001 census will be very similar to the 1991 census, but a number of questions will be asked for the first time. A general health question will be included, in which respondents will be asked to assess whether their own health in the preceding 12 months has been 'Good', 'Fairly good' or 'Not good'. Respondents will be asked if they provide unpaid personal help for a friend or relative with a long-term illness, health problem or disability, and the time spent each week in providing such care. This will provide information about the number of carers. An ethnic origin question (discussed in Chapter 4) will be asked in Northern Ireland. The census white paper proposed a question on religion, which will probably be included, and a question on income, which was subsequently dropped. Further information on the 2001 census can be found on the census web site, the address of which is given at the end of this chapter.

The data are used for a wide range of purposes by many different groups of people. The census is used as a basis for revenue distribution to local authorities. They, in turn, use data from it in planning public services, such as education, transport and health. In addition to this, the census acts as a 'gold standard' against which other social surveys can be judged. Detailed information about the way the census was undertaken in 1991 and the questions asked can be found in *A Census user's handbook*[1] and *The 1991 census user's guide*.[2]

Despite the size and scope of the census, it is now accepted that approximately 1.2 million people living in Britain avoided being included in the 1991 census.[3] The OPCS discovered this when it compared the census count with the updated mid-year population estimates and found a shortfall which could not be accounted for by deaths or out-migration. Unfortunately, but not surprisingly, the same people also managed to avoid enumeration in the official census validation survey carried out shortly after the census in order to establish its accuracy. Thus, relatively little is known with great certainty about the nature of the 'missing million'. The 'Estimating with confidence' project at the universities of Manchester and Southampton has established a 'gold standard' estimate of the likely geographical distribution of these people.[3] The estimates can be accessed on the MIMAS, formerly known as MIDAS, computer system at Manchester University, and the contact address is given at the end of this chapter. Because the 'missing million' are not a random sample of the population, studies which ignore this group are likely to produce biased results. Young men and elderly women were particularly likely to be missed by the 1991 census. Thus, the effects of this omission need to be taken into account.[3]

In the UK, three organizations are responsible for censuses. The ONS, formerly the OPCS, takes censuses in England and Wales. Censuses for Scotland and Northern Ireland are taken by the General Register Office for Scotland (GRO(S)) and the Northern Ireland Statistics and Research Agency (NISRA), of which the Census Office Northern Ireland (CO(NI)) is part. The first census was taken in 1801, and a decennial census has been conducted ever since, with the exception of 1941. Individual records of nineteenth-century censuses are available for historical research and family histories.[4]

The nineteenth full census was held on Sunday, 21 April 1991 and the twentieth will take place on Sunday, 29 April 2001. These dates are not as arbitrary as they might seem. The enumeration year is fixed, but the day is flexible, and experience has shown that picking a date in April produces the best response. The optimum date is one when people are likely to be at their usual address, with reasonable weather and daylight hours, and avoiding local and national elections. The day should also be reasonably consistent with previous censuses and in time to produce the results by a specified deadline.

The scale of the survey is reflected in the fact that it took some 118 000 enumerators to distribute the forms for the 1991 census. Expenditure on the census over the 10-year period from 1986–87 to 1995–96 was estimated to be £117 million. At the peak of work, it was estimated that as many as one in 400 people in Britain were being paid to work on the census, and the completed census forms took up some 12 miles of shelving space.[5]

Between censuses, mid-year population estimates are derived from the previous census, birth and death registration data, data about internal migration, which are collected by the NHS Central Register when people change their general practitioners, and data about international migration, which are taken from the International Passenger Survey, as well as claims for political asylum. At times of rapid change, for example when many people are moving around the country in search of work, population estimates for particular areas can become inaccurate. In many decades there have been demands for

5-yearly censuses and in 1966 a mid-term sample was undertaken. Others were planned for 1976 and 1986, but fell victim to public expenditure cuts.

Health information and the census

From 1851 onwards, attempts were made to collect information about the 'infirmities' which we now describe as problems with seeing and hearing, mental illness and learning difficulties. Due to the problems which affected reporting rates, not least the stigma attached to these conditions, the question was dropped in 1921.[6] In the 1971 census, only temporary sickness from work was recorded as illness. In 1981, 'permanently sick or disabled' was added as a residual category of economic activity, but it was not possible for children or people who had retired to be included in this category. The absence of this information for 1981 is particularly unfortunate in areas with high proportions of retired people.[7] The 1991 census was the first which asked everyone in the population, 'Do you have any long-term illness, health problem or handicap which limits your daily activities or the work you can do? Include problems which are due to old age'. The aim of this question was to collect information about morbidity and the need for health and social services at a local level, instead of using death rates as a proxy measure.[7]

As the census is a unique source of data at a very local level, it is used by all levels of government for resource allocation. If the censuses were not taken, the process of resource allocation would be even more uncertain than it is.[8] The piloted version of the limiting long-term illness question correlated well with general practitioner consultation rates and so it has been proposed as a nationally consistent indicator of health service needs.[9] Despite the fact that they are the most comprehensive available, census data should not be interpreted uncritically. There has been no definitive study of how the census measure of limiting long-term illness compares to surveys which use interviews or clinical examinations. Because the word 'limiting' was used in the question, some people who might otherwise classify themselves as ill might have been deterred from ticking this census box.

The wording of the census question is crucially important. It aims to collect data about chronic illness. Any condition from asthma to arthritis could be included. Of course, some people with either of these conditions may not consider them serious enough to answer 'yes', while other people with conditions which a medical practitioner might not describe as an illness may have been inclined to do so. As with all self-reported measures of illness, therefore, we need to be aware of the 'iceberg of disease' concept. This refers to the large proportion of symptoms and disease which is not reported to medical practitioners. Because of differences in the way people perceive and report symptoms, measures of illness can vary independently of the prevalence of disease.[10]

There are additional reasons to be wary of self-reported data. Self-reporting of limiting long-term illness has been found to vary by social group,[10] for example by age and social class. When these groups are unevenly distributed geographically, this may lead to bias.[11] There may also be gender differences in reporting.[12] It may also be the case that the reporting of limiting long-term illness may reflect local labour market conditions. In areas of high long-term unemployment, higher rates of positive response to this question occurred, even after controlling for deprivation and regional difference.[13] This casts doubt on the use of this measure as an objective indicator of health care needs which can be used for resource allocation at the national level. Changes to the benefit system and sick-pay may also affect reporting. Similarly, a person's knowledge about the system for allocating resources may affect the way they answer questions.[7]

As well as information about the health of individuals, the census also collects data on the number and characteristics of people living in institutions or 'communal establishments'. The definition covers a wide range of institutions, including long-term homes for elderly people, psychiatric and other long-stay hospitals, hostels, barracks and prisons.[2] In the 1991 census, an important distinction was drawn between NHS or local authority hospitals or homes and non-NHS or local authority hospitals, nursing homes and residential care. A total of 186 136 people aged 85 years and over reporting a limiting long-term illness was enumerated in non-household establishments.[14] Of these, 8 per cent were living in a NHS hospital or home, 22 per cent in local authority homes, 30 per cent in non-NHS nursing homes and non-local authority homes, and 37 per cent in residential homes. Also in 1991, people sleeping rough were enumerated separately by category, but only small numbers were found. For example, in Great Britain, only thirty-six 16 to 17 year olds sleeping rough were enumerated.[15] This gross underenumeration is discussed in Chapter 6.

The housing tables also include information about types of dwellings, distinguishing, for example between flats and houses and whether dwellings are permanent or non-permanent. Non-permanent accommodation is that which is not constructed of permanent building materials such as brick or concrete. In most cases, non-permanent accommodation refers to static caravan parks or houseboats, although travellers living under plastic sheets would also count if that were their permanent home.

A final point to remember when interpreting census data is whether results are reported at the individual or household level. For example, people aged over 45 suffering from a limiting long-term illness were more likely than others to be living in a household with others with a limiting long-term illness. Thus, the household as well as the individual frequency of illness may need to be considered, especially for the allocation of resources.[16]

Accessing published census data

Census data for England, Wales and Scotland are published jointly, whereas Northern Ireland data are published separately. Despite their drawbacks, census data are undoubtedly an invaluable source of information about the population. Data from the census are published in two ways, by area and by subject. Tabulations are produced for a range of geographical areas, including counties, former regional health authorities, and parliamentary constituencies. The county volumes are often available in the offices of local councils and in some public libraries. Reports are also produced containing national data on a wide range of topics including a specific report on *Persons with limiting long-term illness*. The content of tables from this report is shown with examples in Table 2.1. The following reports on specific topics include data about 'long-term illness' in one or more tables. Some useful tables from these volumes are listed in Table 2.2.

Persons living in communal establishments
Children and young adults
Persons aged 60 and over
Housing and the availability of cars
National migration
Regional migration
Household and family group
Report for England, regional health authorities.

The most detailed information about health is found in *Limiting long-term illness, Communal establishments,* and the *Report for England, regional health authorities,* Parts I and II.

The following volumes may also contain information relevant to health issues:

Historical tables
Sex, age and marital status
Ethnic group and country of birth
Usual residence
Economic activity
Workplace/transport
Qualified manpower.

The information presented in these tables is somewhat daunting at first sight, but the basic arrangement is consistent throughout. In most of the tables, information is tabulated by age, sex, marital status, region, economic position, social class, ethnic group, long-term illness, housing conditions including amenities and tenure, employment and education.

For people such as researchers interested in statistics about a large number of very small areas, electronic datasets are available. The 1991 census is the first for which anonymised individual records were made available. The sample of anonymised records (SARs) consists of a 2 per cent sample of the population and a separate 1 per cent sample of households. Researchers are given access to the individual records, which allow analyses to be done more flexibly to answer specific questions. For instance, how more or less likely is a woman born in Bangladesh to be ill than a woman born in Scotland and does this vary by age and/or by current district of residence?

Table 2.1 Examples of data in the *'Limiting long-term illness'* volume of the 1991 census

Table number	Geographical area	Examples
1. Age, sex and marital status: number of residents in household with a limiting long-term illness	Great Britain, England and Wales, England, regions, metropolitan counties, Inner London, Outer London, regional remainders, Wales and Scotland	In Great Britain, 583 372 people aged 85 and over were enumerated; of these, 364 161 (or 62%) had a limiting long-term illness
2. Communal establishments: number of people with a limiting long-term illness by age and sex	Great Britain, England and Wales, England, Wales, Scotland	In England, 43 459 people were classed as camping or sleeping rough at the census; of these, 11 321 reported a limiting long-term illness
3. Ethnic groups: number of people with limiting long-term illness by age, sex and nine ethnic groups	Great Britain, England and Wales, England, Wales, Scotland	To answer the question 'Which ethnic group reported the highest proportion of ill children?': on average, only 2% of children aged between 0 and 4 years reported a limiting long-term illness, ranging from almost 4% of Black African children to only 1.3% of Chinese children
4. Economic activity: number of people with limiting long-term illness by age, sex and economic situation	Great Britain, England and Wales, England, Wales, Scotland	In Great Britain, among men in the age group 40–44 who were retired, 33% suffered from a limiting long-term illness, compared to 3.5% for the male population as a whole in this age group

5. Tenure and amenities: number with limiting long-term illness by household, age, sex, region and tenure	England and Wales, England, Wales	For Great Britain as a whole, 42% of households with no bath, shower or inside toilet and no central heating contain someone with a limiting long-term illness, compared with 25% of households which possess these amenities
6. Housing: number with limiting long-term illness by household, age, sex and type of housing	Great Britain, England and Wales, England, Wales, Scotland	Less than 0.5 per cent of households lived in non-permanent accommodation, but 30% of these had at least one ill person in the household .
7. Household composition: households with residents with limiting long-term illness, by age, sex, household type, economic activity of the head of household and number of dependants	Great Britain, England and Wales, England, Wales, Scotland	There were 6 674 358 households enumerated in Great Britain with a least one resident with a limiting long-term illness; of these, 1 058 284 (16%) have one or more dependent children

Source: Office of Population Censuses and Surveys 1991 census. *Limiting long-term illness, Great Britain*. London: HMSO, 1993.

Table 2.2 Other tables from the 1991 census containing data about limiting long-term illness

	Table
OPCS 1991 census. Report for England. *Regional health authorities* (Part I, Volume 1). London: HMSO, 1993	12. Limiting long-term illness in households by age, sex, regional health authority 13. Limiting long-term illness in communal establishments by age, sex, regional health authority 14. Limiting long-term illness by economic position, age, sex, regional health authority
OPCS 1991 census. Report for England. *Regional health authorities* (Part I, Volume II). London: HMSO, 1993	29. Dependants and limiting long-term illness by age, economic activity and regional health authority 45. Households with pensioners: housing; household composition by number of households up to 0.5 persons per room, facilities and limiting long-term illness by regional health authority
OPCS 1991 census. *Topics report for health areas. Great Britain.* Volume I. London: HMSO, 1993	11. Limiting long-term illness of residents in households by age, sex, marital status and regional health authority 12. Limiting long-term illness and ethnic group: by sex, age and regional health authority 13. Limiting long-term illness by household composition, sex, age, number of children in the household and regional health authority 16. Limiting long-term illness in communal establishments – persons 60 and over with limiting long-term illness 19. Cars and pensioners – households with residents by age, sex, marital status, number of cars and persons with limiting long-term illness
OPCS 1991 census. *Communal establishments. Great Britain.* Volume I. London: HMSO, 1993	3. Type of establishment, migrants and limiting long-term illness; the table contains information on numbers of ill people in various establishments by sex, age, resident/visitor, staff/non-staff and countries (England and Wales, England, Wales, Scotland)

OPCS 1991 census. *Communal establishments Great Britain.* Volume II. London: HMSO, 1993

4. Breakdown of communal establishments by ethnic group, age, sex, status as resident/visitor, staff/non-staff, and also by region (five categories)
5. Economic position as above, but regions given by county, eight age groups, and includes a category for the 'permanently sick' (in the 'economically inactive' category)
6. Establishment size includes number of residents, staff etc.
7. Number of establishments by region.

OPCS 1991 census. *Children and young adults. Great Britain.* Volume I. London: HMSO, 1993

1. Residents aged under 16: migrants and persons with limiting long-term illness in households and communal establishments by sex and age (0–15 years), and by county
2. Residents aged 16 to 29: migrants and persons with limiting long-term illness in households and communal establishments by sex and age (0–15 years), by county
3. Economic position includes a category for 'permanently sick'

OPCS 1991 census. *Persons aged 60 and over. Great Britain.* London: HMSO, 1993

2. Limiting long-term illness: numbers ill by age, sex, marital status by region
5. Limiting long-term illness in communal establishments and in households; the table gives figures for type of establishment by age, sex and status as residents/visitors

OPCS 1991 census. *Ethnic group and country of birth. Great Britain.* Volume II. London: HMSO, 1993

8. Communal establishments – categories of interest, as listed before
10. Economic position includes a category for the 'permanently sick'

The Office for National Statistics Longitudinal Study

The ONS Longitudinal Study, formerly known as the OPCS Longitudinal Study, links the census records of a 1 per cent sample of the population of England and Wales with birth, death and cancer registrations. It started in 1971, and the sample is made up of people born on four dates during any year. Using the National Health Service Central Register, it links census data with births and deaths, taking into account immigration and emigration. Records of Longitudinal Study members have now been linked with 1971, 1981 and 1991 census data. The structure of the Longitudinal Study is shown in Fig. 2.1. It has an advantage over most cohort studies in that the sample size is over 500 000 and much non-response is avoided, although there may be some problems with the linking of data and sample bias.

The Longitudinal Study was set up to be used for a wide range of mortality and fertility analyses based on the demographic, social, economic and environmental factors recorded at the census. This allows an assessment of the association between factors such as social class, employment status and adult mortality rates, or between parents' social circumstances and birth spacing and infant mortality.

The inclusion of cancer registrations was intended to enable analysis by occupation at different stages in the life cycle. Data on subjects such as occupation, employment status and housing conditions can now be linked over a 20-year period, from 1971 to 1991, and are currently being linked to mortality data for the 1990s. These data will eventually be linked to the 2001 census. The inclusion of a question identifying people from ethnic minority groups in the 1991 census offered the potential to ask questions such as how work and housing conditions for ethnic minorities relate to, for example, cancer incidence in these groups. In addition, the question on long-term illness should lead to an analysis of how its incidence among people with various census characteristics is associated with subsequent mortality. At the time of writing, data from the 1991 census, and hence records on long-term illness, have been added relatively recently, so extensive analyses of this information have yet to be published.

The complexity and confidentiality requirements of the Longitudinal Study mean that people who wish to analyse data have to make a specific application, but support is provided to people who do so. Contact details can be

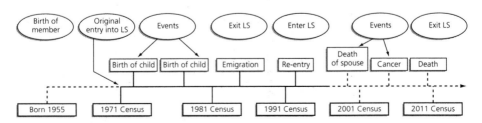

Fig. 2.1 The events in the life of a member of the ONS Longitudal Study (LS). (Source: Office for National Statistics.)

found at the end of this chapter. A detailed description of the Longitudinal Study data together with an assessment of the quality and completeness of the data was published by OPCS in 1995.[17] Information about the Longitudinal Study can be obtained through the Longitudinal Study User Group and Longitudinal Study Support Programme and there are also Longitudinal Study Working Papers and User Guides.[18–21]

Longitudinal Study data and publications cover a wide range of topics, including general and methodological, social and economic change, demographic studies, migration, gerontological studies, ethnicity, housing, inequalities in health and mortality, and cancer studies. Findings are published in the Longitudinal Study series listed below, as well as in articles in a wide range of journals. A review of the Longitudinal Study was published in 1999 and it included a comprehensive list of publications containing analyses of the data.

The Longitudal Study series

Fox AJ, Goldblatt PO. *Longitudinal Study 1971–1975: socio-demographic mortality differentials.* Series LS No 1. London: HMSO, 1982.

Fox AJ. *Longitudinal Study 1971–1977: social class and occupational mortality.* Series LS No 2. London: HMSO, 1982.

Leon D. *The social distribution of cancer.* Series LS No 3. London: HMSO, 1988.

Grundy E. *Women's migration: marriage, fertility and divorce.* Series LS No 4. London: HMSO, 1989.

Kogevinas M. *Longitudinal Study: socio-demographic differences in cancer survival.* Series LS No 5. London: HMSO, 1990.

Goldblatt P, ed. *Mortality and social organisation.* Series LS No 6. London: HMSO, 1990.

Hattersley L, Creeser R. *The Longitudinal Study: 1971–1991: history, organisation and quality of data.* Series LS No 7. London: HMSO, 1995.

Dale A, Williams M, Dodgeon B. *Housing deprivation and social change.* Series LS No 8. London: HMSO, 1996.

Gleave S and Hattersley, eds. *Migration analysis using the Office for National Statistics Longitudinal Study.* Series LS No 9. London: TSO, 2000.

Office for National Statistics. *Review of the ONS Longitudinal Study.* London: ONS, 1999.

Health topics in other general surveys

The General Household Survey

The General Household Survey is an annual survey conducted since 1971 by the OPCS and now by the ONS. For funding reasons, it was suspended for 1997–8. After pressure from a wide range of users inside and outside government, it was decided to reinstate the survey in 1998. Data were collected in 1998–9 but not in 1999–2000. The suspensions mean that there has been a break in the continuous nature of the survey and that its long-term future was in doubt.[22] After a review and much lobbying by its many users, the ONS has since announced plans to continue the General Household Survey for 5 years from 2000–1 onwards.

In the General Household Survey, information is collected on a wide range of subjects, including household composition, accommodation, migration, employment, education, travel and health. The sample of approximately 17 000–20 000 is different every year, rather than a being a panel or cohort study. There is a multistage sampling process, with electoral wards as the primary sampling units. It is designed to produce representative results over a spectrum of social and geographical conditions. The sample covers England, Wales and Scotland. Reports are published annually. Since 1994, they have had the title *Living in Britain*. Northern Ireland has a similar survey, the Continuous Household Survey.

In the General Household Survey, people are asked 'Do you have any long-standing illness, disability or infirmity?', wording which is somewhat different from that in the census. Those who reply positively to this question are then asked, 'Does this illness or disability limit your activities in any way?'. There is also a question on acute sickness or restricted activity, referring to whether the respondent has had to cut down on the things he or she usually does due to illness or injury in the preceding 2 weeks. The survey therefore produces three different statistics on self-reported illness, long-standing illness or disability, limiting long-standing illness or disability and restricted activity in the 14 days prior to the interview.

Use of health services is also covered in the form of a question on consultations with a general practitioner in the preceding 2 weeks, attendance at outpatient services at hospital visits, excluding ante-natal or post-natal over the previous 3 months, and in-patient hospital stays over the previous year. It also asks, in some years, about private health insurance and use of private health care. The association between self-reported illness and health service use can thus be investigated. Other health-related questions, such as those about smoking and birth-control, are not asked every year. While the General Household Survey obviously has a much smaller sample size than the census and cannot tell us about illness at a small area level, it can be used for monitoring regional differences and national trends. From 2000 onwards, there will be a continuous element and a number of additional sections, varying from year to year.

Questions asked every year:

Long-standing illness or disability prevalence

Acute sickness: prevalence and duration of restricted activity

Health in general in 12 months before interview

GP consultations in 2 weeks before interview, including site of consultation
Whether a prescription was given

Out-patient attendances in 3 months prior to interview

Stays in hospital as in-patient in the last 12 months.

Asked every 2 years or less often:

Contraception: current use of contraception

Whether woman/partner has been sterilised

Whether women/partner would have difficulties in having more children

Health behaviours: personal rating of own drinking behaviour

Prevalence of cigarette, pipe and cigar smoking

Number and type of cigarettes smoked

Whether ever smoked cigarettes, cigars and pipes regularly

Dentistry: whether has any natural teeth

Whether goes to dentist for check-ups or only when having trouble

Elderly people: use of health and social services by persons over 65

Difficulties with sight or hearing in persons aged 65 or over, which has been asked intermittently.

Health topics included 1971 to 1996:

Family information/fertility: marriage, cohabitation, childbirth, contraception, sterilisation and infertility

Chronic health problems: chronic sickness including long-standing illness or disability, prevalence, effects, contact with health services. Health in general in 12 months prior to interview

Short-term health problems in 14 days prior to interview: prevalence and effects

Use of health services: GP consultations, reason for the consultation and outcome, out-patient attendances, day-patient visits, in-patient spells, mobility aids

Accidents: accidents at home

Elderly people: social support and elderly people, informal carers

Sight and hearing: tinnitus

Dental health: natural teeth, visits to dentists

Drinking and smoking.

General Household Survey publications

Office for National Statistics. *Living in Britain: results from the General Household Survey*. Series General Household Survey. London: TSO, published annually.
Office for National Statistics. *Living in Britain: preliminary results*. London: TSO, published annually.

The Labour Force Survey

The Labour Force Survey (LFS) was first undertaken in 1973 by the Department of Employment. It is now commissioned by the Department for Employment and Education and undertaken by the ONS. Its primary aim is to gather information about employment and unemployment among men aged 16–64 years and women aged 16–59, using definitions compatible with other European countries. It also covers many health-related topics, as well as information about housing and education. The questions asked about employment and unemployment in the Labour Force Survey are described in Chapter 5. The socio-demographic information collected includes nationality and housing tenure. Until recently, the Labour Force Survey was the only major survey to gather information about people's self-defined ethnic group. From time to time, as part of the survey, supplementary or trailer surveys are undertaken on topics of particular interest. In the past, the topics have included detailed questions on housing, asked in 1988 and 1991, and questions on occupational health, asked in 1990 and 1993/4. Both are described in Chapter 6. The Labour Force Survey, therefore, collects useful information about work, social circumstances and health of people of working age.

The size of the health-related component of the Labour Force Survey expanded during the 1990s. The survey asks whether respondents are limited in the type of work they can do and, if so, the type of health problem or disability they have. In 1993/4, a new question was introduced, asking respondents whether they expected the problem to last more than a year. The aim was to provide a reliable measure of long-term illness or disability. This question has been used to collect information about employment and disability.[23] In addition, by including a question about whether respondents suffered from any illness or disability that was caused or made worse by work, the survey is now a major source of information about occupational health.[24–26] This is discussed in more detail in Chapter 6. Questions about sickness absences are routinely included. In 1997, new disability questions were introduced to monitor the 1995 Disability Discrimination Act.

The Labour Force Survey was conducted biannually until 1983 and then annually between 1984 and 1991. Since 1992, it has been undertaken quarterly. The sample now consists of a quarterly survey of approximately 15 000 private households in Great Britain, with a 'booster' survey carried out between March and May of over 44 000 private households in Great Britain and 4000 in Northern Ireland. Thus, the spring quarter is based on over 60 000 private households. As well as private households, people living in NHS accommodation and students in halls of residence are also sampled. Information about the students is obtained by proxy from their parents when they are interviewed as part of the normal survey. People at the 12 000 sample addresses are interviewed on five separate occasions at quarterly intervals. Respondents may not always be interviewed directly, and informants from the same households may be used as proxies. The first interviews are face to face, but subsequent interviews are carried out by telephone.

Labour Force Survey publications

Office for National Statistics. *Labour Force Survey quarterly supplement*.
London: TSO.
Office for National Statistics. *Labour market trends* (formerly *Employment gazette*)
London: TSO, published monthly.
Includes studies of special groups such as ethnic minorities, people with
disabilities and self-employed people.
Office for National Statistics. *Labour Force Survey*, historical supplement. London:
TSO, 1997.
Health and Safety Commission. *Health and safety statistics*, Health and Safety
Executive books. Published annually from 1992/3 onwards.

Health-related topics in other general surveys

Of the seven continuous large-scale surveys undertaken by the ONS, the
National Food Survey, the National Travel Survey, the Omnibus Survey, the
Family Expenditure Survey and the Family Resources Survey contain ques-
tions related to health, either on a regular or ad hoc basis. These are shown in
Table 2.3; some are discussed elsewhere in this book. A programme of
National Diet and Nutrition Surveys is described in Chapter 6. The Depart-
ment of the Environment, Transport and the Regions' English House Condi-
tion Survey also covers health-related topics.

Table 2.3   Health-related topics in ONS' continuous surveys

Survey		Topics
National Food Survey	Chapter 6	Consumption and expenditure on different types of food
National Travel Survey	Chapter 7	'Transport disabled'; journeys made on foot and by bicycle
Omnibus Survey		Prevalence of back pain; adult drinkers' behaviour and knowledge; residual medicines
Family Expenditure Survey	Chapter 5	Expenditure on private medical insurance, private medical, nursing, dental and optical fees; NHS charges
Family Resources Survey 1996/7	Chapter 4	Prevalence of disability and take-up of disability benefits
English House Conditions Survey	Chapter 6	Illness and disability; use of aids and adaptations

Publications from ONS' continuous surveys

Ministry of Agriculture, Fisheries and Food. *National Food Survey*. London: TSO, published annually.

Department of the Environment, Transport and the Regions. *National Travel Survey*. London: TSO, published annually.

Dodd T. *The prevalence of back pain in Great Britain in 1996*. A report on research for the Department of Health using the Omnibus Survey. London: TSO, 1997.

Office for National Statistics. *Family Spending*. London: TSO, published annually.

Department of Social Security. *Family Resources Survey*. London: TSO, published annually.

Department of the Environment, Transport and the Regions. *English House Condition Survey*. London: TSO, published annually.

Population surveys focusing specifically on health and illness

Health surveys for England and Scotland, the Health and Well Being Survey for Northern Ireland, and the Welsh Health Survey

The Health Survey for England, which started in 1991, is an annual survey series commissioned by the Department of Health. It is designed to monitor progress towards two 'Health of the Nation' targets relating to blood pressure and obesity, to estimate the proportions of people in England with specified health conditions, to estimate the prevalence of risk factors associated with these conditions, and to examine differences between population subgroups, notably those defined by age, sex, region and social class. Since 1995, the survey has been used to measure the heights of children at different ages, replacing the National Study of Health and Growth. The coverage and topics for surveys are shown in Table 2.4.

The 1997 survey concentrated on young people aged between 2 and 24 years. The survey collected self-reported information about health-related behaviours such as smoking and drinking, self-reports of health conditions and symptoms, reports of doctor-diagnosed conditions and use of services.

The survey's scope has expanded over the years. For 1991 to 1994, it measured height, weight, blood pressure and waist and hip circumference. From 1995 to 1997, lung function was included. Blood samples were also obtained from people aged 11 upwards. In 1996, saliva samples from children were analysed for cotinine, an indicator of smoking. The 1998 survey returned to cardiovascular disease as the main topic. In 1999, the survey continued to concentrate on cardiovascular disease, diabetes, physical activities and respiratory disease and also focused on ethnic minorities. From 1991 to 1993, the surveys were undertaken by the OPCS. Following market testing, responsibility for the survey then transferred to the Joint Health Survey Unit of Social and Community Planning Research, now known as the National Centre for

Table 2.4   Topics in the Health Survey for England

Year	Sample	Coverage	Topics
1991–4	1991: about 3000 1992: about 4000 1993: about 16 000 1994: about 16 000	16 years and over	Cardiovascular risk factors
1995–1996	16 000 adults 3600 children	2 years and over	General health, smoking, drinking and blood pressure, respiratory conditions, accidents and, in 1995, disability
1997	8000 adults 8000 children		Children and young people
1998	16 000 adults 3600 children		Cardiovascular disease
1999	8000 adults 8000 adults from ethnic minorities 4000 children from ethnic minorities		

Social Research, and the Department of Epidemiology and Public Health at University College, London.

The 3-yearly Health Survey for Scotland is similar to the Health Survey for England. It was first undertaken in 1995–6 by Social and Community Planning Research and the Department of Epidemiology and Public Health at University College, London. The 1995 survey involved interviews with over 7900 adults aged 16–64 and concentrated on cardiovascular disease, health behaviours and risk factors.

The Northern Ireland Health and Well-Being Survey was first undertaken in 1997. As well as collecting similar information to that in the Health Survey for England, the Northern Ireland survey also investigates perceptions of health and mental health.

Wales has its own Welsh Health Survey, which was first undertaken in 1994–5 and covered different topics from the Scottish and English surveys. This survey was undertaken by the South East Institute of Public Health. The report covers a number of areas, including the use of and satisfaction with hospital, general practitioners and community services, and illness treated by a doctor, including heart disease, diabetes, chest conditions and mental illness. Questions were also asked about lifestyle factors, including smoking, diet and exercise, whether an individual was a carer, improvements to the NHS, purchase of 'over the counter' medicines and knowledge of first aid. In addition, the survey used the questions from a standardized health and well-being questionnaire, the SF36. A special feature of the survey was the inclusion of an additional sample of people with learning disabilities. The Welsh

Survey was a postal survey with a sample size of 50 000, of which approximately 28 000 were returned. It was repeated in 1998.

Data sets from the surveys are deposited at the Data Archive at the University of Essex. The address of the archive is given at the end of this chapter.

Publications from Health Survey programmes

White A, Nicolaas G, Foster K, Browne F, Carey S. *Health Survey for England 1991*. London: HMSO, 1993.

Breeze G, Maidment A, Bennet N, Flatley J, Carey S. *Health Survey for England 1992*. London: HMSO, 1994.

Bennett N, Dodd T, Flatley J, Freeth S, Bolling K. *Health Survey for England 1993* London: HMSO, 1995.

Calhoun H, Prescott-Clarke P. *Health Survey for England 1994*. London: TSO, 1996.

Prescott-Clarke P, Primatesta P. *Health Survey for England 1995*. London: TSO, 1997.

Prescott-Clarke P, Primatesta P. *Health Survey for England 1996*. London: TSO, 1998.

Prescott-Clarke P, Primatesta P. *Health Survey for England: the health of young people 1995–7*. London: TSO, 1998.

Health Survey for England, adult reference tables 1997. On the internet at http://www.open.gov.uk/stats/hsl2697/intro.htm.

Dong W, Erens R, eds. *Scotland's health: Scottish Health Survey 1995*, Vol. 1. Edinburgh: TSO, 1997.

Dong W, Erens R, eds. *Scotland's health: Scottish Health Survey 1995*, Vol. 2. Edinburgh: TSO, 1997.

The Welsh Office. *The Welsh Health Survey 1995*. Cardiff: HMSO, 1996.

National Assembly for Wales. *The Welsh Health Survey, 1998*. Cardiff: National Assembly for Wales, 1999.

Other population survey series focusing on health and illness

The government has commissioned a number of other health surveys on specific topics. These are shown in Table 2.5. Surveys of adult and children's dental health are undertaken every 10 years and include an examination by a dentist, in addition to interviews. From 1975 onwards, OPCS undertook an 'infant feeding' survey every 5 years. The sample is identified from birth registrations and mothers are sent a series of questionnaires. As well as asking how their children are fed at various stages of the first year of life, questions are asked about the mothers' lifestyles, including smoking and drinking habits, and also about their socio-economic background. In 1995, the survey included a separate survey of Asian parents.

A biennial survey of smoking among secondary school children has been undertaken since 1982. Children aged between 11 and 15 years are asked about their smoking behaviour and complete a diary in which they record all

Table 2.5 Survey series focusing on health and illness

Title	Geographical areas	Status	Sample size	Topics covered
National Diet and Nutrition Survey Programme	England, Wales and Scotland	Ongoing programme for different age groups; adults, children and elderly people	About 2500 in each group	Dietary intake by social class and other socio-demographic variables; dental examination in elderly people and in children
Smoking among secondary school children	England, Wales and Scotland	Biennial series since 1982	About 3500 in each country	Children aged 11–15; how much they smoke, where they get cigarettes, and smoking behaviour of family and friends; alcohol included from 1994
Children's attitudes to smoking	England	Annual since 1997	About 4000 aged 11–15 years	Attitudes to smoking and awareness of anti-smoking campaigns
Health Education Monitoring Survey	England	Annual since 1995	5000–8000 adults	Attitudes to general health, smoking, drinking, physical activity, nutrition, sexual behaviour, social support and civic engagement
Adult Dental Health Survey	UK	Decennial since 1968	About 7000	Dental experiences, attitudes and knowledge of dental care, loss of teeth, use of dentures, condition of teeth
Children's Dental Health Survey	UK	Decennial since 1973	17 000 children aged 5–15 years	Dental inspection plus survey of dental history, dental experience and dental care
Infant Feeding Survey	England, Wales, Scotland and Northern Ireland	5-yearly since 1975	11 000	Proportion of mothers who breast feed and how long for; at what age solid foods are introduced

Publications from surveys of health and health-related behaviour

National Diet and Nutrition Survey Programme

Gregory J, Foster K, Tyler H, Wiseman M. *The Dietary and Nutritional Survey of British Adults*. London: HMSO, 1990.

Gregory J, Collins DL, Davies PSW, Hughes JM, Clarke PC. *National Diet and Nutrition Survey: children aged 1.5 to 4.5 years*. Vol. I *Report of Diet and Nutrition Survey*. London: HMSO, 1995.

Gregory J, Hinds K. *National Diet and Nutrition Survey: children aged 1.5 to 4.5 years*. Vol. II *Report of the Dental Survey*. London: HMSO, 1995.

Finch S, Doyle W, Lowe C, Bates CJ, Prentice A, Smithers G, Clarke PC. *National Diet and Nutrition Survey: people aged 65 years and over*. Vol. I. London: TSO, 1998.

Steele JG, Sheiham A, Marcenez W, Walls AWG. *National Diet and Nutrition Surveys: people aged 65 years and over*. Vol. 2 *Report of the oral health survey*. London: TSO, 1998.

Smoking among secondary school children

Jarvis L. *Smoking among secondary school children 1996, England*. London: TSO, 1997.

Barton J, Jarvis L. *Smoking among secondary school children 1996, Scotland*. London: TSO, 1997.

Jarvis L. *Teenage smoking attitudes in 1996*. London: TSO, 1997.

Goddard E. *Young teenagers and alcohol*. Vol. I, *England*. London: TSO, 1997.

Goddard E. *Young teenagers and alcohol*. Vol. II, *Scotland*. London: TSO, 1998.

Children's attitudes to smoking

Dawe F, Goddard E. *Smoking-related behaviour and attitudes*. London: TSO, 1997.

Barton J. *Young teenagers and smoking in 1997*. London: TSO, 1998.

Office for National Statistics. *Teenage smoking attitudes in 1998*. London: ONS, 2000.

Health Education Monitoring Survey

Bridgwood A, Malbon G, Lader D, Matheson J. *Health in England 1995. What people know, what people think, what people do*. Office for National Statistics. London: HMSO, 1996.

Hansbro J, Bridgwood A, Morgan A, Hickman A. *Health in England 1996. What people know, what people think, what people do*. Office for National Statistics. London: TSO, 1997.

Bridgwood A, Rainford L, Walker A. *All change? The Health Education Monitoring Survey one year on*. London: The Stationery Office, 1998.

Office for National Statistics. Health in England 1998: *Investigating the links between social inequalities and health*. London: TSO, 2000.

Adult dental health survey

Office for National Statistics. *Adult dental health survey: oral health in the United Kingdom 1998*. London: TSO, 2000.

Children's dental health survey

O'Brien M. *Children's dental health in the UK 1993*. Office of Population Censuses and Surveys. London: HMSO, 1994.

Infant feeding survey

Foster K, Lader D, Chessbrough S. *Infant feeding 1995*. London: TSO, 1997.

Thomas H, Avery V. *Infant feeding in Asian families*. London: TSO, 1997.

cigarettes smoked in the previous week. Saliva samples are also taken. From 1994 onwards, questions were also asked about drinking behaviour.

The Health Education Monitoring Survey is an annual series first carried out in 1995. It was designed to monitor trends in the health-related knowledge, attitudes and behaviour of adults aged 16–74 in England as part of measuring progress towards 'Health of the Nation' targets. Adults were asked about general health, prevention of skin cancer, smoking, drinking, physical activity, nutrition and, in the group aged 16–54 years only, sexual health. A section on drug use and attitude to drugs was included in 1995.

Occasional surveys: the psychiatric morbidity surveys and other ad-hoc surveys

In 1992–3, OPCS did a series of surveys of psychiatric morbidity in adults. The sample included people aged 16–64 years living in England, Scotland and Wales in private households and in institutions, as well as homeless people, which included people in night shelters and people sleeping rough. To date, this is the only large-scale official survey of mental illness in Great Britain. The aim was to estimate the prevalence of various types of mental illness, to identify the nature

Surveys of psychiatric morbidity and the health of prisoners

Surveys of psychiatric morbidity in Great Britain

Meltzer H, Gill B, Petticrew M, Hinds K. *Report 1. The prevalence of psychiatric morbidity among adults living in private households.* London: HMSO, 1996.

Meltzer H, Gill B, Petticrew M, Hinds K. *Report 2. Physical complaints, service use and treatment of adults with psychiatric disorders.* London: HMSO, 1996.

Meltzer H, Gill B, Petticrew M, Hinds K. *Report 3. Economic activity and social functioning of adults with psychiatric disorders.* London: HMSO, 1996.

Meltzer H, Gill B, Petticrew M, Hinds K. *Report 4. The prevalence of psychiatric morbidity among adults living in institutions.* London: HMSO, 1996.

Meltzer H, Gill B, Petticrew M, Hinds K. *Report 5. Physical complaints, service use and treatment of residents with psychiatric disorders.* London: HMSO, 1996.

Meltzer H, Gill B, Petticrew M, Hinds K. *Report 6. Economic activity and social functioning of residents with psychiatric disorders.* London: HMSO, 1996.

Meltzer H, Hinds K, Petticrew M, Hinds K, Gill B. *Report 7. Psychiatric morbidity among homeless people.* London: HMSO, 1996.

Foster K, Meltzer H, Gill B, Hinds K. *Report 8. Adults with psychotic disorders living in the community.* London: HMSO, 1996.

Surveys of the health of prisoners

Bridgwood A, Malbon G. *Survey of the physical health of prisoners, 1994.* London: HMSO, 1995.

Singleton N, Meltzer H, Gatward R, Cold J, Deasy D. *Psychiatric morbidity among prisoners.* London: TSO, 1998.

and extent of social disabilities associated with mental illness, to investigate the use of health, social and voluntary care services, to examine recent stressful life events which are associated with mental illness, and to investigate the relationship between mental illness and the use of tobacco, alcohol and drugs.

The survey used a standardised questionnaire of psychiatric morbidity, the revised Clinical Interview Schedule, which covers such topics as sleep problems, fatigue, worry, irritability and depression. Eight reports and two bulletins have been published covering the prevalence of mental illness, characteristics of people suffering from mental illness, medication, treatment and use of services, use of alcohol and drugs and the social and financial circumstances of people with mental illness.

In 1997–8, a survey of psychiatric morbidity was undertaken among prisoners. The sample was drawn from all prisons in England and Wales and included men and women on remand as well as sentenced prisoners. Topics covered included prevalence of mental health problems, deliberate self-harm, use of alcohol and drugs and background characteristics and lifetime experiences. This complemented the survey of the physical health of 1000 prisoners in thirty-two prisons in England and Wales which was undertaken in 1994. In this survey, health and health-related behaviour of sentenced male prisoners was compared to those of the general population. Blood pressure, respiratory function, height and weight were measured.

In the mid-1980s, a series of disability surveys was undertaken by the OPCS. These are described in detail in Chapter 4.

Contact addresses and web sites

Census Division
Office for National Statistics
Segensworth Road
Titchfield
Hampshire PO15 5RR
Census general enquiries, telephone
01329 813800
Census internet page:
http://www.statistics.gov.uk

General Register Office for Scotland
Census and Population Statistics
Division
Ladywell House
Ladywell Road
Edinburgh EH12 7TF
Telephone: 0131 334 0380
Web site: http://www.gro-scotland.gov.uk/

The census in Northern Ireland is dealt with by:

Northern Ireland Statistics and Research Agency
McAuley House
2–14 Castle Street
Belfast BT1 1SA
Telephone: 028 9034 8100
Web site: http://www.nisra.gov.uk/

The most accessible way for researchers to get further information about the census datasets is through MIMAS (Manchester Information and Associated Services) at Manchester University. This has a user-friendly interface called 'Casweb' for the 1991 Census Area Statistics.
Web site: http://www.mimas.ac.uk

Information on the 2001 census can be obtained from Office for National Statistics and details are published in *2001 census information papers* and at:
Web site: http://www.statistics.gov.uk/

Longitudinal Study
For academic users, access to the longitudinal study can be obtained through the Longitudinal Study User Group and Longitudinal Study Support Programme based at:
Centre for Longitudinal Studies (CLS)
6th Floor
Institute of Education
20 Bedford Way
London WC1H 0AL
Web site: http://www.cls.ioe.ac.uk
Email: ls@cls.ioe.ac.uk

General Household Survey and other Office for National Statistics surveys
Information about published data is available from:
Social Survey Division enquiries
Office for National Statistics
1 Drummond Gate
London SW1V 2QQ
Telephone: 020 7533 5500

Health Survey for England
Web site: http://www.doh.gov.uk

Academic users can access raw data from:
The Data Archive
University of Essex
Wivenhoe Park
Colchester
Essex CO4 3SQ
Telephone: 01206 872001
Fax: 01206 872003
or through BIRON: http://dawww.essex.ac.uk

Labour Force Survey
Quantime Bureau Service, disk and on-line services
Quantime Ltd
Maygrove House
69–70 Maygrove Road
London NW6 2EG
Telephone: 020 7625 7111

National Online Manpower Information System (NOMIS)
Unit 1L Mountjoy Research Centre
University of Durham
Durham DH1 3SW
Telephone: 0191 374 2468

References

1. Openshaw S, ed. *A census user's handbook*. London: Longman, 1995.
2. Dale A, Marsh C, eds. *The 1991 census user's guide*. London: HMSO, 1993.
3. Simpson S, Dorling D. Those missing millions: implications for social statistics of undercount in the 1991 census. *Journal of Social Policy* 1994; **23**(4): 543–67.
4. Higgs E. *A clearer sense of the census: the Victorian censuses and historical research*. Public Record Office Handbooks, No. 28. London: HMSO, 1996.
5. Mahon B, Pearce D. The 1991 Census of Great Britain. *Social Trends*, 21. London: HMSO, 1991.
6. Charlton J, Wallace M, White I. Long-term illness: results from the 1991 census. *Population Trends* 1994; **75**: 25.
7. Martin S, Sheldon T, Smith P. Interpreting the new illness question in the UK census for health research on small areas. *Journal of Epidemiology and Community Health* 1995; **49**: 634–41.
8. Diamond I. The census. In: Dorling D, Simpson S, eds. *Statistics in society*. London: Arnold, 1998, pp. 9–18.

9. Dale A. The content of the 1991 census: change and continuity. In: Dale A, Marsh C, eds. *The census user's guide*. London: HMSO, 1993.
10. Blane D, Power C, Bartley M. Illness behaviour and the measurement of class differentials in morbidity. *Journal of the Royal Statistical Society* 1996; **159**(1): 77–92.
11. O'Donnell O, Propper C. Equity and the distribution of UK NHS resources. *Journal of Health Economics* 1991; **10**: 1–19.
12. MacIntyre S, Hunt K, Sweeting H. Gender differences in health: are things really as simple as they seem? *Social Science and Medicine* 1996; **42**(4): 617–24.
13. Haynes R, Bentham G, Lovett A, Eimermann J. Effect of labour market conditions on reporting of limiting long-term illness and permanent sickness in England and Wales. *Journal of Epidemiology and Community Health* 1997; **51**(3): 283–8.
14. Office of Population Censuses and Surveys 1991 Census. *Persons aged 60 and over, Great Britain*. London: HMSO, 1993.
15. Office of Population Censuses and Surveys 1991 Census. *Communal establishments, Great Britain*, Vol. I. London: HMSO, 1993.
16. Glaser K, Murphy M, Grundy E. Limiting long-term illness and household structure among people aged 45 and over, Great Britain 1991. *Ageing and Society* 1997; **17**(1): 3–19.
17. Hattersley L, Creeser R. *Longitudinal Study 1971–92: history, organisation and quality of data*. Series Longitudinal Study No. 7. London: HMSO, 1995.
18. Office of Population Censuses and Surveys Census 1971–81. *The Longitudinal Study: linked census data England and Wales*. London: HMSO, 1988.
19. Rosato M, Harding S, McVey E, Brown J. Research implication of improvements in access to the Office for National Statistics Longitudinal Study. *Population Trends* 1998; **91**: 35–42.
20. Office of Population Censuses and Surveys, City University (London, England) Social Statistics Research Unit. *Office of Population Censuses and Surveys Longitudinal Study user manual*. London: Social Sciences Research Unit, City University, London, 1990.
21. Goldblatt P, ed. Series LS, No. 6. *Mortality and social organisation*. London: HMSO, 1990.
22. Owen C. Government Household Surveys. In: Dorling, D, Simpson, S, eds. *Statistics in society*. London: Arnold, 1999, pp. 19–28.
23. Sly F, Duxbury R. Disability and the labour market: findings from the Labour Force Survey. *Labour Market Trends* December, 1995; **103**: 439–59.
24. Health and Safety Statistics 1989–1990, *Employment Gazette* Occasional Supplement No. 1, 1991; **99** No. 9, September.
25. Health and Safety Statistics 1990–1991, *Employment Gazette* Occasional Supplement No. 1, 1992; **100** No. 9, September.
26. Stevens G. Workplace injury: a view from Health and Safety Executive trailer to the 1990 Labour Force Survey. *Employment Gazette* 1992; **100** No. 12.

Matters of life, death and illness

3

BIRTHS, CONGENITAL ANOMALIES, DEATHS, CANCER AND COMMUNICABLE DISEASES

Alison Macfarlane, Azeem Majeed, Neil Vickers, Phil Atkinson and John Watson

Registration and notification of vital events

Births, congenital anomalies and abortions

Death statistics

Cancer registration

Monitoring communicable diseases

This chapter describes and discusses the data that are derived from the registration and notification of specific life events. These include civil registration of births and deaths and notification of abortion and of specific diseases or conditions, notably congenital anomalies, cancer and communicable diseases. The chapter ends by describing some of the ways in which these data are used as proxy indicators to monitor the health of the population and the performance of the National Health Service (NHS).

Registration and notification of vital events

The origins of civil registration

The civil registration of births, marriages and deaths is a major source of statistics. In England and Wales, registration started in July 1837. Its primary purpose was legal, but statistics have always been an important by-product. Before this time, the only records of births, marriages and deaths were in the parish registers maintained by the established church and in records held by other churches.

The General Register Office for England and Wales was established in Somerset House in London to co-ordinate the work of local registrars of births, marriages and deaths and to set up systems for deriving statistics from the records they sent in. The office was headed by a Registrar General,[1] but the statistical system was set up by the first 'compiler of abstracts', William Farr,[2] an early member of the Statistical Society of London, which later became the Royal Statistical Society.

Following two further Acts of Parliament, registration began in Scotland in 1855 and in Ireland in 1864, and separate General Register Offices were set up in Edinburgh and Dublin. After partition, a further office was set up in Belfast. Registration is still organized separately in Scotland and Northern Ireland. The General Register Office for England and Wales is part of the Office for National Statistics (ONS) and the General Register Office for Northern Ireland is part of the Northern Ireland Statistics and Research Agency (NISRA).

Initially, birth registration was restricted to live births. Stillbirth registration did not start until 1927 in England and Wales, 1939 in Scotland and 1961 in Northern Ireland.[3] In England and Wales, death registration was compulsory from the outset, with a fine of £10 if the person officiating at the burial did not report the death to the registrar within 7 days. Birth registration did not become compulsory until 1874. This means that births and also infant deaths were under-reported in the mid-nineteenth century.

The legal requirement to register births, marriages and deaths means that the data are now likely to be complete. Most are of good quality, as registrars have specific questions to ask and receive training from the ONS. On the other hand, the system is inflexible in that many of the questions asked at registration need an Act of Parliament to change them. Until the review of civil registration in 1999, politicians have showed little interest in legislating on this subject. In 1990, the Office of Population Censuses and Surveys (OPCS) published a White Paper 'Registration: proposals for change'.[4] Since then, only two of the proposals have been enacted, both through private members' bills. The first, which came into effect in October 1992, lowered the gestational age criterion for registering a fetal death as a stillbirth from 28 to 24 weeks. The second enabled marriages to take place in premises other than register offices and religious premises. Some other modifications have come about without primary legislation. It is likely that new legislation will make major changes to the registration system.[5]

Civil registration is not the only source of data about births and deaths. They are also collected through special notification systems and through 'confidential enquiries', which are described later.

Notifications of specific conditions

Most of our attempts to monitor the incidence of diseases rely on indirect measures, such as consultations with general practitioners or admissions to hospital. For monitoring communicable diseases, cancer and congenital anomalies, however, there are specific notification or registration systems.

The statutory requirement to notify certain infectious diseases came into being towards the end of the nineteenth century. Diseases such as cholera, diphtheria, smallpox and typhoid had to be reported from 1891 onwards in London and from 1899 in the rest of England and Wales.

Cancer registration was introduced in the 1930s, as treatments began to develop. The notification of congenital malformations, or anomalies as they are now called, developed in the 1960s in response to severe limb malformations among babies born to women who had taken a drug, thalidomide. These systems are described later in this chapter, while the notification of industrial diseases and injuries is described in Chapter 6.

For a disease or injury to be notified and thus appear in the statistics depends on a chain of events taking place. The Communicable Disease Surveillance Centre, which monitors communicable diseases in England, represents this as a pyramid. It points out that for someone's illness to appear in statistics, they must first see a doctor. Many episodes of communicable disease are not brought to the attention of a doctor. The extent to which this occurs varies from disease to disease. For example, most people with an influenza-like illness will not see their doctor, whereas it is most unlikely that people with meningitis would not be be cared for by the health service.

Next, the doctor must make the correct diagnosis. Clinical diagnoses are subjective, as different doctors diagnose different conditions based on the same symptoms. The degree of subjectivity varies by type of infection. Microbiological confirmation also varies with type of infection. For example, most viral infections causing gastrointestinal upsets will not be investigated microbiologically as they are self-limiting diseases requiring no specific treatment.

The person will not appear in the statistics unless the episode is reported. When a communicable disease is diagnosed, it is obligatory to report the case only if it is one of a list of statutorily notifiable infectious diseases. Even among this list of diseases, there is considerable under-reporting and the extent of this will also vary from disease to disease.

Consequently, an understanding of the issues involved in the diagnosis and reporting of individual communicable diseases is necessary when examining routinely collected statistics. For most purposes, complete reporting of every case of disease is not necessary if the objective of surveillance is to monitor the trends in the occurrence of the disease. Provided that diagnosis and reporting practice remain approximately constant, significant changes in the occurrence of the disease can be determined by observation of the trends in reported cases. On the other hand, there are some diseases for which reporting of every single case is essential in order to initiate local action. Similar considerations apply to the notification of congenital anomalies and the registration of cancer.

Births, congenital anomalies and abortions

Birth statistics

Births must be registered at the register office in the district where they occur. Live births must be registered within 42 days in England, Wales and Northern Ireland and within 21 days in Scotland. A baby born dead after 24 or more completed weeks of pregnancy must be registered as a stillbirth. A certificate of cause of stillbirth, completed by a doctor, is needed for registration. The registrar issues a birth certificate and makes a 'draft entry' in the register. Most register offices now do this by computer, using standard software. Information collected at registration includes the place where the birth occurred, the mother's usual address, and her country of birth.

Concern about the decline in the birth rate in the 1930s generated demands for additional data to interpret these rates. Under the Population (Statistics) Acts of 1938 and 1960, additional information is collected in confidence, including the mother's date of birth and the number of previous live births and stillbirths by her current and any previous husband. The father's date and place of birth and his occupation are recorded for births within marriage and for those outside marriage registered jointly by both parents. For births outside marriage registered by the mother on her own, the mother's occupation is recorded.

Since 1986, the mother's occupation can be recorded for any birth, but the data are not routinely published as they are incomplete.[3] The registrar allocates the baby's NHS number and sends this, together with a copy of the 'draft entry', to the director of public health in the NHS district in which the birth occurred. This means that there is some delay before the baby's NHS number is passed on to clinical staff, making it difficult to link babies' records to their mothers' records. For this reason, the system is changing and by 2001 NHS numbers will be allocated at birth via a computer linked to the NHS Central Register.

Birth registration is not the only system used to collect data about new babies, as the diagram in Fig. 3.1 shows. Births must also be notified to the district director of public health within 36 hours of occurrence. In practice, since the start of the internal market in 1991, the notification has gone to the community trust. The midwife who delivers the baby usually notifies the birth, but occasionally births are notified by the father, the mother or a doctor. The notification form includes identification details such as the mother's name, place of birth, and place of usual residence, the gestational age and the birthweight of the baby as well as any congenital anomalies apparent at birth. The amount of other information varies from place to place.

At the time of writing, the health authority or community trust extracts the NHS number from the draft entry and sends the baby's birthweight back to the registrar of births and deaths. The registrar adds the birthweight to the 'draft entry' and sends a copy to the ONS for processing with other birth registration records, and another to the NHS Central Register at Southport to open a record for the baby. In England, most data from birth notification are not analysed or

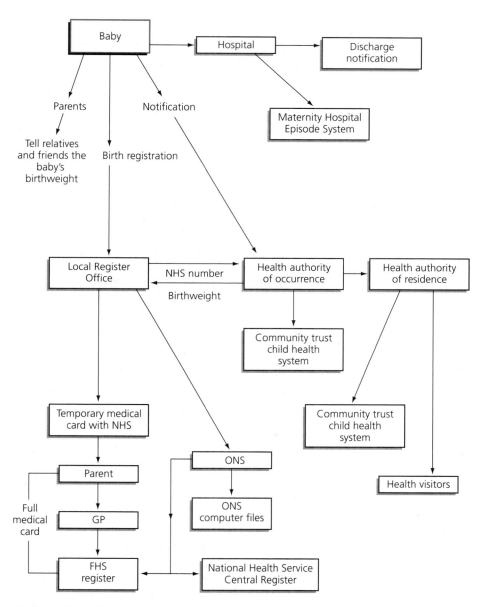

Fig. 3.1   Flows of data about live births in England in 1999. (Reproduced from: Birth counts, statistics of pregnancy and childbirth.)[3]

published, but the notification is usually used to set up a record for the baby in a local child health computer system, whose main purpose is to administer appointments for immunisation and tests of children's health and development. In Wales and Northern Ireland, this process is now being developed as a basis for compiling some basic national data about maternity care.

ONS publishes birth data in *Birth statistics, Series FM1* and in a number of its other series. Some birth data usually appear in conjunction with data about infant mortality in *Mortality statistics, Series DH1* and *Series DH3*, which are described later. The main publications containing birth data for England and Wales are listed in Table 3.1. The ONS publishes the data in the DVS series on CD-ROM and the FM1 monitors about 6 months after the end of the year to which they apply, then publishes fuller tables in its annual reference volumes. In 1999, the ONS replaced the monitor series with reports in its existing quarterly journal, *Population trends,* and a new journal, *Health statistics quarterly.* Birth statistics for Northern Ireland are published in the *Annual report of the Registrar General for Northern Ireland* and those for Scotland appear in the *Annual report of the Registrar General for Scotland.*

As Fig. 3.1 shows, there is a third stream of data collection about births. Hospital and community case notes contain a considerable amount of information about the clinical aspects of the labour and delivery. In England, a 'minimum dataset' of data items extracted from these is aggregated nationally through the Hospital Episode System (HES), which is described in Chapter 8. In addition to the admitted patient record for all hospital births, there is a 'maternity tail' containing data about labour and delivery. This minimum dataset was specified in the early 1980s by the Steering Group on Health Services Information.[6] It should also be collected for home births and births in private hospitals, but only about a quarter of home births and virtually no births in private hospitals find their way into the system. The resulting data are often referred to as Körner data, after Edith Körner, the chair of the group. Unfortunately, the maternity information in the Hospital Episode System is incomplete and generally of poor quality, even though some hospitals collect good quality data locally.[7,8] Furthermore, if a baby is ill and admitted to a special or intensive care unit, the data collected about this are not linked routinely to the Hospital Episode System birth record.

The system started in 1988, but before 1997 few data been published. Attempts are now being made to improve the situation. Key data, such as trends in induction and caesarean rates up to 1994–5, together with comments on data quality, were published in a Department of Health statistical bulletin late in 1997.[7] Data for subsequent years should appear annually. Regular publication should provide an incentive to hospitals to send in data and improve their quality. Nevertheless, progress was hampered by the dismantling of many of the regional databases which existed before the NHS regions were abolished. Thus, in England, there is considerable duplication of effort in collecting birth statistics, but no single system containing reliable data about the care given to women and their babies and no way of linking these with data about their social background.

In Scotland, high quality data about maternity care are collected through the SMR2 Maternity Discharge Sheet and published annually in *Scottish health statistics.* Data for the years 1976–95 were summarised in a special publication, *Birth in Scotland.*[9] Wales and Northern Ireland have now started to collect maternity data via child health computer systems using data from birth notification. Data for Wales have been published by the Welsh Health Information Services in a series of reports, *Maternity data/information aspects of the child*

Table 3.1 Publications containing birth statistics

Series	Title	Coverage	Content
FM1	Annual reference volume, *Birth statistics*, review of the Registrar General on births and patterns of family building	Annual volume with many 10 year comparisons; mainly England and Wales as a whole, but with some tables for regions and districts	Characteristics of live and stillbirths, including seasonality, place of delivery, multiplicity; characteristics of the parents, including ages, occurrence in or outside marriage, previous children, country of birth of parents, and fathers' social class
VS and PP1	Annual reference volume, *Key population and vital statistics*	England and Wales, local authorities and health authorities	Birth rate, births occurring inside and outside marriage, sex of child, infant deaths and stillbirths
	Annual report of the Registrar General for Scotland	Scotland and local authorities	Live and stillbirths, fertility rates
	Annual report of the Registrar General for Northern Ireland	Northern Ireland and local government districts	Live and stillbirths, fertility rates
FM1	Monitor/tables in *Population trends*: live births in England: local and health authority areas	Single years; local and health authorities in England and Wales	Live births and general fertility rates
FM1	Monitor/tables in *Population trends*: conceptions in England and Wales	Single years; local and health authorities in England and Wales	Overall numbers and rates of conceptions leading to registrable births or legal abortions; under-age conceptions

Table 3.1 Continued

Series	Title	Coverage	Content
DVS1	Births and deaths summary data on CD-ROM	England and Wales, local authorities and health authorities	Summary figures of births, fertility rates; comparative numbers and rates
DVS2	Births data on CD-ROM	England and Wales, local authorities and health authorities	Births by age of mother, number of children, type of institution in which the birth occurred and birthweight
DVS4	Births and deaths by wards	Electoral wards	Live births, stillbirths and deaths by sex
DVS5	Infant mortality	England and Wales, local authorities and health authorities	Live births, stillbirths and infant deaths; live and stillbirths by birthweight and stillbirths by gestational age

health system.[10,11] In Northern Ireland, the data are aggregated separately by each of the four health and personal social services boards, but data are sometimes collated for the province as a whole.

Congenital anomalies

Until recently, congenital anomalies were known as congenital malformations. The system for monitoring them in England and Wales was set up in 1964. The aim was to identify promptly any increases in anomaly rates so that early action could be taken, but false alarms, caused by improvements in the rate of reporting and other factors, have occurred more often than real increases. The system, which is voluntary, is linked to the birth notification. The notification form requests information about any anomalies and the health authority extracts details of these and forwards them to the ONS. Each month, the ONS compares the numbers of particular types of anomalies reported from each area with recent trends reported from that area and informs the health authority of any increases. When compiling annual tables, the ONS also uses data from death and stillbirth registrations.

Under-reporting has always been a problem with this system, despite a number of attempts to improve it. Originally, all anomalies, no matter how minor, were notifiable, but in 1990 an exclusion list was introduced. Additionally, the system was originally restricted to anomalies detected within 10 days of birth, although even these were not all notified. By definition, anomalies which do not become apparent until later, for example cardiovascular anomalies, could not be recorded. Since 1 January 1995, the upper time limit no longer applies.

Other improvements have come from a review of the system by a working party whose recommendations were published in 1995.[12] To improve the completeness of data, it suggested that health authorities should collect data from laboratories and hospital departments dealing with babies who have congenital anomalies and monitor abortions carried out because a malformed baby is expected. It also suggested that health authorities should develop systems of electronic data capture. Perhaps most importantly, it recommended that if there was a local register of anomalies, data from this should be forwarded to the ONS, to avoid duplication of effort by using parallel sets of notifications. This is now beginning to happen and the ONS is working with local registers through the British Isles Network of Congenital Anomaly Registers (BINOCAR).

The main publication for England and Wales is an annual reference volume, *Congenital anomaly statistics, Series MB3,* details of which are shown in Table 3.2. Until 1993, its title was *Congenital malformation statistics.* In 1999, the ONS issued a guide for data users and suppliers, which, as well as describing the notification system, lists regional registries and international organisations concerned with surveillance of anomalies.[13]

Table 3.2 Publications containing congenital anomaly statistics

Series	Title	Coverage	Content
MB3	Congenital anomaly statistics, notifications: a statistical review of notifications of congenital anomalies received as part of the England and Wales National Congenital Anomaly System	Usually a single year England and Wales	Rates, by conditions, usual area of residence of mother, birthweight, age of mother, parity, father's occupation, father's social class, and abortions on grounds of fetal anomaly
	Congenital malformations in Scotland	Scotland	
	Annual report of Chief Medical Officer for Northern Ireland	Northern Ireland	

There are separate notification systems for Scotland and Northern Ireland. In Scotland, data on congenital anomalies come from three sources, the SMR2 maternity record, records of hospital in-patient stays by babies, and the still-birth and neonatal death records. The data are published by the Information and Statistics Division (ISD) of the NHS in Scotland in *Congenital malformations in Scotland*. In Northern Ireland, congenital anomalies are monitored by the Regional Medical Genetics Centre at Belfast City Hospital and published in the *Annual report of Chief Medical Officer for Northern Ireland*.

Abortion notifications

Pregnancies terminated under the 1967 Abortion Act must be notified on the prescribed form to the chief medical officers of England, Wales and Scotland within 7 days. The 1967 Abortion Act does not apply to Northern Ireland. Abortions must be carried out by a registered medical practitioner in an NHS hospital or other premises approved by the Secretary of State. Information about the woman, the grounds for abortion, the method used and the type of premises is recorded. By arrangement with the chief medical officers, the ONS undertakes the statistical processing and analysis of abortion statistics for England and Wales. The statistics are published in annual volumes (Table 3.3). Up to 1998, provisional data were published in quarterly and annual monitors. In 1999, the monitors were discontinued and some of the tables were incorporated into *Health statistics quarterly*. Abortion statistics for Scotland are published by the Information and Statistics Division in an annual *Health briefing* and then in *Scottish health statistics*.

Table 3.3 Publications containing data about legal abortion

Series	Title	Coverage	Content
AB	Annual reference volume: *Abortion statistics, England and Wales*	Annual since 1969/England and Wales, some tables for health authorities	Statutory grounds, age parity, length of stay, marital status, area of residence, type of premises, procedure used, complications and deaths, abortions carried out on medical grounds such as rubella or congenital anomalies
AB	Annual monitor/tables in *Health statistics quarterly*: legal abortions, residents of regional and district health areas	Annual/England and Wales, health authorities	Marital status, age group, parity, operations type of premises, gestation
AB	Quarterly monitor/tables in *Health statistics quarterly*: legal abortions, residents of regional and district health areas	Quarterly/England and Wales, health authorities	Marital status, age group, parity, operations, type of premises, gestation
AB	Annual monitor/tables in *Health statistics quarterly*: legal abortion in England and Wales	Annual/England and Wales	Purchaser, marital status, age group, parity, operations, type of premises, gestation
	Health briefing	Annual/Scotland	Age, parity, gestational age at termination

Death statistics

Death registration

When a death occurs, a doctor issues a medical certificate of 'cause of death'. The next of kin are required to take the certificate to the register office in the locality where the death has occurred and register the death, within 5 days. The registrar then completes a 'draft entry' in the register, although most register offices now do this by computer. The information recorded is the person's date of birth, date of death, place of death, place of residence, causes of death given on the medical certificate and the person's last occupation. A death certificate is issued and a copy of the 'draft entry' is sent to the director of public health for the NHS district in which the death occurred.

In England and Wales, further copies are sent to the ONS for data processing and to the National Health Service Central Register to remove the person from his or her general practitioner's list. The ONS uses the information on the 'draft entry' to do statistical analyses and to compile registers of individual death records. Causes of deaths are coded according to the International Classification of Diseases (ICD), using special software, and an 'underlying cause' is derived. Prior to 1993, this was done manually, using slightly different coding rules. The change caused discontinuities in the data. The problems are documented in OPCS and ONS publications containing death data for 1993 and in an article in *Population trends*.[14,15]

If further information is received from coroners or pathologists, the ONS amends the cause of death on its own records, but not on the public records. It has two computerised databases, one with public records and one with the amended data. The process of death registration and the way statistics are derived from it have been described in detail in an article in *Health statistics quarterly*.[16]

The ONS has copies of all entries of deaths since 1837 and can provide copies of death certificates for individuals for epidemiological research or family histories. These records can be obtained from local register offices or the Family Records Centre in London. (The address is given at the end of the chapter). Separate but similar registration systems exist in Scotland and Northern Ireland.

Measures of mortality

In these publications, death rates are expressed in a number of different ways. The most common are summarised in Table 3.4. Most of the publications contain fuller explanations and definitions. Crude death rates do not allow for differences in the age structure of populations. A social group or geographical area with a high proportion of elderly people is likely to have a higher overall death rate than one with a high proportion of young people, even if the death rate at each age is lower in the first group. The most common methods of standardisation used to compensate for this are described in Table 3.4.

Table 3.4 Death rates and standardised death rates

Crude death rate	Number of deaths per 1000 people
Age-specific death rate	Number of deaths per 1000 people in a specific age group, for example 65–74 year olds
Standardised mortality ratio (SMR)	Indirect standardisation uses a set of national or reference death rates and applies them to the structures of groups within the country. Thus, SMR compares the 'expected deaths', which would occur in a population if it had the same mortality rate as a 'reference' population, often England and Wales as a whole, and the 'observed' deaths, which actually occurred in the population or category of people. It expresses the 'observed' deaths as a ratio of the 'expected' deaths. The SMR for the 'reference' group is 100. A population with an SMR under 100 has fewer deaths than expected and a population with an SMR over 100 has more deaths than expected
Age-standardised mortality rates	Direct standardisation takes a standard age structure for a population and applies to this the death rates of each of the groups being compared. This gives an 'expected' number of deaths, which is divided by the total number of people in the standard population. These rates are called age-standardised mortality rates. ONS tends to use the *European standard population* for calculating age-standardised rates, as it has a similar structure to that of England and Wales and the resulting rates can be compared internationally
Years of life lost	The number of years of life lost due to death at a 'premature' age. ONS takes 85 years as a 'cut-off' and subtracts the age of death from this. Deaths from causes which tend to occur at an early age, such as accidents, contribute more than others to years of life lost
Years of working life lost	The numbers of years of life lost if death takes place before the end of the assumed working life. ONS takes this as 65 years of age

Uses of mortality statistics

Mortality statistics not only form the cornerstone for monitoring the health of populations, but are also used extensively and sometimes fallaciously in resource allocation, in planning and in monitoring services.

A very common use of mortality data is to monitor and describe disease patterns, for example the increase in deaths attributed to acquired immune deficiency syndrome (AIDS) and epidemics such as influenza. Mortality data may be linked with other data to explore possible explanations for disease outbreaks, such as clusters of leukaemia around power stations.

Death statistics are also used to monitor the outcomes of health care. There have been many attempts to use death statistics to monitor the effectiveness of health services. For example, there are hospital league tables and clinical effectiveness indicators that attempt to use death rates to compare the performance of hospitals. This is despite the fact that statisticians from Florence Nightingale and her contemporaries onwards have pointed out that mortality in hospitals is strongly influenced by factors such as the proportion of people admitted who are severely ill and whether terminally ill people are discharged home or elsewhere to die. Furthermore, the statistical validity of rankings, especially when based on small numbers of events, is very questionable. In Scotland, better facilities for record linkage have meant that some of these factors can be taken into account when devising statistical indicators, and they are not usually published in rank order.

Mortality rates are often used to monitor the health of the population. For example, the Department of Health's *Public health common dataset* contains many mortality rates. These are often used as proxy measures of morbidity in public health initiatives, notably the Conservative government's *Health of the nation* and the Labour government's successor *Our healthier nation*. Using mortality rates in this way ignores the fact that people who suffer severe morbidity, for example a stroke, are increasingly likely to survive and die later from some other cause.

Mortality rates are used as proxy measures of social deprivation or morbidity in formulae used to allocate NHS resources. Standardised mortality ratios (SMRs) are thought to be correlated both with measures of illness or morbidity and with measures of social deprivation. They are therefore used as proxy measures of 'need' for health care or social care in formulae used to allocate resources to both health authorities and local authorities. There is a major flaw in this, as the conditions from which people die are very often not those for which they need either acute hospital treatment or long-term care. Furthermore, the measure used for allocating resources to health authorities is the square root of the standardised mortality ratio for people aged 0–74 years. In fact, the association between social deprivation and standardised mortality ratio is usually strongest among people in the 0–64 age group. There is reluctance to use this standardised mortality ratio in resource allocation, however, as doing so would mean transferring resources from more affluent areas to inner cities.

Publications

Mortality statistics are published by the ONS in volumes in its DH series, for individual years, tabulated by age, sex, area of residence and certified cause of death (Table 3.5). In England and Wales, special publications are devoted to perinatal and infant mortality and to accidents and violence. The published geographical breakdown is by region, local authority and health authority.

Table 3.5 Annual publications containing mortality data

Series	Title	Coverage	Content
DH1	*Mortality statistics, general, England and Wales*	Some time series, otherwise single year/ England and Wales, some tables for regions	Deaths and death rates by age, sex, marital status; SMR for specific causes; place of death by age and cause; place of death registration and place of birth; years of life lost
DH2	*Mortality statistics, cause, England and Wales*	Some time series/England and Wales	Deaths by age, sex and ICD code; SMR; age-standardised rates
DH3	*Mortality statistics, childhood, infant and perinatal, social and biological factors, England and Wales*	England and Wales, some tables by region	Stillbirths and infant mortality in relation to occupation of parents, area of residence, country of birth of mother, duration of pregnancy, cause of death, place of confinement, age of mother, birthweight and multiple births
DH4	*Mortality statistics, injury and poisoning, England and Wales, known as Mortality statistics, accidents and violence up to 1989*	England and Wales	Information obtained from coroners' inquests; deaths deaths by sex, age and month of occurrence, and by cause, type and place of accident, including fire, road traffic accident, violence and poisonous substances
DH5	*Mortality statistics, area, England and Wales, discontinued after 1992*	England and Wales, standard regions, Greater London, Metropolitan and non-metropolitan counties, RHA, DHA	Covered same subjects as DH2 on microfiche; some tables now appear in DH1, others on disc as table VS3
DH6	*Mortality statistics, childhood, England and Wales; separate volumes for years 1986–92*	England and Wales, some tables by region, 1986–92 only	Stillbirths, early and late neonatal deaths; deaths at 28 days to 14 years by cause, sex and age group; from 1993 onwards, combined with DH3
	Annual report of the Registrar General for Scotland	Scotland and local authorities	Deaths by cause, sex, age at death; stillbirth and infant mortality rates
	Annual report of the Registrar General for Northern Ireland	Northern Ireland and local government districts	Deaths by cause, sex, age at death; stillbirth and infant mortality rates

Up to 1998, death data for England and Wales for each year appeared first in monitors in the DH series, followed later by fuller annual reference volumes (Table 3.6). In 1999, the monitor series was replaced by tables in ONS's quarterly journal, *Population trends* and in its new *Health statistics quarterly*. In the aftermath of a major reorganisation of OPCS' computing arrangements in the early 1990s, some annual volumes contained data for more than 1 year. The changes were summarised in the introductory section of *Mortality statistics, Series DH1, No. 28*, which covered the 3 years 1993–5 and was published by ONS in 1997, and were described in articles in *Population trends* and *Health statistics quarterly*.[14-16]

Mortality statistics for Northern Ireland are published in the *Annual report of the Registrar General for Northern Ireland* and those for Scotland appear in the *Annual report of the Registrar General for Scotland*.

As well as monitors and annual reference volumes, the ONS provides summaries for local and health authorities on CD-ROM. Data can also be supplied for other geographical areas, down to electoral wards. Health authorities can obtain individual records for their geographical area. Aggregated mortality data, along with data on other subjects, are available for all health authorities in England in the *Public health common dataset*, described later in this chapter.

Many health authorities also obtain computerised files of individual records of deaths of their residents. This allows them to use postcodes to analyse data for small areas, such as enumeration districts. By linking these with data in family health services' age–sex registers, mortality rates can also be computed for individual general practices.

In 1997, the ONS published 95 years of data on a CD-ROM, *Twentieth century mortality*.[17] This contains counts of numbers of deaths in each year from 1901 to 1995, tabulated by International Classification of Diseases code, in 5-year age bands. The corresponding population estimates are given to allow rates and time trends to be calculated. It also published a two-volume review on paper, *The health of adult Britain, 1841–1994*.[18] The associated data were published on a further CD-ROM in 1998.

Decennial supplements

Every 10 years, when census data are analysed, they are compared with data from death registration in England and Wales to produce 'decennial supplements'. These compare the characteristics of people who die in the years immediately before and after the census with those of the population enumerated in the census. Analyses of death rates by area of residence and occupation have been done since the 1850s. These have highlighted geographical areas and occupations with high mortality rates. Their use in monitoring occupational health is described in Chapter 6, and analyses of inequalities in decennial supplements are described in Chapter 4.

Since 1911, the occupations have been grouped into the Registrar General's social classes, which are listed and discussed in Chapter 4. These have shown wide disparities between the mortality of the least and most privileged

Table 3.6 Mortality data published up to 1998 in ONS monitors, and as reports in *Health statistics quarterly* from 1999 onwards

Series	Title	Coverage	Content
DH2	Mortality cause by quarter	England and Wales, counties, regions	Cause by age and sex
DH3	Infant and perinatal mortality, social and biological factors	England and Wales, health authorities, regions	Live births, stillbirths, neonatal, post-neonatal and infant deaths; live births weighing less than 1500 g and 2500 g
DH3	Infant and perinatal mortality, social and biological factors	England and Wales	Stillbirth and infant mortality rates by birthweight, cause of death, mother's age, country of birth and marital status, father's social class
DH3	Sudden infant deaths	Current year and previous 4 years/ England and Wales	Sudden infant deaths by sex, age at death, month of occurrence, birthweight, mother's age, country of birth and marital status, father's social class and other causes mentioned on death certificate
DH4	Deaths from injury and poisoning by quarter	England and Wales	Transport accidents, accidents at home, suicide, homicide by age group
DH4	Fatal accidents occurring during sport and leisure activities	England and Wales	Generated from coroners' reports; deaths from air sports, athletics, ball games, horse riding, motor and water sports, cycling, mountaineering, and among spectators by age

occupational groups. The fact that these widened during the 1970s caused embarrassment to the Conservative government, which ensured that few social class analyses related to the 1981 census were published on paper, while the rest were released on expensive and unreadable microfiches. Since then, however, there has been a change of policy and the decennial supplements have become much wider ranging documents. They now include analyses of data from other sources, notably the OPCS Longitudinal Study (described in Chapter 2), to complement the traditional decennial supplement analyses. The decennial supplements published since this policy was established are listed in Table 3.7. Work started in 1998 on a geography supplement linked to the 1991 census, but the many boundary changes during the 1990s have made analyses difficult and the supplement is not planned to appear until the year 2000.

Confidential enquiries

Deaths in a few special categories are examined through a process known as 'confidential enquiry'. In these, anonymised information from case notes and reports from professionals who gave care to the people who died are gathered together and examined by panels of relevant professionals. The panels attempt to assess whether the death was 'avoidable' or, more recently, whether there are elements of substandard care, and draw lessons from them. The process has been criticised for failing to make comparisons with care given to groups of people who did not die, and they have now started to introduce these.

At the time of writing, there are four confidential enquiries: the Confidential Enquiry into Maternal Deaths (CEMD), the National Confidential Enquiry into Peri-operative Deaths (NCEPOD), the Confidential Enquiry into Suicide and Homicide by People with Mental Illness (CISH) and the Confidential Enquiry into Stillbirths and Deaths in Infancy (CESDI).[19] The National Confidential Enquiry into Peri-operative Deaths began in 1988 and is contracted out to the Royal College of Surgeons. It audits deaths occurring within 30 days of any surgical or gynaecological operation. It is very incomplete, with over a fifth of surgeons and anaesthetists failing to take part. The Confidential Enquiry into Suicide and Homicide by People with Mental Illness was set up in 1991 to audit suicide and homicide among people who have been in contact with the mental health services. The other two enquiries are described on the following pages.

Table 3.7 'New style' decennial supplements for England and Wales

Series DS, number	Title	Year of publication
9	Mortality and geography, a review in the mid-1980s	1990
10	Occupational health, decennial supplement	1995
11	The health of our children	1995
12	The health of adult Britain, Volumes 1 and 2	1997
13	Inequalities in health	1997

for the use of cancer data, which far surpassed the traditional uses of monitoring time trends and geographical variations. The working party's vision included the use of cancer statistics in the management of resources required for the preventative, curative and laboratory services for cancer, and planning and evaluation of services, particularly screening programmes. It advocated the planning and evaluation of clinical management and treatment based on accurate, unbiased survival data and clinical trials.

The working party also proposed that the data could be used for research into the causes of cancer, involving case-control studies and the 'flagging' of cohorts of people at the NHS central register, and that information could be provided for health education and health promotion. If linked with other databases, it was thought that the system could enable evaluation of the quality of care and quality assurance and that cost could be related to clinical outcome.

The introduction of the NHS internal market in 1991 and the subsequent abolition of regional health authorities put a question mark over the future of cancer registries and put a brake on implementation of the working party's recommendations.

Cancer registration has never been compulsory. An executive letter from the NHS Executive, EL(92)95, was issued in December 1992 instructing all NHS providers to supply data for the contract minimum dataset from July 1993.[32] This makes it mandatory in the NHS, but the private sector is under no obligation to supply data. A study of cancer registration in south east England found that people dying in private hospitals were significantly more likely to be registered by DCO.[33] In view of private institutions' increased share in the health care market, it is essential that they, too, be required to provide data.

Which data are collected?

Each registry attempts to record data on every malignant tumour diagnosed on its territory and on some in-situ tumours. Data items can be grouped under four headings: personal data, data on the tumour, treatment data and outcome variables. Since 1993, cancer registries have collected a common minimum dataset. Its content reflects a change in focus in cancer registration, from epidemiology to contracting. The items are listed in Table 3.9. The data collected on the tumour include its site, or position in the body, its morphology, or tissue of origin, its microscopic structure, its behaviour in terms of whether it is benign, *in situ*, or malignant, and its stage, or how advanced it is in its natural history.

In 1997, a new core contract for cancer registration was agreed by the registries in consultation with the Department of Health.[34] This set ambitious targets for data quality, by standardising the data collected and introducing benchmarks for quality.

Prior to 1993, a more restricted dataset was available. Registries did not all collect the same variables. Personal data typically included the patient's name, address, date of birth, date of diagnosis, address and postcode, marital status, occupation and NHS number. Data were also collected on the tumour itself, including site, morphology, behaviour, stage and the basis of the diagnosis, whether by histology, cytology, clinical opinion or post-mortem. Most

Table 3.9 The contract minimum dataset for cancer registration

Contract details	Provider code
	Date of first registration
Patient details	Surname
	Forenames
	Date of birth
	Address
	Sex
	Marital status
	NHS number
	Ethnicity
	Occupation
	Date of death
Tumour details	Date of diagnosis
	Tumour site
	Tumour morphology
	Pathology verification
	Behaviour code in ICD-10
	Tumour stage
Spell details	Admission date
	Discharge date
Episode details	Patient identifier
	Specialty
	Consultant
	Diagnosis
	Treatment
	Date of treatment
	Case note number

registries also collected information on the mode of presentation, whether by screening, autopsy or symptoms.

Treatment was followed up for a limited period, usually 6 months. Any treatments initiated within the follow-up period were recorded using OPCS operation codes. District of residence was recorded, along with district of treatment, provider code, the name and address of the patient's general practitioner and the name of the consultant under whose care the person was treated. A few outcome variables were collected, including cause, place and date of death. Information is sometimes available on whether a post-mortem examination was made.

Who can access cancer registration data?

Until 1991, a major function of registries in England and Wales was to provide information on cancer to regional and district directors of public health to use in their annual reports and for monitoring cancer in their local populations.

As a consequence of the introduction of the NHS internal market from 1991 onwards, the registries' role switched to providing data to purchasing authorities. These include new health authorities and private sector purchasers. Since the abolition of regional health authorities, a health authority has been appointed 'lead purchaser' for each registry. The lead purchaser co-ordinates the commissioning of cancer registry data on behalf of all NHS authorities in its area, is responsible for cancer registration in the region, and is accountable to the regional office for these functions.

Most regional registries publish annual reports containing many of the most important data in summary form. Obtaining clinical case notes can take over a year and, consequently, reports of cancer incidence in a given year cannot be completed for at least 2 years. In the late 1990s, registries started to forge electronic links with NHS-wide networks, with the aim of curtailing such delays. In Scotland, the way registry data are linked to hospital activity databases tends to make retrieval speedier.

Researchers can also obtain registry data on diskette. A fee may be payable and usually larger fees are charged to commercial users than to researchers. Registered users of the census can obtain regional cancer registry data and link postcodes to enumeration districts to generate profiles of incidence, treatment and survival by census variables, such as car ownership, housing tenure, unemployment or deprivation scores such as the Carstairs, Jarman and Townsend indices. Some regional registries may also provide data on social class according to the occupation as recorded on the death certificate.

The main printed publications at national level in England and Wales are in the MB1 series (Table 3.10). The annual publications in this series include extensive commentary about the registration scheme and the changes it has undergone. They also include articles on international trends in cancer incidence and mortality, cancer registration, risk and survival patterns at the main sites, such as breast and lung cancer. The detailed tables of registrations by region are issued on diskette, with those for earlier years being on microfiche. Up to 1998, incidence and survival data were also published in the OPCS's and ONS's monitor series. Since 1999, these tables and some commentaries have been published in the ONS's *Health statistics quarterly*. In the mid-1990s, the reorganisation of the system in England and Wales delayed publications.

Table 3.10 Publications containing cancer registration statistics

Series	Title	Coverage	Content
MB1	*Cancer statistics registrations, registration of cancer diagnosed in England and Wales*	Annual/England and Wales, England, Wales	Incidence and mortality ratios by sex and site, cumulative risk of registration; registrations by sex and site; standardised registration ratios and age-standardised rates
	Cancer statistics, Scotland	Scotland	

This was followed by a spate of the publications in the late 1990s. In 1999, the ONS published a CD of cancer registrations, containing records of both new cases and deaths. It also published a major book, *Cancer survival trends in England and Wales, 1971–1995: deprivation and NHS region*, accompanied by a CD-ROM.[35,36]

Monitoring communicable diseases

The Communicable Disease Surveillance Centre (CDSC) of the Public Health Laboratory Service (PHLS), which was set up in 1977, is responsible for the collection, collation and dissemination of information on communicable disease in England and Wales. The Communicable Disease Surveillance Centre is responsible for running a range of special surveillance systems for communicable diseases, including AIDS and human immunodeficiency virus (HIV) infection, monitoring the childhood immunisation programme in England and Wales, and co-ordinating European-wide systems for legionnaires' disease and *Salmonella* infection.

The Communicable Disease Surveillance Centre publishes the weekly Communicable Disease Report, *CDR weekly*, in which information on a rotating cycle of infections is published. This is supplemented by the monthly *CDR Review*, recently replaced by the journal *Communicable Disease and Public Health*, with more detailed reports on specific infections, original papers, extended review articles and outbreak reports covering food, water, and blood-borne infections including HIV/AIDS.

The Communicable Disease Surveillance Centre also publishes a range of ad-hoc reports and standard papers in peer-reviewed journals relating to the occurrence of various communicable diseases and will provide data on the occurrence of disease from both routine surveillance and special surveillance systems. No charge is usually made for this information, although requests for detailed information which is not readily available may incur a charge. The Communicable Disease Surveillance Centre publications are available by subscription and can usually be found in medical and public libraries. The *CDR weekly* is supplied free to people working in public health, communicable disease control and microbiology.

Developments in information technology, including access to the internet, are likely to provide opportunity for the provision of data in a more publicly and readily available form in the future. The Public Health Laboratory Service worldwide web site already contains some communicable disease data, including AIDS/HIV quarterly surveillance tables, laboratory and outbreak reports of gastrointestinal diseases, the *Influenza weekly bulletin*, recent influenza activity data and notification data for England and Wales. This site is under review, and will contain a wider range of information is being added.

The Scottish Centre for Infection and Environmental Health (SCIEH) in Ruchill Hospital, Glasgow, is responsible for the collection, collation and dissemination of information on communicable disease in Scotland. It collects information on a wide variety of communicable diseases, including HIV and AIDS, and returns from genitourinary clinics providing details of new cases of sexually transmitted disease. Information is in the form of weekly reports and published in *Scottish health statistics*. The Information and Statistics Division also publishes a health briefing, *Cases seen at genito-urinary medicine clinics*.

Communicable disease statistics in Northern Ireland are collected by the Department of Health, Social Services and Public Safety. Infectious disease statistics and sexually transmitted disease statistics based on new patients seen in genitourinary clinics were published in *Health and personal services statistics for Northern Ireland* and are now published in the Department of Health, Social Services and Public Safety's volumes of *Community statistics*. At the time of writing, data from the system of notifying sexually transmitted diseases are incomplete, following the collapse of the computer system in the largest clinic in the Royal group of hospitals. AIDS and HIV data can be found in the *Annual report of the Chief Medical Officer for Northern Ireland*.

Data from the European surveillance schemes and outbreak reports of interest to the European community are published in *EuroSurveillance Weekly*.

Sources of information on communicable disease

The two major types of information on communicable disease in England and Wales are notifications of infectious diseases to proper officers of local authorities, forwarded to the Public Health Laboratory Service Communicable Disease Surveillance Centre, and reporting of microbiologically confirmed infections by NHS, private and public health laboratories to the Public Health Laboratory Service Communicable Disease Surveillance Centre.

These two sources account for the large majority of data on communicable disease in England and Wales. Other sources include reports of consultations with general practitioners in the Royal College of General Practitioners Weekly Returns Service, or in the similar scheme organised by the Welsh Unit of the Communicable Disease Surveillance Centre, special surveillance systems for particular diseases or groups of diseases such as HIV/AIDS and illness in schools that are part of the Medical Officers of Schools Association (MOSA). Hospital Episode System data relating to reports of clinical activity during admissions to NHS hospitals and death registration also contain data on communicable diseases.

Notification of communicable diseases

Over the century since notification was first introduced, the list of notifiable diseases has enlarged, with some differences between the countries of the UK. The current list for England and Wales, as defined by the Public Health Act 1984, is shown in Table 3.11.[37]

Medical practitioners are statutorily obliged to report notifiable diseases to the 'proper officer' of the local authority, normally the consultant in communicable disease control, in which the disease is identified or suspected. In 1999, they were paid £2.65 for each reported notification.[38]

Table 3.11   Diseases currently notifiable

Acute encephalitis	Paratyphoid fever
Acute poliomyelitis	Plague
Anthrax	Relapsing fever
Cholera	Rubella
Diphtheria	Scarlet fever
Dysentery	Smallpox
Food poisoning	Tetanus
Leprosy*	Tuberculosis
Leptospirosis	Typhoid fever
Malaria	Typhus
Measles	Viral haemorrhagic fever
Meningitis	Viral hepatitis
Meningococcal septicaemia	Whooping cough
Mumps	Yellow fever
Ophthalmia neonatorum	

*Notified directly to the Director of the Public Health Laboratory
Service Communicable Disease Surveillance Centre.

Notifiable diseases are reported on clinical suspicion, with or without microbiological support for the diagnosis. Accuracy of diagnosis is of secondary importance. If a diagnosis later proves to be incorrect, the notification can always be changed or cancelled. For some diseases, the clinical manifestations are very specific, but for others they are not. For example, many cases of rash appearing in children are reported as measles, but only a small proportion of these are now found to be due to infection with the measles virus.[39]

The standard notification report form records only a limited amount of information, but some local authorities have designed their own form to record additional data items such as those shown in Table 3.12.

Each week, the proper officer is required to provide a weekly statistical return to the Public Health Laboratory Service Communicable Disease Surveillance Centre giving information on the type of disease, and the exact age and sex of individual notifications that have been received during the week. This is followed at quarterly intervals by a statistical return incorporating any corrections to the original weekly figures. Although individual records are collected centrally, neither names nor addresses are included in the details submitted by proper officers.

The prime purpose of the notifications system is *speed* in detecting possible outbreaks and epidemics. Unfortunately, considerable reporting delays and under-notification occur, although the degree of under-notification varies with disease type. A review of national neonatal meningitis data in England and Wales during the years 1975–91 found that neonatal meningitis was seriously under-notified.[40] The ratio of laboratory reported cases to cases notified ranged from 12 : 1 in 1985 to 4 : 1 in 1989. A study in the 1970s used several different sources of data, including statutory notifications, to identify cases of acute bacterial meningitis in childhood in a defined population.[41] Only half the cases of meningococcal meningitis and less than one-quarter of other types of bacterial meningitis had been notified.

Notifications of tuberculosis (TB) are more complete than notifications of

Table 3.12 Common data items on 'standard' and 'amended' notification forms used at local level

Data items on 'standard' notification form
Name
Address
Age
Date of birth
Sex
Disease
Onset date
Notification date
Additional data items on some 'amended' notification forms
Postcode
Ethnic group
Country of birth
Tuberculosis smear positivity
Occupation, and/or place of work
Vaccination status
Risk group
Laboratory confirmed
Local general practitioner

meningitis, yet an audit of tuberculosis in east London found 15 per cent of identified cases were not notified.[42] Even bank holidays can cause a drop by 15 to 30 per cent in the number of weekly notifications, and the shortfall may not be made up in succeeding weeks. Notifications may not give precise estimates of the incidence of individual infectious diseases, but they do provide crude indicators of change in incidence in the community.

National notification statistics were originally collected at the General Register Office, later part of the OPCS and now part of the ONS. In 1997, the responsibility for administering the notification system transferred to the Communicable Disease Surveillance Centre. Notification data collected before 1997 were published by OPCS, then ONS in Series MB2. This had a weekly, a quarterly and an annual publication cycle. Since 1997, the Communicable Disease Surveillance Centre has published weekly data in the *CDR weekly* and quarterly and annual data in special reports. Data down to district level are now available on the Public Health Laboratory Service worldwide web site. In Scotland, data are notified to the Information and Statistics Division. They are published weekly by the Scottish Centre for Infection and Environmental Health and annually in *Scottish health statistics*.

Laboratory reports

Microbiologists report positive infectious disease isolates from microbiologists to the Public Health Laboratory Service Communicable Disease Surveillance Centre. The concept of a network of microbiology laboratories reporting to a national centre dates back to 1939. In 1996, the Communicable Disease

Surveillance Centre received approximately 250 000 reports from 370 laboratories in England, Wales and Northern Ireland and some from laboratories in the Irish Republic. Laboratories in Scotland report to the Scottish Centre for Infection and Environmental Health.

The organisms to be reported can be summarised as those of public health importance, and are laid down in the 'reporting guidelines' document issued to all laboratories in England and Wales.[43] These include the 'high profile' organisms, well known to the general public, and listed in Table 3.13. Laboratory reporting tends to take place in a reasonably timely fashion, allowing the data to be used by epidemiologists for the early recognition of outbreaks. A great deal of information is often available about the organism, normally genus and species and often type, making it possible to do detailed epidemiological studies into the changing patterns of infection.

Reporting is voluntary for NHS laboratories and, unfortunately, not all participate in the surveillance scheme. Non-reporters tend to be the larger laboratories in urban areas, such as London. Participating laboratories do not always report all isolates of requested organisms or all requested data items. The level of under-reporting varies from laboratory to laboratory and organism to organism.

Tuberculosis, which has a particularly high incidence in London, is poorly reported. For example, when a comparison was made between laboratory reports and notifications in 1993, it was found that for every one laboratory report there were four notifications.[44] In 1996, laboratories in the Thames regions reported just under 1600 positive isolates of gonorrhoea compared with 5800 diagnoses of gonorrhoea from genitourinary clinics in the same regions, a ratio of 1 : 4.[45]

Other than the type of organism, the information collected is very limited. It usually consists of age, sex, site of microbiological specimen, and type of test. Virtually no geographical data are recorded on the location of the infected person.

Data based on laboratory reporting are routinely published in the *CDR weekly* and the *Communicable disease and public health journal*. They are also available on the Public Health Laboratory Service web site.

Royal College of General Practitioners' weekly returns service

Since 1967, diagnoses of common infectious diseases have been reported to the Royal College of General Practitioners' weekly returns service by a cohort of general practices. The surveillance system currently involves around

Table 3.13 'High profile' organisms reported to the Communicable Disease Surveillance Centre

Escherichia coli O157	Methicillin-resistant Staphylococcus aureus (MRSA)
Salmonella	Legionella
Campylobacter	Influenza
Cryptosporidia	Hepatitis

eighty practices distributed throughout England and Wales. The practices report the diseases shown in Table 3.14 on a weekly basis, some electronically and some using paper forms. The participating general practitioners are provided with 'diagnostic guidelines'. Although these are not the same as strict diagnostic criteria, they may be effective in achieving some degree of standardisation. Diagnoses are not substantiated by diagnostic test, but the weekly returns service claims it has evidence that individual doctors are consistent in their use of diagnostic terms.[46]

The reporting practices serve 600 000 people, about 1 per cent of the population of England and Wales. The sparse geographical distribution of the practices precludes their use as markers for pattern and spread of disease at a local and regional scale. Despite the small population base, trends in key conditions show close similarity with trends from other surveillance systems, with changes often appearing several weeks before laboratory report and notifications. Data from the weekly returns service are reported in the special Communicable Disease Surveillance Centre quarterly and annual reports and in peer-reviewed journals.[46] Influenza reports can be found on the Public Health Laboratory Service worldwide web pages.

Special surveillance systems

The reporting system for AIDS was first established in 1982 when dermatologists, venereologists and microbiologists were asked to provide confidential reports to the Public Health Laboratory Service Communicable Disease Surveillance Centre. The report form asks information about the patient's demography, risk group, clinical presentation and type of care. Studies have shown that, despite sometimes considerable reporting delay, a very high proportion of all AIDS cases is reported.[47,48]

AIDS was more formally defined in 1985 and this definition was revised further in 1987 and 1993. These revisions have not had a substantial impact on recorded trends. It has become clear, however, that the introduction of effective antiviral therapy has had a marked effect in delaying progression to AIDS in people who are treated before an AIDS-defining condition develops and in delaying death in people who already have AIDS. The AIDS dataset tells us little about recent transmission patterns, because of the long delay between infection and diagnosis.

Table 3.14   Common infectious disorders reported by the Royal College of General Practitioners' weekly returns service

Infectious intestinal disease	Infectious hepatitis
Whooping cough	Mumps
Scarlet fever	Infectious mononucleosis
Chicken pox	Scabies
Herpes zoster	Meningitis
Measles	Hand, foot and mouth disease
Rubella	Other infectious diseases in the ICD classification, such as warts and candida

Laboratories began reporting newly identified HIV infections to the Communicable Disease Surveillance Centre when the tests became available in 1984. This surveillance system is voluntary, too, but most laboratories participate. The Public Health Laboratory Service AIDS and Sexually Transmitted Diseases Centre estimates that at least three-quarters of all laboratory-diagnosed infections are reported. Information associated with each HIV report includes basic demographic and risk group data, but there is no information on place of residence. HIV test data are biased towards those people who perceive themselves to be at risk or who are ill and therefore go for or are recommended to take an HIV test.

The report of laboratory diagnosis of HIV infection is supplemented by a comprehensive programme of anonymous testing for HIV in attenders at genitourinary medicine clinics, injecting drug users, pregnant women, women having abortions, and babies. The main aim of the programme is to monitor the prevalence and associated risks of HIV in accessible groups. Some of these groups are made up of people whose behaviour makes them vulnerable to infection, while others are more representative of the general population. About 650 000 specimens are tested each year.[49] They all have patient-identifying details permanently removed before testing so that there is no possibility that individual test results can be traced back to the source person. The programme also allows the proportion of HIV infections which remain undiagnosed to be estimated. HIV-infected pregnant women are particularly unlikely to have their HIV infection diagnosed clinically.[50]

AIDS and HIV data are published in AIDS/HIV quarterly surveillance tables, a monthly insert in the *CDR weekly*, and a number of surveillance system specific annual reports.[51] In Scotland, HIV and AIDS are reported to the Scottish Centre for Infection and Environmental Health and published annually in *Scottish health statistics*. In Northern Ireland, data are published in the *Annual report of the Chief Medical Officer for Northern Ireland*.

The *KC60 sexually transmitted disease surveillance system* collects data from all NHS genitourinary medicine clinics in England. It is based on the KC60 statistical return, which collects aggregate data on the number of diagnoses of key conditions each quarter, subdivided by sex and, for males, by sexual orientation. Diagnoses rather than individuals are counted, so that some people may be counted more than once in a quarter.

While the KC60 data are the mainstay of sexually transmitted infection surveillance in England, they are limited. Important epidemiological information on age, ethnic group, area of residence, and location of care is not available for individuals. Reporting systems which collect disaggregated data, based on individuals, from genitourinary medicine clinics have been implemented in Scotland[52] and the Thames regions.[53] These systems have already produced useful epidemiological data.[54] The possibility of extending these disaggregated systems to the whole country is now being investigated. Despite the limitations of the KC60 dataset, it is comprehensive, as all genitourinary medicine clinics have a statutory obligation to report to the Communicable Disease Surveillance Centre.

The Department of Health published annual data from the KC60 aggregate return for 1994 onwards in a statistical bulletin *Sexually transmitted diseases, England. New cases seen at NHS GUM clinics.* Information about trends in the main diseases in England was also included. In 1997, responsibility for collecting KC60 data transferred to the Communicable Disease Surveillance Centre. Routine output is now published in a special CDR bulletin. Similar statistics for Scotland are published by the Information and Statistics Division in a briefing, *Cases seen at genito-urinary medicine clinics* and in *Scottish health statistics.*[55] Data for Northern Ireland are now published in the Department of Health and Social Services' *Community statistics* and were formerly published in *Health and personal social services for Northern Ireland.* Similar data are now found in *Health statistics Wales,* while those for years before 1995 appeared in *Health and personal social services statistics for Wales.*

Surveillance for Creutzfeldt-Jacob disease (CJD) started in 1990 and is undertaken by the National CJD Surveillance Unit in the Western General Hospital, Edinburgh. An annual report describing the work of the unit and the results of the surveillance programme, with an epidemiological commentary is available from the unit. Since 1996, the statistics for confirmed cases of new variant Creutzfeld-Jacob disease and other referrals to the unit have been published quarterly. National surveillance programmes have been established in many countries of the European Union, and the unit has a grant from the European Union to co-ordinate common diagnostic criteria and methodologies.

Data about people with communicable diseases who are admitted to hospital as either an in-patient or a day case are collected through the hospital data collection systems described in Chapter 8. The quality of the information on diagnoses given to episodes of illness in patients in hospital is dependent not only on the diagnosis itself and the accuracy of the junior doctors entering the information on the hospital reporting forms, but also on the validity of the coding of the information provided by hospital clerks. The accuracy of diagnostic coding has been subject to criticism, but has improved over the last few years. In general, data quality is higher in Scotland than in the other countries of the UK.

Only severe cases of communicable diseases are admitted to hospital. Thus, this dataset represents a small and extremely biased sample of true disease incidence. Furthermore, in England, hospital providers do not always submit an Hospital Episode Statistics record for each and every episode of treatment. Attempts are made to estimate the magnitude of the shortfall using 'grossing factors'. On the other hand, episode data which are submitted have to conform to certain standards, so information in the Hospital Episode Statistics data fields tends to be both valid and complete.

It is important to remember that each record details a single episode of care within a particular consultant specialty at a single hospital provider. Therefore if, during a spell of treatment, a patient is transferred to another consultant and/or a different provider, a new episode record is generated. It is estimated that about 5 per cent of 'in-patient spells' consist of more than one episode and so generate more than one record. Despite all these problems, ad-hoc analyses of communicable disease data from this source are sometimes published in medical journals.[56]

Communicable disease is likely to be under-represented in published analyses of registered deaths tabulated according to their 'underlying cause'. Frequently, infections may have contributed to death but are not coded as the underlying cause. In addition, an infection may cause a death but not be mentioned on the death certificate, because the appropriate investigations have not been carried out. Influenza is a particularly good example of this. Influenza appears on the death certificate in only about 15 per cent of the 'excess' deaths attributed to influenza during epidemics.

The Medical Officers of Schools Association has a scheme whereby diagnoses of a range of illnesses in children in the participating schools are reported to the Public Health Laboratory Service Communicable Disease Surveillance Centre. These include clinically diagnosed infectious diseases. The range of diseases is not comprehensive, however, and, as the schools are mostly boarding schools, they may be unrepresentative of all school-age children in the population.

The information that is currently available from occupational health service records or from certification of illness for social security purposes is now very limited, due to changes in regulations and the facility for self-certification that has been available in recent years. It is therefore no longer usable for charting epidemics of communicable diseases.

Use of registration and notification data for monitoring NHS performance and the health of the population

From the mid-1980s onwards, there has been an increasing tendency to use data from registrations and notifications as proxy measures of either the 'performance' of hospital or other services or as measures of the health of the population. In England, a large database was compiled of hospital 'performance indicators', later renamed 'health service indicators'. These were released on disc and subsequently on CD-ROM.

Many of these indicators were based on small numbers, but confidence intervals were not used to indicate statistical variability. They were rarely adjusted to take account of the characteristics of the local population or the way people in it were referred to hospital. Bringing together data about a hospital for comparative purposes is a useful exercise, if the data are interpreted with caution. On the other hand, in England there was a tendency to rank them into 'league tables' and interpret the rankings as measures of the quality of care provided. In Scotland, record linkage made it possible to provide more useful data and strenuous efforts were made to avoid ranking the data.[57]

The requirement for directors of public health to produce annual reports prompted the compilation of the public health common dataset, based in geographically defined populations. This brought together data on births, abortions, deaths and cancer registration with data about hospital treatment and census data for health authority areas. The development of the *Health of the nation* strategy from 1990 onwards led to its targets being added to the dataset.

Following a consultation in 1995, the Department of Health has been rationalising the many sets of indicators into one structured dataset.[58]

The many changes in the boundaries of health authorities in the 1990s and the change in coding of underlying cause of death in 1993 led to many discontinuities, and in 1996, a special CD-ROM was issued giving time trends in indicators based on 1996 boundaries.

The change of government in 1997, brought a new enthusiasm for performance measurement, with the development of a 'performance framework'[59] and new sets of high-level indicators and clinical indicators, this time using aged-adjusted rates and with confidence intervals for the clinical indicators.[60,61] The current government prefers to use small sets of indicators as proxy measures of much wider aspects of health. Thus, *Saving lives: our healthier nation*,[62] the White Paper setting out a health strategy for England, has only four national targets, with suicide rates being used as a proxy measure of the whole field of mental health.[59] The clinical indicators issued in 1999 contained only six items.[60] The validity of this is clearly open to question. Meanwhile, Scotland continues to exercise caution, issuing its indicators with the warning that: 'It is stressed that no direct inferences about the quality of care should be drawn from the indicators. They are intended to highlight issues which may require further investigation'.[57]

Contact addresses and web sites

Office for National Statistics
1 Drummond Gate
London SW1V 2QQ
General enquiries:
Telephone: 020 7533 6262
Web site: http://www.statistics.gov.uk/
Published tables and specific enquiries, Telephone:

Births and fertility	01329 813758
Mortality	01329 813379
Cancer	01329 813759

Topic enquiries, telephone:

Abortions	020 7533 5112
Conceptions	020 7533 5137
Congenital anomalies	020 7533 5641
Infant and perinatal mortality	020 7533 5205

StatBase web site http://www.statistics.gov.uk/statbase/mainmenu.asp

Family Records Centre
1 Myddelton Street
London EC1R 1UW
Telephone: 020 8392 5300

General Register Office for Scotland
Ladywell House
Ladywell Road
Edinburgh EH12 7TF
Telephone: 0131 314 4254
Web site: http://www.gro-scotland.gov.uk/

General Register Office for Northern Ireland
Oxford House
49–55 Chichester Street
Belfast BT1 4HL
Telephone: 028 90 252031/2
Web site: http://www.nisra.gov.uk/gro/

Public Health Laboratory Service
Communicable Disease Surveillance Centre
61 Colindale Avenue
London NW9 5EQ
Telephone: 020 8200 6868
Web site: http://www.phls.co.uk

Scottish Centre for Infection and
Environmental Health
Clifton House
Clifton Drive
Glasgow G3 7LN
Telephone: 0141 300 1142
Web site: http://www.show.scot.nhs.
uk/ghi/scieh.htm

National Assembly for Wales, formerly
the Welsh Office
Health statistics, telephone:
029 20 825080
Statistical publications:
Publications Unit
Statistical Directorate 5
National Assembly for Wales
Cathay's Park
Cardiff CF10 3NQ
Email: Statswales@gtnet.gov.uk

Information and Statistics Division
Common Services Agency of the NHS
in Scotland
Trinity Park House
South Trinity Road
Edinburgh EH5 3SQ
Telephone: 0131 552 6255
Web site: http://www.show.scot.nhs.
uk/isd/index.htm

Department of Health, Social Services
and Public Safety
Regional Information Branch
Annexe 2
Castle Buildings
Stormont
Belfast BT4 3UD
Telephone: 028 90 522800
Web site: http://www.dhssni.gov.uk/
hpss/statistics/index.html

References

1. Nissel M. *People count*. London: HMSO, 1987.
2. Eyler JM. *Victorian social medicine. The ideas and methods of William Farr*. London and Baltimore: Johns Hopkins University Press, 1979.
3. Macfarlane AJ, Mugford M. *Birth counts, statistics of pregnancy and childbirth*, Vol. 1, Text. 2nd edn. London: The Stationery Office, 2000.
4. Office of Population Censuses and Surveys. *Registration: proposals for change*. London: HMSO, 1990.
5. Office for National Statistics. *Registration: modernising a vital service*. London: ONS, 1999.
6. Steering Group on Health Services Information. *Supplement to the first and fourth reports to the Secretary of State*. London: HMSO, 1985.
7. Department of Health. *NHS maternity statistics, England: 1989–90 to 1994–95*. Statistical bulletin 1997/28. London: Department of Health, 1997.
8. Macfarlane AJ. At last – maternity statistics for England. Editorial. *British Medical Journal* 1998; **316**: 566–7.
9. Information and Statistics Division. *Birth in Scotland, 1976–1995*. Edinburgh: ISD, 1997.
10. Andrews J, Cotter M, Richards R, Lewis D. *Report on maternity data/information aspects of the child health system*. Cardiff: Welsh Health Information Services, 1996.
11. Andrews J, Cotter M, Richards R, King J, Lewis D, Davies M. *Maternity data/information aspects of the child health system*. Second report. Cardiff: Welsh Health Information Services, 1998.
12. Office of Population Censuses and Surveys. *The OPCS monitoring scheme for congenital malformation: a review by a working group of the Registrar General's Medical Advisory Committee*. Occasional Paper 43. London: OPCS, 1995.

13. Office for National Statistics. *The national congenital anomaly system. A guide for data suppliers.* London: Office for National Statistics, 1999.
14. Office for National Statistics. *Mortality statistics, England and Wales, 1993, 1994 and 1995.* Series DH1, No. 28. London: TSO, 1997.
15. Rooney C, Devis T. Mortality trends by cause of death in England and Wales 1980–94: the impact of introducing automated cause coding and related changes in 1993. *Population Trends* 1996; **86**: 29–35.
16. Devis T, Rooney C. Death certification and the epidemiologist. *Health statistics quarterly* 1999; **1**: 21–33.
17. Office for National Statistics. *Twentieth century mortality, England and Wales, 1901–1995.* CD-Rom, with 1996 update disc. London: ONS, 1997.
18. Charlton J, Murphy M, eds. Office for National Statistics. *The health of adult Britain, 1841–1994.* Series DS, Nos. 12 and 13. London: TSO, 1997.
19. Department of Health. *Action to strengthen confidential enquiries – Baroness Jay.* Press Release 98/225. London: Department of Health, 1998.
20. Department of Health, Welsh Office, Scottish Office Home and Health Department, Department of Health and Social Services, Northern Ireland. *Report on Confidential Enquiries into Maternal Deaths in the United Kingdom, 1994–96.* London: TSO, 1998.
21. Hawkins MM, Swerdlow AJ. Completeness of cancer and death follow-up obtained through the National Health Service Central Register for England and Wales. *British Journal of Cancer* 1992; **66**: 408–13.
22. Swerdlow AJ, Douglas AJ, Vaughan Hudson G, Vaughan Hudson B. Completeness of cancer registration in England and Wales: an assessment based on 2,145 patients with Hodgkin's disease independently registered by the British National Lymphoma Investigation. *British Journal of Cancer* 1993; **67**: 326–9.
23. Gulliford MC, Bell J, Bourne HM, Petruckevitch A. The reliability of cancer registry records. *British Journal of Cancer* 1993; **67**: 819–21.
24. Gulliford MC, Petruckevitch A, Burney PG. Survival with bladder cancer, evaluation of delay in treatment, type of surgeon, and modality of treatment. *British Medical Journal* 1991; **303**: 437–40.
25. Pollock AM, Vickers N. The reliability of Thames cancer registry data on 673 cases of colorectal cancer: the effect of registration. *Quality in Health Care* 1995; **71**(3): 637–41.
26. Chouillet AM, Bell CMJ, Hiscox JG. Management of breast cancer in southeast England. *British Medical Journal* 1994; **308**: 168–71.
27. Basnett I, Pollock AM, Gill M. Collecting data on cancer [letter]. *British Medical Journal* 1994; **308**: 791.
28. Basnett I, Gill M, Tobias JS. Variations in breast cancer management between a teaching and a non-teaching district. *European Journal of Cancer* 1992; **28A**: 1945–50.
29. Pollock AM, Vickers N. Reliability of cancer registry records [letter; comment]. *British Journal of Cancer* 1993; **68**: 1045–6.
30. Swerdlow AJ. Interpretation of England and Wales cancer mortality data: the effect of inquiries to certifiers for further information. *British Journal of Cancer* 1989; **59**: 787–91.
31. OPCS. *A review of the National Cancer Registration system in England and Wales,* Series MB1, No.17. London: HMSO, 1990.
32. NHS Executive. Executive letter EL(92)95. London: Department of Health, 1992.
33. Pollock AM, Vickers N. Why are a quarter of cancer deaths in South East England registered by 'death certificate only' (DCO)? Factors related to DCO registrations in the Thames Cancer Registry between 1987 and 1989. *British Journal of Cancer* 1995; **71**: 637–41.

34. NHS Executive. Executive letter EL(96)97. Annex A. London: Department of Health, 1997.

35. Coleman MP, Babb P, Damiecki P, Grosclaude P, Honjo S, Jones J, Knerer G, Pitard A, Quinn MJ, Sloggett A, De Stavola BL. *Cancer survival trends in England and Wales, 1971–1995: deprivation and NHS region.* Studies in Medical and Population Subjects No. 61. London: The Stationery Office, 1999.

36. Coleman MP, Babb P, Mayer D, Quinn M, Sloggett, A. *Cancer survival trends in England and Wales, 1971–1995: deprivation and NHS region (CD-ROM).* London: Office for National Statistics, 1999.

37. *Public Health (Control of Disease) Act 1984.* London: HMSO, 1984.

38. Advance Letter (MD) 2/98 NHS Executive, 9 March 1990. Fees and allowances payable to doctors for sessional work in the community health services, medical services to local authorities (under collaborative arrangements), medical examinations of prospective national health services employees, and notification of infectious diseases and food poisoning.

39. Surveillance of measles since the vaccination campaign. *Communicable Disease Report Weekly* 1995; **5**, 8.

40. Synnott MB, Morse DL, Hall SM. Neonatal meningitis in England and Wales: a review of routine national data. *Archives of Diseases in Childhood* 1994; **71**(2): F75–F80.

41. Goldacre MJ, Miller DL. Completeness of statutory notification for acute bacterial meningitis. *British Medical Journal* 1976; **2**(6034): 501–3.

42. Evans T, Packe GE. Audit of tuberculosis notifications. *Thorax* 1997; **52** (Suppl. 6): Abstract.

43. *Reporting to the Public Health Laboratory Service Communicable Disease Surveillance Centre: a reference for laboratories.* Colindale: Public Health Laboratory Service, 1997.

44. Mangtani P, Rodrigues L, Watson J. Laboratory reports of opportunistic and other mycobacterial infections and their relationship to notifications of tuberculosis in England and Wales. *Tubercle and Lung Disease* 1995; **76**(3): 201–4.

45. Atkinson P, Humphrey J. Under-reporting of sexually transmitted infections from laboratories in the Thames regions. 23rd Annual Conference of the Public Health Laboratory Service, University of Warwick, 7–9th September 1998 (Abstract).

46. Fleming DM, Crombie DL. The incidence of common infectious diseases: the Weekly Returns Service of the Royal College of General Practitioners. *Health Trends* 1985; **17**: 13–16.

47. Evans BG, McCormick A. Completeness of reporting cases of acquired immune deficiency syndrome accounting for reporting delay. *Journal of the Royal Statistical Society* [A] 1994; **157**: 31–40.

48. Hickman M, Aldous J, Gazzard B, Ellam A. AIDS surveillance: a direct assessment of under-reporting. *AIDS* 1993; **7**(12): 1661–5.

49. Unlinked anonymous HIV prevalence monitoring programme England and Wales. *Report from the unlinked anonymous surveys steering group. Data to end of 1995.* London: Department of Health, 1996.

50. Gibb DM, MacDonagh SE, Tookey P, Duong T, Nicoll A, Goldberg DJ, Hudson CNN, Peckham CS, Ades AE. Uptake of interventions to reduce mother to child transmission of HIV in the United Kingdom & Ireland. *AIDS* 1997; **11**: F53–8.

51. Mortimer JY, Evans BG, Goldberg DJ. Surveillance of HIV infection and AIDS in the UK: an overview from the Public Health Laboratory Service AIDS Centre. *Communicable Disease Review* 1997; **7**(91): R118–20.

52. Noone A, Chalmers J, Young H. Surveillance of sexually transmitted infections in Scotland. *Eurosurveillance* 1998; **3**(6): 65–8.

53. Maguire H, Davidson F. Regionwide surveillance of sexually transmitted infections in a Thames region. *Irish Journal of Medical Science* 1994; **163**, Suppl. 13 (Abstract).

54. Hughes G, Catchpole M. Surveillance of sexually transmitted infections in England and Wales. *Eurosurveillance* 1998; **3**(6): 61–65.

55. Information and Statistics Division Scottish Health Service. *Genitourinary Medicine Statistics Scotland Annual Report 1995/96*. Edinburgh: Common Services Agency, 1997.

56. Ryan MJ, Ramsay M, Brown D, Gay NJ, Farrington CP, Wall PG. Hospital admissions attributable to rotavirus infection in England and Wales. *Journal of Infectious Diseases* 1996; **174** (Suppl 1): S12–18.

57. Kendrick S, Cline D, Finlayson A. *Clinical outcome indicators for Scotland: lessons and prospects*. Paper for the Third International Conference on Strategic Issues in Health Care, University of St Andrews, April 2–4 1998.

58. National Centre for Health Outcomes Development. *Compendium of clinical and health indicators*. London: National Centre for Health Outcomes Development, published annually.

59. Department of Health. *A national framework for assessing performance*. London: Department of Health, 1998.

60. Department of Health. *Quality and performance in the NHS. Clinical indicators*. Leeds: NHS Executive, 1999.

61. Department of Health. *Quality and performance in the NHS. High level performance indicators*. Leeds: NHS Executive, 1999.

62. Department of Health. *Saving lives: our healthier nation*. Cm 4386. London: Department of Health, 1999.

4 Looking at health inequalities

SOCIAL CLASS, ETHNIC ORIGIN AND PEOPLE WITH DISABILITIES

Alison Macfarlane, Mel Bartley, Susan Kerrison and Jenny Head

> Measuring the health effects of affluence and disadvantage
>
> Why disability surveys cannot count
>
> Ethnic minorities and migrant groups

For over 150 years, official statistics have revealed inequalities in health, mortality and life expectancy between the populations of geographical areas and between social and occupational groups within each population. A persistent finding is the strong tendency for more affluent and privileged groups to have better health than those that are less advantaged. This chapter describes how such groups are classified, the methods used to assess inequalities in health and sources of official data. In doing so, it takes a critical look at social and 'ethnic' classifications and at statistics collected about people with disabilities.

In many analyses of differences between the health of people living in different types of geographical areas, the areas are classified using census variables, grouped together to form various types of 'deprivation indices'. Unfortunately, census questions change infrequently, so over the years, the data collected can lose their relevance as indicators of deprivation. As the census is undertaken only every 10 years, the indices can quickly become out of date. In addition, such analyses are limited as only censuses, counts of people claiming benefits and statistics about hospital in-patient treatment aim to cover everyone and can therefore be disaggregated to a local level. As Chapter 2 shows, many health surveys are based on samples which are not large enough to derive estimates at a local level.

When groups of individuals are compared, they are usually placed in categories that are often based on their occupation, and reflect their status or position within society. Differences between these groups can be assessed using data from people who die or experience ill-health and data about the population as a whole.

Official surveys which ask questions about disability are of two types:

surveys that ask non-specific questions about ill-health or 'limited activity', and those that focus specifically on people with disabilities. The most prominent surveys in this latter group are the series of surveys undertaken by the Office of Population Censuses and Surveys (OPCS) in the mid-1980s. The surveys used questions based on the International Classification of Impairment, Disability and Handicap (ICIDH). Organisations of disabled people argue that the methods used in these surveys are biased, as they preclude any exploration of how social, economic and environmental barriers affect impaired people. A further criticism is that the need to constrain government expenditure means that the findings of official surveys all tend to underestimate the numbers of disabled people and their needs.

All surveys of disability require people to classify themselves as disabled at some stage in the study. People's willingness to do this is affected by the circumstances of the study and their individual characteristics, such as age. This problem makes the studies of disability very sensitive to small changes in the methods used. With a few exceptions, samples for general surveys are drawn from private households and therefore little information is available about people with disabilities living in institutions. A further deficiency is that the surveys tend to concentrate on adults, so there is very little information about numbers of or needs of children with disability. Information about the financial circumstances of disabled people, employment and use of services is also sparse.

After much research and political debate, the government decided to include a question on ethnic origin in the 1991 census, but developing categories for ethnic groups which are valid, reliable, acceptable to respondents and yet can take into account changing ethnic identities is not a simple matter. The categories chosen have been heavily criticised as too broad, disguising the heterogeneity of populations descended from migrants from the Indian subcontinent and from Africa, who differ in language, religion and diet. They also provide little information about significant ethnic groups within the majority 'white ' population, such as the Irish. The new questions developed for the 2001 census answer some, but not all, of these criticisms.

Despite their limitations, the categories are used in an increasing number of datasets which focus on health or have a health component. Similar questions have been used in the Labour Force Survey since 1981 and in the General Household Survey since 1983. In 1995, ethnic group was collected for the first time as part of the dataset for the hospital episode statistics and also included in cancer registrations. Ethnic group is not recorded at death registration, so death rates, often used as proxy measures of health, cannot be tabulated by ethnic group. Instead, the country of birth is recorded on the death certificate and is often used as a proxy measure of the person's ethnic origin, but this has obvious limitations. All these problems mean that the available data are of limited usefulness in disentangling the relationship between ethnic origin and health and that they may even be misleading.

Measuring the health effects of affluence and disadvantage

The inequalities between the health and life expectancy of affluent and deprived areas and the inequalities between social groups feature extensively in debates about resource allocation, health promotion and, more fundamentally, in political debates about social justice. Under the Conservative government, health inequalities were either ignored or described as 'health variations' in policy documents. Since May 1997, they have been back on the agenda, although it remains to be seen whether the policies being adopted will be adequate to tackle them.

This section outlines the methods used to produce the statistics about inequalities in health, concentrating on data from reference books and other published sources. Although data are now much more widely available to researchers for 'secondary analysis' on a personal computer than they were 10 years ago, producing and analysing statistics on inequalities can be very complex, and anyone doing so will need further help.

There are two ways of looking at health inequality. Comparisons can be made either between the health of people in areas with different levels of affluence or poverty, or between the health of groups of people with different levels of privilege or disadvantage.

Differences between the health of populations of geographical areas

To compare the mortality of geographical areas, two types of data are needed. The first is a measure of death rates in the areas and the second is a means of classifying areas as socially advantaged or disadvantaged. National death rates and local rates for areas as small as electoral wards are published each year by the Office for National Statistics (ONS) and by the General Register Offices for Scotland and Northern Ireland.

After each census, more detailed analyses are done, using census data to group areas according to their characteristics, as a number of data items collected can be regarded as social and economic measures. As described in Chapter 3, these analyses are usually published in a decennial supplement on area mortality for England and Wales. The supplement for the 1981 census contained a wider range of analyses than its predecessors and had the broader title 'Mortality and geography'. At the time of writing, the ONS is producing a similar supplement to the 1991 census. It is a particularly difficult task, because of the large number of changes in both local government and health authority boundaries during the 1990s. In addition, many researchers produce their own analyses.

Census measures often used in these analyses include characteristics of households, as well as of individual people within them. Household measures include housing tenure, in other words whether people own or rent their homes, whether or not a car is available to members of the household,

Key official publications

Area mortality decennial supplements for England and Wales
General Register Office. *Registrar General's statistical review. Decennial supplement, England and Wales, 1961. Area mortality tables.* London: HMSO, 1967.
Office of Population Censuses and Surveys. *Area mortality. The Registrar General's decennial supplement for England and Wales, 1969–1973*, Series DS No. 4. London: HMSO, 1981.
Office of Population Censuses and Surveys. *Mortality and geography. A review in the mid-1980s in England and Wales.* Series DS No. 9. Britton M, ed. London: HMSO, 1990.

whether the household is overcrowded and whether amenities such as a kitchen or a bathroom are shared with other households.

As time goes on, measures can gain and lose in usefulness or their meaning can change. Up to the 1960s and 1970s, knowing whether a household had an inside toilet was a useful piece of information, but it is now rare to be without one. The significance of being an owner-occupier paying a mortgage rather than rent is also changing as a measure of inequality. In the past, it was considered an advantage, but many home 'owners' are now under considerable financial stress.

It is possible, by combining data items from the census, to derive measures of the overall level of deprivation or affluence of geographical areas. This measure can then be used to group similar areas and their mortality can be compared. Four such 'deprivation indexes' are commonly used: the Jarman index[1,2] the Townsend index,[3] the SCOTDEP index,[4] devised and commonly used in Scotland, and the Department of the Environment Index of Local Deprivation.[5,6] Others have been compiled for specific purposes.

Despite their important role in political debates on health inequality, these deprivation indices can be misleading, even though there is a general likelihood of relatively poor health in areas that rank highly on these indices. Although an area which is economically disadvantaged may have high mortality overall, the disadvantaged individuals within it may not have a higher than average rate of death.

The one major advantage of looking at health inequality by using area statistics is that mortality rates for areas are available every year, while statistics on differences in mortality between social groups rely on using data from the census, which is taken only at 10-year intervals. The measures used to classify the area as affluent or disadvantaged also tend to rely on census data and these may change from census to census. Other local authority statistics, such as numbers of children receiving free school meals or numbers of people receiving housing benefits, are collected continuously and are used in the Department of the Environment's index. Up to the present, little use has been made of such data to investigate inequalities in mortality, however.

The same approach can be used to look at morbidity, or ill-health. In addition to the difficult problem of defining just what counts as illness, there are few data which can be used at a very local level. From 1911 to 1981, the only question on ill-health included in the census asked if people were not working, permanently or temporarily, because of ill-health. This measure cannot, therefore, be used to investigate the health of people with no paid employment, for example if they look after the home or because of their age. For the first time, in 1991 (as described in Chapter 2), everyone was asked if they suffered a long-term illness which limited their activities in any way.

Data about hospital treatment (described in Chapter 8) can also be analysed by area of residence. Apart from in Scotland, where data can be linked, they refer to episodes of hospital care rather than the people who receive it. This means that they can be used to calculate operation rates, but not the proportion of people in the population with given conditions. This problem is particularly serious for conditions for which people are likely to have more than one hospital stay. In addition, differences in hospital admission rates can reflect differences in access and clinical practice as well as differences in morbidity.

The General Household Survey collects data about self-reported ill-health and about use of services, as Chapter 2 explains. It can be disaggregated by country of Great Britain and by region within England, but its sample is not large enough for data to be used at local level. As described in Chapter 2, the Health Survey for England and the Health Survey for Scotland provide information about factors that are thought relevant to heart disease, such as breathlessness and angina, diet, smoking and exercise. There is also information on stress and psychological well-being. Again, the sample is not large enough to provide data for areas below regional level.

This means that the census is the only data source from which person-based data can be derived for small areas. As well as being collected only at 10-yearly intervals, the data in it are not very specific. Nevertheless, the 1991 census did identify differences in illness rates for more and less disadvantaged areas.

Differences between the health of social groups

There are several ways in which individuals can be classified into groups with more and less privilege or disadvantage, in economic and social terms. The measure used depends upon what is thought to be the most important aspect of privilege and disadvantage. Opinion is divided about the relative importance of, for example, income, the sort of conditions people have at work, and the level of status or prestige accorded to a person by others.

The classification most often used in health inequality statistics is the Registrar General's social class classification shown in Table 4.1. This allocates jobs into six 'social classes' based on occupation.[7] This is described in official reports as a measure of a 'general standing in the community', in other words, status, and also of 'occupational skill level'. In the past, before each census, a committee of senior civil servants and outside advisors revised the classification by deciding which job went into which class. This is a rather 'unscientific' procedure, without any clear grounds for making the decisions;

Table 4.1   Social class according to occupation

Group	Description	Example
I	Professional	Doctors, lawyers
II	Managerial and technical occupations	Teachers, most managerial and senior administrative occupations
IIIN	Skilled occupations, non-manual	Clerks, shop assistants
IIIM	Skilled occupations, manual	Bricklayers, coal miners below ground
IV	Partly skilled occupations	Bus conductors, traffic wardens
V	Unskilled occupations	General labourers
Others	Armed forces	
	Unclassified	People about whom there is no information or whose occupations do not fit into the classification, students
	Unoccupied	Unemployed people are only classified as unoccupied if they are not seeking paid employment, or are on a government employment or training scheme

people in the same class do not necessarily have jobs with similar levels of skill or prestige. Although there are differences between the mortality rates of classes, there are also considerable differences between the occupational groups within each social class.

The other measure which is commonly used in official reports is the 'socio-economic group' (SEG). This is described as a measure of status which groups together people with similar lifestyles.[7] Again, the extent to which it does so has not been explicitly validated.

These criticisms of the Registrar General's social classes prompted development of other classifications with a firmer base in sociological theory, notably the Erikson–Goldthorpe or CASMIN scheme[8] and Eric Olin Wright's scheme.[9] The CASMIN scheme attempts to group people according to the type of work they do and their relationship to their employment. This includes whether they are self-employed or employees, whether they are supervisors or managers, and whether or not their job has security and a career structure.

For the 2001 census, the OPCS and the Economic and Social Research Council commissioned a research project at the University of Essex to produce a better defined classification, to be known as National Statistics socio-economic classes (SEC).[10] This classification, shown in Table 4.2, attempts to classify jobs in a similar way to the CASMIN schema.

Mortality differences between social groups, defined in any of these ways, can be calculated using data about people who die and data about the population as a whole. As mentioned above, this can be done only at 10-year intervals, when the census can be used as a source of data about the number of people in each occupation and hence each social class.

One of the series of 'decennial supplements' produced for England and Wales following each census analyses mortality according to social class. In the past, this was called the *Decennial supplement on occupational mortality*, because data on mortality were analysed by individual occupations, as well as by social classes. After the 1991 census, two separate volumes were

Table 4.2   National Statistics Socio-economic
Classification to be used from 2001 onwards

1. Higher managerial and professional occupations
   1A   Employers and managers in large
        establishments
   1B   Professionals
2. Lower managerial and professional occupations
3. Intermediate occupations
4. Small employers and own account workers
5. Lower supervisory, craft and related occupations
6. Employees in semi-routine occupations
7. Employees in routine occupations

Never worked and long-term unemployed
Not stated

Source: *The Economic and Social Research Council
review of government social classifications,* 1998.

produced; one, on *'occupational mortality'*, focused on specific occupations, while the second, on *'health inequalities'*, contained analyses by social class. Each was a wide-ranging review, covering analyses from the Longitudinal Study and other relevant datasets, along with the traditional decennial supplement analyses and appendices explaining the techniques and classifications used.

Decennial supplements consistently report sizeable differences in mortality between the Registrar General's social classes for men of working age. The differences in women's mortality are less apparent if women are allocated to classes according to their own occupations, but equally clear when married

Key official publications

Decennial supplements containing analyses by social class
Office of Population Censuses and Surveys. The Registrar General's Decennial supplement for England and Wales, 1961. *Occupational mortality tables.* London: HMSO, 1971.
Office of Population Censuses and Surveys. *Occupational mortality 1970–1972.* Decennial supplement. Series DS, No. 1. London: HMSO, 1978.
Office of Population Censuses and Surveys. *Occupational mortality.* Decennial supplement 1979–1980 and 1982–83. Part 1, Commentary. Series DS No. 6. London: HMSO, 1986.
Office of Population Censuses and Surveys. *Occupational mortality.* Decennial supplement 1979–1980 and 1982–83. Part 2, Microfiche tables. Series DS No. 6. London: HMSO, 1986.
Office of Population Censuses and Surveys. *Occupational mortality.* Decennial supplement 1979–1980 and 1982–83. Childhood supplement. Series DS No. 8. London: HMSO, 1988.
Drever F, Whitehead M, eds. Office for National Statistics. *Inequalities in health.* Series DS No. 15. London: TSO, 1997.

women are classified according to the 'social class' of their husbands. There are a number of serious problems about measuring inequalities in women's mortality. One is that when a married woman's death is registered, an occupation is not always put on her death certificate. Another is that the very classification of individual jobs into classes takes little account of the differences in men's and women's jobs and typical work histories. For example, men still tend to receive higher pay for similar work and are less likely to have to take the major responsibility for care of home, children and elderly people. In addition, the range of jobs done by women is different from the range of jobs done by men.

Classifying babies and children is also difficult. Normally, they are classified according to their fathers' social class, except for children whose births were registered by their mother on her own. In fact, babies and children can be classified by the characteristics of their mother, their father, the couple jointly, or their household, and the extent to which each should be used is unclear.[11]

Another important source of data on health inequalities is the OPCS, now the ONS, Longitudinal Study, which is described in Chapter 2. The Longitudinal Study makes it possible, for example, to analyse mortality in women according to an occupation they had 10 or 20 years earlier, although they may be out of the labour market at the time of death. It can do the same for men who were unemployed at the time of a previous census. Use of the Longitudinal Study also makes it possible to analyse mortality according to the wider range of socio-economic characteristics recorded in the census but not on death certificates. These include household tenure and car ownership. It is also possible to do analyses by educational level, but these are of limited value. The question used in the 1981 and 1991 censuses was designed to ascertain how many people had higher level qualifications. This means that the data cannot be used to subdivide the majority of the population whose highest qualification is at A level or below.

Analyses of data from this study are available in the OPCS's and the ONS's 'Series LS' volumes, which are listed in Chapter 2. The Longitudinal Study was also used extensively in the decennial supplement 'Health inequalities' and is frequently used in other work on health inequalities.

As with mortality, the illness rates of social groups can be compared. This is usually done using the Registrar General's social classes, but the General Household Survey uses socio-economic groups, and other surveys use several different measures.

There may be disagreement about what counts as a serious illness, as the impact of the same illness can vary between social groups. For example, vertigo may have less effect on the working life of a stockbroker or university lecturer than on a building worker. The advantage of looking at inequalities in morbidity is that the sample surveys used to collect these data are done each year. In addition, the sample surveys ask everyone their occupation, which means they can be allocated to a social class, and the percentages of people in each class who are ill can easily be calculated. Although the General

Household Survey samples are too small to produce reliable differences between small areas, their samples of around 15 000 people per year make them sufficiently large to give reliable estimates of differences in health between the six 'social classes'.

As well as the other surveys, the third and fourth studies of *Morbidity statistics from general practice,* described in Chapter 8, coded patients' social classes and other socio-economic factors, and extensive analyses have been published.[12,13] In contrast, neither the General Practice Research Database nor hospital-based systems, such as Hospital Episode Statistics in England, Patient Episode Database Wales, SMR1 in Scotland or the Hospital Inpatients System in Northern Ireland, code social class and all record very little socio-economic information about patients.

In Scotland, mortality and morbidity are not often analysed by social class, but most data are tabulated by the deprivation score of people's area of residence. This reflects the influence of an article published in the mid-1980s by two Scottish researchers, who attacked social class as 'an embarrassment to epidemiology'.[14]

How is health inequality measured?

Rather than using 'crude rates', that is, the total number of deaths or cases of illness divided by the size of the population, the various methods of 'standardisation' described in Chapter 3 are often used in analyses of inequality. This is because crude death rates can mask differences in age or social class distributions of populations. For example, comparing health in Liverpool with that in Bournemouth without taking account of the age distribution of people in these two areas might suggest that Bournemouth, despite its middle-class population, clean air and high rate of home ownership, has many more deaths per head of population each year than Liverpool. This reflects the fact that Bournemouth is popular as a retirement area, precisely because of its good climate, clean air and amenities, so the proportion of elderly residents is much higher than in Liverpool.

To allow for such differences, standardisation is used extensively in published analyses of data about mortality and cancer incidence. Until recently, standardisation tended not to be used in survey reports, for example those on the General Household Survey. On the other hand, rates of illness were tabulated by broad age groups. Standardised rates are now sometimes used in reports using these data.

The conventional standardised mortality ratio (SMR) has been developed over the years. It is quite likely that its development has been influenced by a number of different social and political interests. It is certainly not the 'one and only' way of dealing with the problem. In the mid-nineteenth century, William Farr, who devised this method, used the healthiest and therefore usually the most affluent districts, with the lowest mortality as the 'standard'. Data from these were used to calculate 'expected' death rates. These are the rates which the other 'unhealthy' and also more disadvantaged districts would have had if their death rates in each age group had been the same as those for the 'healthy districts'.[15] The difference between these 'expected' and actual death rates gave a much bigger-looking 'health effect' than would have been seen if the whole population had been used as the comparison. There is no real reason why data should not be analysed in this way as well as in the more conventional manner.

There are circumstances in which it may not be appropriate to calculate an overall measure such as a standardised mortality ratio, as this can obscure trends within specific groups. For example, human immundeficiency virus (HIV)-related deaths have little effect on the standardised mortality ratios for the population as a whole, but mortality among men in the younger age groups has increased since the mid-1980s. Finally, the choice of populations as the standard for calculating standardised rates can be somewhat arbitrary. The population used can be that of the UK, Great Britain, England and Wales or the individual countries of which they are made up. Increasingly, 'European standard populations' are now being used. Each can give slightly different results. Appendices A and B of the 1991 decennial supplement *Health inequalities* summarises clearly the types of standardisation used in the supplement.

Like all statistics, those on health tend to be used, and even designed, to defend one or other political position during specific historical periods. It can be helpful to be aware of the political context in which a set of statistics is being used, or in which it was invented in the first place. This can happen, for example, when one group is trying to justify an increase in the resources given to it by government, and another group is competing for those resources, or the government itself is trying to justify a cut in resources. Since the publication and attempted suppression in 1980 of the report on *Inequalities in health*, better known as the 'Black report',[16] statistics on health inequality have been used in campaigns against poverty and social injustice.

Statistics on health inequality have, not surprisingly, often been hotly disputed. One early example of this was when public health reformers campaigned for clean water in the nineteenth century. People who resisted this argued that clean water would allow feeble infants to survive and thereby *increase* the adult death rate. This gave rise to a long technical argument. Such arguments have bequeathed to us standardisation as a special way to measure health differences between groups.

Other major sources of information

In addition to the data in the publications described above, further data are available to people with facilities to analyse them. In order to gain access to these data, it is necessary to go through the Economic and Social Research Council's Data Archive at the University of Essex, but this is possible only for people in academic institutions.

A number of reports have brought together data from a multiplicity of sources. The first is the original classic 'Black report'.[16] Only a few copies were printed, as the government of the day did not want it widely read. Fortunately, it was republished in paperback in 1982.[17] It was subsequently reprinted in the early 1990s, together with a second report, *The health divide*, written by Margaret Whitehead to update the information.[18] In 1997, following the precedent set by these, the government commissioned former Chief Medical Officer, Donald Acheson to undertake an independent enquiry into inequalities in health. His report, published in November 1998, was less radical than the earlier reports.[19]

Why disability surveys cannot count

Official surveys of people with disabilities have been the subject of fundamental criticism from organisations of people with disability over many years.[20,21] One problem is that there is a perception that government-funded surveys are often undertaken with one eye on the need to constrain government expenditure and keep the costs down. In other words, they tend to underestimate the numbers of people with disabilities, and the need for services and financial support.[22] As well as this, there is a controversial conceptual issue. The definition used in official surveys which focus exclusively on disability, strongly implies that the disadvantages or 'handicaps' that people with disabilities face are simply caused by their impairments rather than by society's failure to adapt to their needs. Surveys using this type of definition, therefore, individualise the problem and preclude any exploration of how social, economic and environmental barriers affect impaired people. The definitions which are at the centre of the criticism, are in the World Health Organisation International Classification of Impairments, Disabilities and Handicaps, and are shown in Table 4.3.

The International Classification of Impairments, Disabilities and Handicaps was published for trial purposes as a supplement to the ninth revision of the *International classification of diseases* (ICD).[23] The scheme was opposed by organisations of disabled people since its inception,[21] as it appears to suggest that 'handicaps' are caused by 'impairments'. By the tenth edition of *International classification of diseases*, serious reservations were being expressed and there were increasing requests for revision of the definition of handicap so as to place more emphasis on the effects of interaction with the environment. Despite these criticisms and the fact that International Classification of Impairments, Disabilities and Handicap was intended as a pilot, official surveys of people with disabilities in the UK undertaken in the last two decades appear wedded to this definition.

A revision of the International Classification of Impairments, Disabilities and Handicap is now underway. At the time of writing, it has been placed for

Table 4.3   World Health Organisation's definitions of impairment, disability and handicap

Impairment
In the context of health experience, an impairment is any loss or abnormality of psychological, physiological or anatomical structure or function.

Disability
In the context of health experience, a disability is any restriction or lack (resulting from an impairment) of ability to perform an activity in the manner or within the range considered normal for a human being.

Handicap
In the context of health experience, a handicap is a disadvantage for a given individual, resulting from an impairment or a disability, that limits or prevents the fulfilment of a role that is normal (depending on age, sex and social and cultural factors) for that individual.

Source: World Health Organisation 1980.[23]

information and comment on the World Health Organisation's web site. The new classification system, *ICIDIH-2: International classification of functioning and disability* is radically different from the first international classification. The new system does not focus exclusively on disability. Instead, it aims to deal with functional states associated with *health conditions* at body, individual and society level. The term includes disease, injury and health-related states such as ageing, pregnancy, genetic predisposition and stress. Information is organised in three dimensions: the *body* dimension comprises classifications of body systems and body structures, the *activities* dimension covers the range of activities performed by an individual and the *participation* dimension classes areas of life where an individual may or may not be involved. For example, a young person with diabetes who is dependent on insulin has an impairment, may experience no limitations in activities but may experience limitations in participation in social situations where food is central. Because of its breadth, the system is intended for use in all areas of health care, not just in relation to disability. The beta-2 version has been placed on the web for testing and comment before submission to the World Health Assembly in 2001.

Supporters of the original International Classification of Impairments, Disabilities and Handicap argue that there is little intrinsically wrong with the definition itself. They see problems arising because surveys using it have tended to concentrate on estimating the prevalence of 'impairments' and 'disability' rather than on exploring 'handicaps', in other words, environmental barriers.[24] There is no guarantee that the new classification will not suffer a similar fate. It may be that the emphasis will be on recording impairments and activities rather than participation. The problem may not lie with the definition, but with the aims and attitudes of people commissioning such surveys.

Counting people or identifying barriers?

ESTIMATING THE NUMBER OF PEOPLE WITH DISABILITIES: REGISTERS AND OFFICIAL SURVEYS

Since the National Assistance Act of 1948, local authorities have been required to keep registers of people certified as blind or partially sighted, deaf and with physical disabilities. Since the 1989 Children Act, they have also been required to keep a register of children with special needs, including those with disabilities. Health authorities have also set up child health computing systems (CHCS) to record comprehensive information about each child's health, although, since the introduction of the internal market, these have been run by community trusts.

If these registration systems were properly co-ordinated and organised, they could potentially provide comparative local and national information about the prevalence and types of disability. Unfortunately, many of these systems have been neglected and the data are of poor quality. Comparison between local authority disability registers and estimates of prevalence of disability from surveys has suggested that the registers fail to record more than half of the people with disabilities.[21] Using the OPCS's surveys, the Royal National Institute for the Blind estimated that 64 per cent of blind people were not registered.[25] Registers of children with special needs and child health computing systems fare little better. For example, when one such child health system in Northern Ireland was compared with a Northern Ireland Cerebral Palsy Register, only half the children registered on the national register were found to be recorded on the local child health computing system.[26] In general, there appears to be a lack of agreement about collecting, recording and collating information in child health computing systems and this has led to under-recording.[27]

In the absence of reliable data from other sources, survey data are used to estimate the numbers of people with disabilities. Non-specific questions about long-term illness have been asked regularly in three general surveys which cover a variety of topics. The census asked a question for the first time in 1991, the General Household Survey has included a question since 1975, and the Labour Force Survey has included a question biannually since 1993/4. The advantage of these general surveys is that they ask questions about aspects of everyday life, such as use of services, housing and employment. This offers the potential to find out additional information about the circumstances of people with long-term illnesses. In practice, the information in the General Household Survey and Labour Force Survey is often limited by the size of the sample, and data aggregated over several years are needed to provide fuller information. Further information about the General Household Survey can be found in Chapter 2 and further information about the Labour Force Survey can be found in Chapter 5.

The first large-scale survey focusing specifically on disability was undertaken by the OPCS in 1969 and was published as *Handicapped and impaired in Great Britain*.[28,29] This was followed in the mid-1980s by a comprehensive series of surveys undertaken by the OPCS, using questions based on the International Classification of Impairments, Disabilities and Handicap. These will be referred to as the OPCS surveys. Since then, questions based on the International Classification of Impairments, Disabilities and Handicap have been asked as part of the 1995 Health Survey for England and the 1996/7 Family Resources Survey (FRS). A major series of surveys on psychiatric morbidity was undertaken by the OPCS in 1995. A description of these appears in Chapter 2. Nearly all these surveys cover Great Britain only, but Northern Ireland has its own versions of the Labour Force Survey and the General Household Survey, the latter being called the Continuous Household Survey. In addition, surveys were undertaken in Northern Ireland based on the OPCS series. The reports are available from the Northern Ireland Statistics and Research Agency. The details of all these surveys can be found in the list of key official publications at the end of this section.

THE INFLUENCE OF THE OPCS SURVEYS

In the 1969 survey, *Handicapped and impaired in Great Britain*, degree of disability was defined in terms of a series of questions about capacity for self-care, and people who needed assistance in terms of self-care were defined as 'handicapped'. The OPCS surveys were commissioned by the Department of Health and Social Security for planning and benefit purposes and aimed to provide estimates of the prevalence of disability, information about the financial and social consequences of disability, and the use of health and personal social services. They included mental as well as physical disabilities. Children and adults were surveyed in both communal or residential establishments and private households. A set of screening questions about problems in undertaking a number of daily activities was administered to people at 100 000 addresses, and people with at least one problem, some 10 000 people, were interviewed in depth. The findings are published in a series of six separate reports, listed at end of this section.

The OPCS devised questions, based on the International Classification of Impairments, Disabilities and Handicap, to cover all types of disability. Information was obtained about limitations people experience in performing activities in ten different areas, including locomotion, seeing and intellectual functioning. The survey questions were then scaled for severity by panels, which included professionals and people with disabilities, to devise an overall severity scale with ten categories. The OPCS concluded that the method used in both surveys set a low threshold for disability, yet the survey gives one of the lowest estimates of the prevalence of disability.

There have been many criticisms of the basis for this methodology, but it has proved highly influential and has been adapted for use in many other official surveys. The 1995 Health Survey for England (described in Chapter 2) included questions on disability for everyone over 10 years of age. The focus was on disability rather than handicap and the survey did not attempt to investigate the social, economic or other consequences of disability. The Health Survey adapted a standardised protocol based on the International

Table 4.4 Surveys which estimate the percentage of people with disabilities

Survey	Question/definition	Type	Age range surveyed	Sample	Prevalence – adults in private households (%)
Handicapped and impaired in Great Britain [28,29]	Need for assistance with self-care	Single survey	Adults	Households in Great Britain	6
OPCS surveys 1985/6	Postal screening questionnaire then interviews questions based on the International Classification of Impairments, Disabilities and Handicap	Series of surveys	All ages	Households and institutions in Great Britain	13
Health Survey for England 1995	Based on the International Classification of Impairments, Disabilities and Handicaps	Single survey	Aged 10 and over	Households in England	18
Family Resources Survey 1996/97	Screening question for limiting disability/illness as in General Household Survey then OPCS survey questions based on the International Classification of Impairments, Disabilities and Handicap	Single survey	Aged 16 and over	Lower income households in Great Britain	20
Census 1991	Do you have any long-term illness, health problem or handicap which limits your daily activities or the work you can do? Include problems which are due to old age	Decennial, first asked in 1991	All ages	Households and institutions in UK	15
Labour Force Survey 1994/95	Do you have a long-standing health problem or disability which affects the kind of paid work you can do? Do you expect this problem or disability to last more than 1 year?	Asked biannually since 1993/4	Working age: 16–64 men 16–59 women	Households in Great Britain	11 (working age)
General Household Survey 1996	Do you have any long-standing illness, disability or infirmity? Does this illness of disability limit your activities in any way?	Asked annually since 1975	All ages	Households in Great Britain	25

Classification of Impairments, Disabilities and Handicap,[30] developed by the World Health Organisation for use in health surveys.[31] It included questions such as 'Can you walk up and down a flight of twelve stairs without resting?' and 'Can you get in and out of a chair on your own?'.

The Family Resources Survey, a continuous survey of some 25 000 lower income households, asks whether respondents have a limiting long-term illness or disability. In 1996/7, positive answers to this question, or other questions about the receipt of disability benefits, were used to select respondents for a follow-up interview focusing specifically on disability.[31,32] In addition, all respondents aged over 75 received a follow-up interview about disability. This interview uses the same questions as the OPCS surveys to obtain estimates of the prevalence, severity and financial problems of disabled people.

WHAT DO 'DISABILITY' SURVEYS MEASURE?

The disability movement has argued that one of the major problems with surveys based on the International Classification of Impairments, Disabilities and Handicap is that they do not relate functions to their context. Questions which are based on people's functional limitations in undertaking various tasks, such as whether a person can get in and out a chair on their own, or whether they can get to and use the toilet on their own, are meaningful only in relation to the tools available to carry out the tasks or where the toilet is situated.

For example, in the US census,[33] the 'long form' includes these two questions:

Does this person have a physical, mental or other health condition that has lasted for 6 or more months and which limits the kind or amount of work this person can do?

Because of a health condition that has lasted for 6 or more months, does this person have difficulty in going outside the home alone, e.g. to the shop or visit a doctor's office?

The replies suggested that the prevalence of 'work disability' measured by the first of these questions was the same in New York and Seattle, whereas the prevalence of 'mobility limitation' measured by the second was far lower in Seattle. The conventional individualised medical model led to suggestions that there are differences in the abilities of individuals in Seattle and New York. An alternative social explanation is that the higher prevalence of 'mobility limitation' in New York could be explained by its architecture and harsher winters.

Questions directed to exploring the relationship between disability and the environmental, economic or social constraints may highlight similar variations in Britain. One pilot study which has attempted to explore these issues is *Measuring disablement in society*.[34] Its purpose was to develop and test measures of social inclusion and exclusion in areas such as housing, transport, access and employment. The *National travel survey*[35] also estimates the numbers of 'transport disabled' people by collecting data on people's difficulties in using different forms of transport. These are exceptions, and in general few official data are collected on environmental barriers for disabled people.

OTHER METHODOLOGICAL PROBLEMS IN DISABILITY SURVEYS

In these official surveys, estimates of the prevalence of disability vary widely. For example, they range from 18 per cent for adults in private households in the 1995 Health Survey for England to 25 per cent for the same population in the 1997 General Household Survey. There has been a slow upward trend in such estimates. In 1975, when the General Household Survey first asked the question about long-term limiting illness, 15 per cent of people in all age groups responded positively, while 22 per cent did so in 1996.[36] Similarly, the OPCS surveys estimated a prevalence of 13 per cent in adults in the mid-1980s, and the Family Resources Survey, which used a similar method, estimated a prevalence of 20 per cent in 1996/7. As such surveys are known to be highly sensitive to choice of method, it is difficult to know whether this represents a real increase. The rise in the General Household Survey occurred in all age groups and would appear to be real. In contrast, the Department of Social Security, which commissioned the 1996/7 Family Resources Survey, attributed the increase to methodological problems.[32]

Many factors have been found to influence the results. People's unwillingness to identify themselves as disabled has a major effect on the validity and reliability of the findings of all surveys. In particular, elderly people may see disability as the norm. Compared with the Health Survey for England, the General Household Survey might be expected to give higher estimates for the prevalence of disability, as the questions it asks are all-embracing while those in the Health Survey are specific and more limited. The General Household Survey estimates are higher than those in the Health Survey for people in all age groups except those aged over 75. This suggests that elderly people are less likely than younger people with similar impairments to define themselves as disabled.[37] As was mentioned in Chapter 2, self-reported long-term illness appears sensitive to a range of socio-demographic factors. For example, in the 1991 Census, areas of high long-term unemployment had higher rates of self-reported long-term illness than other areas, even after controlling for deprivation and regional difference.[38]

A further problem is that few estimates of the prevalence of disability are based on surveys which include institutions such as hospitals, residential homes and prisons in the sample. The General Household Survey, Labour Force Survey, Health Survey for England and Family Resources Survey sample only from private households and therefore exclude disabled people living in communal establishments and those who are homeless. Data from the 1991 census showed that 71 per cent of people in communal establishments had a long-term illness or disability. The OPCS surveys estimated that around 7 per cent of people classified as disabled, some 420 000, lived in communal establishments. This is of a similar order to the estimate of half a million derived from the 1991 census. A further omission is that, with the exception of the OPCS surveys, official surveys tend to concentrate on adults. Official data on the prevalence of disability in children or the circumstances of disabled children in the 1990s are sparse.

Screening questions are often used to identify the sample for a more detailed survey. People who are aware that answering positively will result in additional interviews may reply negatively when questions are near the margin.[33] In a follow-up of people who replied both negatively and positively to a disability screening question in the 1986 Canadian Census, 20 per cent who replied positively were found not to have a disability and 5 per cent who responded negatively were subsequently classified as having a disability.[33] This gave an estimate of 3.2 million Canadians with a disability, 2 million from the group who initially screened positive and 1.2 million from those who originally screened negative. Both the OPCS surveys and the 1996/7 Family Resources Survey used screening questions. Finally, the Labour Force Survey and the census responses may be by proxy from another member of the person's household. This can lead to an underestimate of the proportion of disabled people in the population.[39]

The circumstances of disabled people

POVERTY AND EMPLOYMENT

One of the major reasons for commissioning surveys of people with disabilities is to inform policy about benefits. Both the OPCS surveys and the 1996/7 Family Resources Survey were commissioned for this purpose. In the OPCS surveys, respondents who were asked whether they spent more or less on a wide range of items as a result of their disability found it difficult to identify the extent of extra spending. Moreover, the sample appeared skewed towards people with less severe disabilities. Organisations of disabled people therefore argued that this survey significantly underestimated the true costs of disability.[20] The data were subsequently re-analysed by the Policy Studies Institute, which used comparative data from 1985 Family Expenditure Survey. More sophisticated methods were used to make detailed comparisons of the standard of living of disabled people and non-disabled people, controlling for factors such as the differences in income, age and household composition.[40] It was concluded that social security benefits do not compensate adequately for the high unemployment, low earnings and high costs associated with disability.

The 1996/7 Family Resources Survey used a different method again.[31] Respondents were asked whether they incurred extra costs, whether they received help towards the extra costs and whether they have gone without items they thought they needed because they could not afford them. These questions were asked about everyday expenditure, such as food and leisure activities, as well as about items related to disability, such as special equipment.

The OPCS data and the long-term illness data from the General Household

Survey have been used in a series of studies of poverty and disabled children.[41] These studies have established that disability is more common in the children of unskilled or semi-skilled manual workers than in other children. When compared with data from the 1983 Poor Britain Survey,[42] they showed that families with disabled children were four times more likely to be living in poverty than other families.

Data from the Labour Force Survey about the employment of disabled people appear from time to time in articles in *Labour Market Trends*.[43] The most comprehensive survey on this subject was published as *Employment and handicap*.[39] First undertaken in 1996, the surveys collect information about employment circumstances and economic activity rates for disabled people.

Information about benefit rates, the numbers receiving benefits targeted for people with disability and appeals can be found in *Social security statistics*.[44] Only the number of people who are both entitled to benefits and claim them are counted, but the rules of entitlement may bear little relationship to need. The OPCS surveys found that only a quarter of people who were classified in the group with the highest level of disability received attendance allowance.

The Department of Social Security Research Branch publishes a range of reports about disability and benefits. A complete list of its publications can be found on its web site, the address of which is given at the end of this section. The *Directory of disability data sources*[45] lists sources of information about studies of the prevalence of disability, the circumstances of disabled people and disability policy.

USE OF SERVICES

Although the use of health and social care services, equipment and adaptations was comprehensively covered in the fourth report of the OPCS surveys, the changes to services since the mid-1980s mean that the findings are outdated. The General Household Survey also contains comparative information about use of services, aids and mobility difficulties for people with a long-term illness or disability. The scanty information available on people living in long-term care institutions is described in Chapter 9.

Government surveys and registers, particularly those whose aim is to identify needs for services or financial support, often appear to be influenced by the need to keep the costs down. For example, there is a disincentive to placing children on local authority registers as identifying such a child places an obligation on the authorities to provide services. Another example is a recent government survey of the need for housing for wheelchair users, published as *Living independently*.[46] This estimated the shortfall in wheelchair housing as some 13 000 places. This is very low, given that previous estimates had ranged from 60 000 to 330 000. Re-analysis of the data by other researchers found mathematical flaws and criteria which excluded many wheelchair users, such as those who would prefer to be owner-occupiers irrespective of their means. These flaws meant that estimates derived from the research lost all credibility as a estimate of need for wheelchair housing.[22]

Key official surveys and other series: people with disabilities

The OPCS surveys of disability in Great Britain
Report 1 The prevalence of disability among adults. London: HMSO, 1988.
Report 2 The financial circumstances of disabled adults living in private households. London: HMSO, 1988.
Report 3 The prevalence of disability among children. London: HMSO, 1988.
Report 4 Disabled adults: services, transport and employment. London: HMSO, 1989.
Report 5 The financial circumstances of families with disabled children living in private households. London: HMSO, 1989.
Report 6 Disabled children: services, transport and education. London: HMSO, 1989.

Northern Ireland Statistics and Research Agency: surveys of disability
The prevalence of disability among adults in Northern Ireland.
The prevalence of disability among children in Northern Ireland.
Disability and employment in Northern Ireland.
Financial circumstances.
Disabled adults: services and transport.
Disabled children in Northern Ireland: services, transport and education.

Bennett N, Dodd T, Flatley J, Freeth S, Bolling K. *Health Survey for England 1995.* London: HMSO, 1996.
Harris A. *Handicapped and impaired in Great Britain.* London: HMSO, 1971.
Office of Population Censuses and Surveys. *1991 Census. Limiting long-term illness.* Great Britain. London: HMSO, 1993.
Office for National Statistics. *Labour Force Survey historical supplement.* London: TSO, 1997.
Office for National Statistics. *Living in Britain: results from the General Household Survey.* Series General Household Survey. Published annually. London: TSO.

Contact addresses and web sites

World Health Organisation
For details of *ICIDH-2 International Classification of functioning and disability, Beta-2 draft*
Web site: http://www.who.int/icidh

Department of Social Security: Social Research Branch
10th floor Adelphi
2–11 John Adam Street
London WC2N 6HT
Web site: http://www.dss.gov.uk/asf/asd5

Ethnic minorities and migrant groups

The problems of categorising ethnicity

The census question on country of birth has been a source of information about immigration since it was first included in 1841. Migration from Ireland has been a constant feature for at least two centuries. In the early years of the century and again in the 1930s and 1940s, many refugees came from eastern Europe. In the latter half of the twentieth century, there has been migration from Britain's former colonies, in particular the Indian subcontinent and the West Indies. People from migrant groups and their children born in the UK now form about 6 per cent of the population of Britain, with some 3.3 million describing themselves as 'non-white' in the 1991 census. There is clear evidence that there are substantial differences between them and the majority population, in terms of their health, employment and housing.

A question on ethnic origin was proposed for the 1981 census, but the idea was dropped after considerable public resistance. The lack of information about ethnic minority groups started to become an important issue in the 1980s, both for the Thatcher government, which wanted tough immigration controls, and for people who wanted to implement and monitor antidiscrimination policies. From 1981, the Labour Force Survey had contained a question asking people to define themselves as White, West Indian, Indian, Pakistani, Bangladeshi, Chinese, African, Arab, 'mixed origin', or 'other'. There was considerable controversy about the proposals to include a similar ethnic question in the 1991 census, and the categories chosen have been heavily criticised for failing to reflect the complexities of ethnic groups in Britain.[47-9]

In sociological terms, part of the population may be considered to constitute an ethnic group when its members share certain characteristics of ancestry or culture. Ethnicity refers to practices and outlooks which distinguish a given group of people.[50] According to this definition, the 'white' majority population of the UK would also have an ethnic identity. Race is a much older term and, although its use has been largely discredited in health research, it remains an important term which is used politically to highlight the social and economic disadvantages caused by racism.[51] The census categories are a mixture of the old racial categories black/white, and national or colonial origins such as Indian, black Caribbean and Pakistani.

These categories are quite meaningless in terms of definitions of ethnicity and there is a continuous debate about the relevance of such categories to understanding the determinants of health and other social issues. There are a number of problems. The categories are considered too broad, disguising the heterogeneity of populations from India and Africa, who differ in language, religion and diet. They also give little information about the 'white' population, particularly people of Irish origin, and little information about people of mixed race. Some 900 000 people described themselves as 'Indian' in the 1991 census, but the extent to which they share an ancestry or culture is highly questionable, as 16 per cent of the group were born in East Africa, 36 per cent in India and 44 per cent in the UK. Conversely, 74 per cent of those born in East Africa described themselves as 'Indian'. A further issue is that the categories appear unacceptable to some groups and there is evidence of inconsistent self-reports, particularly for young people of black African descent who prefer to describe themselves as 'Black British'. [52]

The breadth of the categories limits the usefulness of the data both for targeting services and as an independent variable in health studies.[49] More fundamentally, because of their inadequacy, research using these categories has been criticised for giving misleading and inadequate explanations for the observed health differences between ethnic minority groups and the 'white' populations. Rather than attributing health disadvantages to social or economic inequalities, they are seen as a consequence of 'inherent' cultural or genetic 'weaknesses' in ethnic minority groups. In *Statistics in society*, James Nazroo suggests that the findings are an artefact of the categories and measures used for both social class and ethnic groups.[53] If other categories for ethnic group and other measures of poverty or deprivation are used, then the link between poverty and poor health in ethnic minority groups can clearly be demonstrated.

Despite the problems, the census categories are becoming increasingly used in health datasets such as Hospital Episode Statistics, where ethnic origin has been recorded since 1995. The census question on ethnic group has been modified for the 2001 census and there are proposals to ask a question about religion for the first time in England, Wales and Scotland. While there is evidence to suggest that this will allow better discrimination between ethnic groups, it will in no way deal with all the criticisms.[54]

The next section describes the datasets which include information on either country of birth or ethnic group as defined by the census categories.

Counting migrants and ethnic groups

MIGRATION

The statistics collected on migration present only a partial view of what is a complex and changing phenomenon. There are four main sources of data about migration to the UK. The country of birth of parents is collected when they register the birth of a child. Data are also collected through the census and other surveys, in particular the International Passenger Survey, through Home Office statistics of people applying for asylum and settlement under the 1971 Immigration Act, and through people entering the labour market by registering for National Insurance and work permits. Each of these routes has limitations and many migrants, such as 'temporary' workers, the self-employed, 'students' and illegal immigrants, go unrecorded.[55]

Birth and fertility statistics, published annually by the ONS in *Birth statistics, Series FM 1,* include analyses by country of birth of mother and also a few tabulations by the father's country of birth. The decennial census has included a question about country of birth since 1841. In 1971, as well as asking about country of birth, the census asked a question about people's parents' birth-place. This was used to estimate the number of second-generation migrants. Data derived from these were updated annually using the birth and death registration and migration statistics to produce proxy estimates of the size of ethnic minority groups. Between 1981 and 1991, data from the Labour Force Survey were used for these estimates. The 1991 census asked people when they came to the UK.

For censuses before 1991, demographic statistics by country of birth were published in *Country of birth* volumes and some tables by country of birth were also included in *County and regional reports*. For the 1991 census, tables cross-classifying country of birth and ethnic group are given in the *Ethnic group and country of birth* volumes and also in the *County and regional reports*. The General Household Survey (described in Chapter 2) has included a question on country of birth since 1971, but because of the sample size, country of birth is usually grouped simply into 'born in UK' or 'born outside UK' in published tables.

The International Passenger Survey started in 1964 and is a sample survey of passengers travelling through major air and sea ports of the UK. A migrant is defined as a passenger entering the UK with the declared intention of residing here for at least a year, having lived abroad for at least a year. The sample size of some 250 000 interviews, only 1 per cent of whom are classified as migrants, makes information about the origin and destinations unreliable.[56] Information from this survey is published by the ONS in *International migration, Series MN*. Summaries also appear in *Population trends* and *Social trends*.

The Home Office publishes data on reasons for acceptance for settlement under the 1971 Immigration Act in its *Control of immigration statistics*. These include the numbers granted refugee status or asylum by nationality. Acceptance for settlement statistics are classified by category, for example children, spouse, own right. These statistics include only people subject to immigration control and therefore do not include those with British or European Union passports, for example those from the Irish Republic.

The most useful non-government source is the Policy Studies Institute, which has conducted a series of surveys of minority ethnic groups.[57,58] The surveys include questions about country of birth and year of entry to the UK.

ETHNIC ORIGIN

Apart from the period between 1881 and 1921, when the census contained questions in Yiddish, no questions about religion, race or any other factors which could define groups as culturally distinct were asked in the census for mainland Great Britain until 1991.[56] In Northern Ireland, however, the census has always included a question about religion, but ethnic group was omitted from the 1991 census as this was thought to be of little relevance to local circumstances.[59] A question on ethnic group will be included in 2001.

In the 1991 census, self-reported ethnic origin could be recorded in one of nine categories. The question is shown in Table 4.5. Most published tables use ten categories, which include the nine groups in Table 4.5 plus an additional group, 'Other groups – Asian'. Some tables also include an additional column, 'Born in Ireland'. Details of the coding are in the 1991 census *Ethnic group and*

Table 4.5 The question asked about ethnic group in the census of population, Great Britain, 1991

Ethnic group	
Please tick the appropriate box.	White ☐ 0 Black-Caribbean ☐ 1 Black-African ☐ 2 Black-other ☐ *please describe*
	Indian ☐ 3 Pakistani ☐ 4 Bangladeshi ☐ 5 Chinese ☐ 6 Any other ethnic group ☐ *please describe*
If the person is descended from more than one ethnic or racial group, please tick the group to which the person considers he/she belongs, or tick the 'Any other ethnic group' box and describe the person's ancestry in the space provided.	

Source: OPCS and General Register Office, Scotland. *1991 census. Definitions, Great Britain.* London: HMSO, 1992

country of birth volumes, published by the OPCS and the General Register Office, Scotland, in 1993. Published tables in national, county and regional volumes include the percentages in each ethnic group. In addition, there are tables of ethnic group by age and sex, as well as employment and housing conditions, household composition, higher educational qualifications and long-term illness. More detailed analysis and commentary appears in a series of four books, *Ethnicity and the 1991 census.* These are listed at the end of the chapter.

Prior to the 1991 census, the main source of information on the ethnic composition of the population was the Labour Force Survey, described in Chapter 2. This survey, which started in 1981 as an annual survey of private households, was the first continuous national survey routinely to include questions on ethnicity. Between 1981 and 1991, people were shown a card and asked to say to which ethnic group they considered they belonged. The groups were White, West Indian or Guyanese, Indian, Pakistani, Bangladeshi, Chinese, African, Arab, Mixed origin, Other.

The ethnic question in the quarterly Labour Force Survey is now based on the 1991 census definitions. Figures are published quarterly by ethnicity, but these are not very reliable given the overall Labour Force Survey sample size. It is necessary to aggregate data across several quarterly surveys to provide reliable estimates of population by ethnicity, age and sex for the years between the census. Some summary tables based on aggregated data appear in *Social trends* and in occasional articles in *Population trends.*[60]

The General Household Survey has also included an ethnicity question since 1983, but limited information is given in published volumes. The equivalent survey in Northern Ireland, the Continuous Household Survey, includes a question on religion. This provides important information about differences in households, housing, health and income between protestants and catholics.

A general discussion and estimates of the population by ethnicity before 1991 were published in *Population trends*.[61] Both the 1991 census and the Labour Force Survey have poorer response rates from black and Asian populations than from the white population.[62,63] In addition, as noted previously, there is evidence of inconsistent self-reports, particularly for young people of black African descent.

Monitoring the health of ethnic groups

Controversies over the inadequacies of the ethnic categories do not account for the fact that ethnic differences in health status and health care provision have often been ignored by prevailing health policy makers, and routine data about ethnicity, disease and access to health care are lacking.[64] It is well known that some conditions such as sickle cell anaemia are more common in some ethnic groups than in others, but the lack of high-quality data on mortality and morbidity by ethnic group means that ethnic differences in common conditions, such as heart disease and diabetes, and unequal access to health care by ethnicity are less widely understood.

MORTALITY RATES, COUNTRY OF BIRTH AND ETHNICITY

Death rates provide one of the most robust ways of comparing the health of different groups, but it is not possible to calculate death rates by ethnic group for the simple reason that the census categories are not recorded on death registrations. Instead, the country of birth of the person who has died is recorded, and is used as a proxy for ethnicity. Mortality rates by country of birth can therefore be calculated, using census data on country of birth as the denominator. Rates by country of birth are usually presented for years straddling the census, as these estimates are likely to be more reliable. A number of analyses have been published.[65-7] Their titles reflect the fact that they compare country of birth rather than ethnicity, but the analyses can be misleading.

For some migrant groups, mortality rates are usually calculated for aggregates of several countries. For example, the Indian subcontinent includes all those born in India, Pakistan, Bangladesh and Sri Lanka, and Ireland sometimes includes both Northern Ireland and the Irish Republic. Calculation of separate rates for each of these countries may be misleading. Geographical and political boundaries may change and informants' reporting of country of birth may be incomplete or inaccurate.

Although country of birth is a useful indicator for possible early environmental influences on health, its use as a proxy for ethnicity is also misleading. As previously noted, migrants to the UK from East Africa are not necessarily people of black African descent: many are south Asians. Published tables do not separate these two categories and also, with the exception of mortality rates based on the 1991 census,[67] they group all migrants from West Africa, who are predominantly black African, and from East Africa, who are predominantly south Asian, into one category, Africa. There are important health differences between these groups. For example, migrants of black African descent have higher rates of hypertension and stroke. Cancer mortality varies among the group, with the prevalence of some cancers being high in migrants from both East Africa and West Africa and that of others being high in migrants from West Africa and the Caribbean.[68]

Apart from these limitations, country of birth has served well as a marker for ethnicity in the past, but is becoming less valid for two reasons. First of all, second-generation migrants have now entered the adult population. Thus, their country of birth no longer reflects the ethnic origin of people below the age of 40.[66,69] Secondly, the census now uses self-defined ethnicity as the preferred measure of ethnic group. Thus, ethnic group definitions will now no longer remain congruent between mortality and census data.

ROUTINE MORBIDITY DATA

It is only recently that major routine disease reporting systems have started to collect information about ethnicity. Of reporting systems, *cancer registration* is likely to provide most information. Information for the registration of new cancers (described in Chapter 3) is collected from hospital case notes. Routine recording of ethnic origin on all patients admitted to National Health Service (NHS) hospitals began in April 1995. This means that, in the future, NHS records may provide a valuable source for examining the incidence of cancer among ethnic groups, although there are currently no routine analyses of cancer incidence or disease experience by ethnic group. Currently, the only data about cancer groups are cancer mortality rates by country of birth. For rapidly fatal cancers, these may provide a fair approximation of disease incidence.

Congenital anomaly notifications (described in Chapter 3) include a unique identifier so that the child can be identified if necessary, but ethnicity is not included in the data held by the ONS. Nevertheless the decennial supplement *The health of our children*[70] contains a chapter on congenital anomalies and ethnic minorities mainly based on analyses by country of birth. *Communicable disease notifications* (described in Chapter 3) do not routinely include ethnicity. To obtain the ethnic group of people notified, it is necessary to conduct special surveys.[71]

In terms of survey data, the census report *Limiting long-term illness* can be used to compare age-standardised morbidity rates, both nationally and for each locality. Many other major government health survey datasets do collect details of ethnic group, but the sample size is usually too small for reliable analyses by ethnic group. The decennial National Morbidity Survey (described in Chapter 8) interviewed patients attending for a general practitioner consultation. In 1991, ethnic group was recorded for all consultations, again using census categories.[72] Data are published for Indian, Pakistani/Bangladeshi and black Afro-Caribbean people, as the numbers of people in the other groups are too small for meaningful analyses.

In the Health Survey for England (described in Chapter 2) respondents are asked to assign themselves to an ethnic group, again using the census categories. Due to the representative nature of the sampling techniques, very few people from minority ethnic groups are included, and published reports have not presented any data by ethnic group.[37] Several years' data have to be aggregated to monitor the health of specific minority groups. In 1999, however, the health of ethnic groups was the focus of the Health Survey for England. Thus, a larger sample of people from ethnic minority groups was included in this survey.

The General Household Survey and the Labour Force Survey include questions on general self-reported health, long-standing illness and limiting long-standing illness. Ethnicity is now self-assigned, using the census categories, but the data from several years' surveys have to be aggregated to obtain reliable information.

The fourth of a series of national surveys of ethnic groups was undertaken by the independent Policy Studies Institute in 1993 and 1994. This included perceptions of general health and also questions about morbidity from heart disease, diabetes, respiratory illness, accidents and the use of health services.[57,73] The introduction to the report of this survey contains a useful overview of data sources on ethnicity and health together with a discussion on their limitations. This survey also covered mental health.[74]

HEALTH AND SOCIAL SERVICES DATA

Since April 1995, the Hospital Episode Statistics (described in Chapter 8) have routinely included information about ethnic group, using the 1991 census categories and ethnic group has been added to many other NHS records in its minimum dataset. Hospital Episode Statistics have the potential to be extremely useful, but there are major concerns about the accuracy and completeness of hospital data about ethnicity, and they must therefore be interpreted with caution. Ethnic group is not among the items of data collected by the Department of Health about the use of local authority social services (described in Chapter 9).

FACTORS ASSOCIATED WITH ILL-HEALTH

The main sources of information about social factors such as unemployment and housing are the 1991 Census, in particular Volume 4 in the series on ethnic groups, and also the Labour Force Survey, General Household Survey and Policy Studies Institute surveys of ethnic groups.[57,58] The data available and where they have been published are summarised in what follows. Some of these topics have been analysed in greater detail in secondary analyses of official statistics and these are listed at the end of this chapter.

Information about education qualifications by ethnicity is included in the reports of the Policy Studies Institute surveys[57,58] and the 1991 census. Information on employment and unemployment can be obtained from the *Census economic activity* volume,[75] where rates are given by ethnicity, age and sex for counties and regions, and from the Labour Force Survey. The Labour Force

Survey quarterly bulletins include economic activity rates and unemployment rates for people over the age of 16 by ethnicity and gender. Four broad ethnic groups – White, Black, Indian, Pakistani/Bangladeshi – are used. There are also regular topic reports from the Labour Force Survey in *Labour Market Trends*, formerly known as the *Employment Gazette*.

Data from the 1991 census about ethnicity are tabulated by social class and socio-economic group in the *Ethnic group and country of birth* volume. Occasionally, Labour Force Survey topic reports include analyses by social class and ethnicity, as described above. The 1991 census county and regional volumes include tables on housing and car ownership by ethnic group. Data from the Survey of English Housing also include ethnic origin. There are very few routinely published data on health-related behaviours by ethnicity. Data on smoking from the 1975, 1976 and 1978 General Household Surveys was published in a special analysis.[65] The Health Education Authority conducted a one-off survey,[69] which included health-related behaviours and ethnicity. The National Food Survey and the National Diet and Nutrition Surveys (described in Chapter 6) could be useful sources of data on dietary habits, but do not collect any data on ethnicity. The 1995 surveys of infant feeding included a specially enlarged sample of Asian babies.[76] Despite the limited published data, there is potential for making fuller use of routine surveys by using data aggregated over several years. For example, this could be done using smoking data from the General Household Survey.

Data from official surveys and the census are available to researchers for further analysis, known as secondary analysis. It is worth looking out for reports of secondary analyses of official data on ethnicity, as these often contain more detailed analyses and useful commentary. For example, the Equal Opportunities Commission has looked at the employment circumstances of women by ethnicity.[77] The Centre for Research in Ethnic Relations at the University of Warwick has produced a series of 1991 Census Statistical papers which present analyses by ethnicity together with commentary. The third in the series examines social and economic circumstances and unemployment rates.[78]

In 1996, the ONS published *Social focus on ethnic minorities*.[79] This provides an overarching view of the ethnicity data from the 1991 census and other data sources. In addition, the decennial supplement *The health of our children*[70] contains a chapter on the health of ethnic minority children.

The future

The categories used to monitor ethnic groups still remain controversial, but developing categories which are valid, reliable, acceptable to respondents and yet can take into account changing ethnic identities is not a simple matter. In preparation for the 2001 census, the ONS has conducted several small-scale tests of modifications of the ethnic question included in the 1991 census. Proposals for the 2001 census were announced in a White Paper[80] published in early 1999 and then tested in a dress rehearsal in April 1999. The census order for England and Wales was approved by a House of Commons Standing Committee in February 2000.[81,82] When the draft census order for Scotland was debated in the Scottish Parliament in February 2000, it decided to include a question on religion and to hold a consultation on the format for this and the ethnic question.[83,84] The census order for Northern Ireland was delayed by the suspension of the Northern Ireland Assembly in January 2000.

A modified version of the 1991 census question will be used in England and Wales. This includes the new categories 'Irish', 'Asian or Asian British', ' Black or Black British' and 'Mixed'. Slightly different forms of the question will be used in Scotland and in Northern Ireland, where it will be the first time that an ethnic question has been included. In addition, if the necessary legislation is passed a question on religion will be asked in England and Wales and in Scotland, partly to help distinguish ethnic minority subgroups from the Indian subcontinent. In Northern Ireland, the form of the ethnic question will be the same as that asked in Britain in 1991, but an additional category 'Irish traveller', will be added.

Whatever categories are chosen, standardised recording of ethnicity on official records such as health and local authority registers is necessary if these routine data sources are to provide meaningful information about the health of ethnic minorities. Estimation of mortality rates for ethnic groups remains a problem, as at present ethnicity is not recorded on death certificates. This is probably not feasible, because of the variability in the recording of ethnicity, and the fact that self-defined ethnicity cannot be recorded after death. Instead, to study mortality by ethnicity, it may be better to utilise datasets which are linked to individuals whose ethnicity is already known. For example, this would be feasible in the Longitudinal Study if the ethnic minority group could be oversampled. Both the quality of the data and the value of the collection will improve in proportion to the use made of them to understand our diverse communities and reduce discrimination.

Key official publications

Office of Population Censuses and Surveys/General Register Office, Scotland. *1991 Census: ethnic group and country of birth*. London: HMSO, 1993.

Coleman J, Salt D, eds. Ethnicity in the 1991 *Census Series, Vol. 1 Demographic characteristics of ethnic minority populations* 1996. London: HMSO, 1996.

Peach C, ed. Ethnicity in the 1991 Census Series, Vol. 2 *The ethnic minority populations of Great Britain* 1996. London: HMSO, 1996.

Ratcliffe P, ed. Ethnicity in the 1991 Census Series, Vol. 3 *Social geography and ethnicity in Great Britain* 1996. London: HMSO, 1996.

Karn V, ed. Ethnicity in the 1991 Census Series, Vol. 4 *Education, employment and housing among ethnic minority populations of Great Britain* 1997. London: HMSO, 1997.

Office for National Statistics. *International migration*, Series MN. London: TSO, published annually.

Home Office. *Control of immigration statistics*, London: TSO, published annually.

Department of Social Security. *Migrant workers*. London: Department of Social Security, published annually.

References

1. Jarman B. Identification of underprivileged areas. *British Medical Journal* 1983; **286**: 1705–9.
2. Jarman B. Underprivileged areas: validation and distribution of scores. *British Medical Journal* 1984; **289**: 1587–92.
3. Phillimore P, Beattie A, Townsend P. Widening inequality of health in Northern England, 1981–91. *British Medical Journal* 1994; **308**: 1125–8.
4. Carstairs V, Morris R. *Deprivation and health in Scotland.* Aberdeen: Aberdeen University Press, 1991.
5. Department of the Environment. *1991 Deprivation Index: a review of approaches and a matrix of results.* London: HMSO, 1995.
6. Department of Environment, Transport and the Regions. *1998 Index of Local Deprivation.* Regeneration research survey no. 15. On the internet at http://www.regeneration.detr.gov.uk
7. OPCS. Standard occupational classification, Vol. 3. *Social classifications and coding methodology.* London: HMSO, 1991.
8. Erikson R, Goldthorpe JH. *The constant flux.* Oxford: Clarendon Press, 1993.
9. Wright EO. *Classes.* London: Verso, 1985.
10. Rose D, O'Reilly K. *Constructing classes. Towards a new social classification for the UK.* Swindon: Economic and Social Research Council/ONS, 1997.
11. Macfarlane AJ, Mugford M. *Birth counts: statistics of pregnancy and childbirth.* Volume 1, text. Second edition. London: The Stationery Office, 2000.
12. Royal College of General Pracitioners, OPCS, DH. *Morbidity statistics from general practice. Third national study: socio-economic analyses,* microfiche. McCormick A, Rosenbaum M, eds. Series MB5 No. 2. London: HMSO, 1990.
13. OPCS. *Morbidity statistics from general practice. Fourth national study, 1991–1992.* McCormick A, Fleming D, Charlton J, eds. Series MB5 No. 3. London: HMSO, 1995.
14. Jones IG, Cameron D. Social class analysis – an embarrassment to epidemiology. *Community Medicine* 1984; **6**: 37–46.
15. Farr W. Letter to the Registrar General. In: *Supplement to the 35th annual report of the Registrar General. Births, deaths and marriages in England 1861–1879.* London: HMSO, 1875.
16. Working group on inequalities in health. *Inequalities in health: report of a research working group.* London: Department of Health and Social Security, 1980.
17. Townsend P, Davidson N. *Inequalities in health: the Black report.* Harmondsworth: Penguin, 1982.
18. Townsend P, Davidson N, Whitehead M. *Inequalities in health: the Black report and the health divide.* Harmondsworth: Penguin, 1992.
19. *Independent Enquiry into Inequalities in Health.* Report. London: TSO, 1998.
20. Abberley P. Disabled by numbers. In: Levitas R, Guy W, eds. *Interpreting official statistics.* London: Routledge, 1996: 166–84.
21. Oliver M. Redefining disability: a challenge to research. In: Swain J, Finkelstein V, French S, Oliver M, eds. *Disabling Barriers – Enabling Environments.* London: Sage, 1993: 61–77.
22. Stewart J, Harris J, Sapey B. Truth or manipulation? The politics of government funded disability research. *Disability and Society* 1998; **13**(2): 297–300.
23. World Health Organisation. *International Classification of Impairments, Disabilities and Handicaps: a manual of classification relating to the consequences of disease.* Geneva: World Health Organisation, 1980.

24. Waddington L. Working towards a European definition of disability. *European Journal of Health Law* 1995; **2**: 3–8.
25. Evans J. *Causes of blindness and partial sight in England and Wales.* Studies on Medical and Population Subjects No. 57. London: HMSO, 1995.
26. Parkes J, Dolk H, Hill N. Does the child health computing system adequately identify children with cerebral palsy? *Journal of Public Health Medicine* 1998; **20**: 102–4.
27. Johnson A, King A. Can routine information systems be used to monitor serious disability? *Archives of Diseases in Childhood* 1999; **80**: 63–6.
28. Harris A. *Handicapped and impaired in Great Britain.* London: HMSO, 1971.
29. Buckle J. *Work and housing of impaired people in Great Britain.* London: HMSO, 1971.
30. World Health Organisation and Netherlands Central Bureau of Statistics. *Third consultation to develop common methods or instruments for health interview surveys.* Voorburg: World Health Organisation, 1993.
31. Craig P. Disability follow up to the Family Resources Survey: aims, methods and coverage. *In-house Social Security Research Report 19.* London: DSS, 1996.
32. Craig P, Greenslade M. *First findings from the Disability Follow-up to the Family Resources Survey.* Research Summary No. 5, Analytical Services Division. London: DSS, 1998.
33. Sampson AR. Surveying individuals with disabilities. In: Spencer BD, ed. *Statistics and public policy.* Oxford: Clarendon Press, 1997: 162–79.
34. Zarb G, Salvage A, Arthur S, Begum N. *Measuring disablement in society, Working Papers 1–5.* London: Policy Studies Institute, 1995.
35. Department of the Environment, Transport and the Regions. *National Travel Survey.* London: TSO, published annually.
36. ONS. *Living in Britain 1996: results from the General Household Survey.* London: TSO, 1998.
37. Prescott Clarke P, Primatesta P. *Health Survey for England 1995.* London: TSO, 1997.
38. Haynes R, Bentham G, Lovett A, Eimermann J. Effect of labour market conditions on reporting of limiting long-term illness and permanent sickness in England and Wales. *Journal of Epidemiology and Community Health* 1997; **51**(3): 283–8.
39. Prescott Clarke P. *Employment and handicap.* London: Social and Community Planning Research, 1990.
40. Berthoud R, Lakey J, McKay S. *The economic problems of disabled people.* London: Policy Studies Institute, 1993.
41. Gordon D, Heslop P. Poverty and disabled children. In: Dorling D, Simpson S, eds. *Statistics in society.* London: Arnold, 1998, pp. 161–71.
42. Mack J, Lansley S. *Poor Britain.* London: Allen and Unwin, 1985.
43. Sly F, Duxbury R. Disability and the labour market: findings from the Labour Force Survey. *Labour Market Trends* 1995; **104**: 5–18.
44. Department of Social Security. *Social security statistics.* London: TSO, published annually.
45. Arthur S, Zarb GA. *Directory of Disability Data Sources.* In-House Report 31. London: Department of Social Security Social Research Branch, 1997.
46. McCafferty P. *Living independently: a study of housing needs of elderly and disabled people.* London: HMSO, 1995.
47. Ahmed WIU. Ethnic statistics – better than nothing or worse than nothing? In: Dorling D, Simpson S, eds. *Statistics in society.* London: Arnold, 1998, pp. 124–31.
48. Fenton S. Counting ethnicity. In: Levitas R, Guy W, eds. *Interpreting official statistics.* London: Routledge, 1996: 143–65.
49. Sheldon TA, Parker H. Race and ethnicity in health research. *Journal of Public Health Medicine* 1995; **14**: 104–10.

50. Bradby H. Ethnicity: not a black and white issue. *Sociology of Health and Illness* 1995; **17**: 405–17.
51. Pfeffer N, Moynihan C. Ethnicity and health beliefs with respect to cancer: a critical review of methodology. *British Journal of Cancer* 1996; **74**: 566–72.
52. Ballard R, Kalra VS. *The ethnic dimension of the 1991 Census: a preliminary report.* Manchester: University of Manchester, 1994.
53. Nazroo JY. The racialisation of ethnic inequalities in health. In: Dorling D, Simpson S, eds. *Statistics in society.* London: Arnold, 1998, pp. 215–22.
54. Southworth J. The religious question: representing reality or compounding confusion? In: Dorling D, Simpson S, eds. *Statistics in Society.* London: Arnold, 1998, pp. 132–9.
55. Singleton A. Measuring international migration: the tools aren't up to the job. In: Dorling D, Simpson S, eds. *Statistics in society.* London: Arnold, 1998, pp. 148–58.
56. Coleman D, Salt J. *The British population: patterns, trends and processes.* Oxford: Oxford University Press, 1992.
57. Modood T, Berthoud R, Lakey J, Nazroo J, Smith P, Virdee S, Beishon S. *Ethnic minorities in Britain: diversity and disadvantage. Fourth National Survey of Ethnic Minorities.* London: Policy Studies Institute, 1997.
58. Brown C. *Black and White Britain. The Third Policy Studies Institute Survey.* London: Heinemann, 1984.
59. Dale A, Marsh C, eds. *The 1991 census user's guide.* London: HMSO, 1993.
60. Haskey J. Population review 8: The ethnic minority and overseas-born populations of Great Britain. *Population Trends* 1997; **88**: 13–30.
61. OPCS. Sources of statistics and ethnic origin. *Population Trends* 1982; **28**: 1–8.
62. Simpson S. Non-response to the 1991 census: its impact on the enumeration of ethnic groups. In: Coleman D, Salt J, eds. *Ethnicity in the 1991 census: demographic characteristics.* London: HMSO, 1996: 63–79.
63. Owen C. Ethnic minorities: Non-response in the Labour Force Survey. *Population Trends* 1993; **72**: 18–73.
64. Chaturvedi N, McKeigue PM. Methods for epidemiological surveys of ethnic minority groups. *Journal of Epidemiology and Community Health* 1994; **48**: 107–11.
65. Marmot MG, Adelstein AM, Bulusu L. Immigrant mortality in England and Wales 1970–78. *Studies in Medical and Population Subjects 47.* London: HMSO, 1984.
66. Balarajan R, Bulusu L. Mortality among immigrants in England and Wales 1979–83: In: Britton M, ed. *Mortality and geography: a review in the mid 1980s.* Series DS, No. 9 London: HMSO, 1990.
67. Harding S, Maxwell R. Differences in mortality of migrants. In: Drever F, Whitehead M, eds. *Health Inequalities.* Decennial Supplement. Series DS No. 15. London: TSO, 1997.
68. Grulich AE, Swerdlow AJ, Head J, Marmot MG. Cancer mortality in African and Caribbean migrants to England and Wales. *British Journal of Cancer* 1992; **66**: 905–11.
69. Rudat K. *Black and minority ethnic groups in England.* London: Health Education Authority, 1994.
70. Botting B, ed. *The health of our children.* Decennial supplement. Series DS No. 11. London: HMSO, 1995.
71. Bhatti N, Law M, Morris JK, Halliday R, Moore-Gillon J. Increasing incidence of tuberculosis in England and Wales: a study of the likely causes. *British Medical Journal* 1995; **320**: 967–9.
72. McCormick A, Fleming D, Charlton G. *Morbidity statistics from general practice fourth national study 1991–1992.* Series MB5, 3. London: HMSO, 1995.

73. Nazroo JY. *The health of Britain's ethnic minorities: Fourth National Survey of Ethnic Minorities.* London: Policy Studies Institute, 1997.

74. Nazroo JY. *Ethnicity and mental health: Fourth National Survey of Ethnic Minorities.* London: Policy Studies Institute, 1997.

75. OPCS. *1991 Census Economic Activity, Great Britain.* London: HMSO, 1993.

76. Thomas M, Avery V. *Infant feeding in Asian families: early feeding practices and growth.* London: TSO, 1997.

77. Equal Opportunity Commission. *Ethnic minority women and the labour market: an analysis of 1991 Census.* Manchester: Equal Opportunity Commission, 1994.

78. Owen D. *Ethnic minorities in Great Britain: economic characteristics.* National Ethnic Minority Data Archive, 1991 Census Statistical Paper No. 3. Coventry: Centre for Research in Ethnic Relations, University of Warwick: 1993.

79. ONS. *Social focus on ethnic minorities.* London: HMSO, 1996.

80. *The 2001 Census of Population.* Cm 4253. London: TSO, 1999.

81. Office for National Statistics, General Register Office Scotland, Northern Ireland Statistics and Research Agency. *Census news, No. 43.* February 2000.

82. *Census, England and Wales. The Census order 2000.* Draft order in council laid before parliament on 10 January 2000.

83. *Census. The census (Scotland) order 2000.* Draft order in council laid before the Scottish parliament on 10 January 2000.

84. General Register Office for Scotland. *2001 census of population, Scotland. Consultation on questions about religion and ethnicity.* Edinburgh: GRO, 2000.

Money matters

5

MEASURING POVERTY, WEALTH AND UNEMPLOYMENT

Paul Johnson, Sarah Tanner and Ray Thomas

Poverty statistics
Wealth statistics
Employment and unemployment

The first two sections of this chapter describe the statistics available on poverty and wealth. There is a long tradition of defining a 'poverty line' as a level of resources below which people are excluded from society. Until the early 1980s, the supplementary benefit level represented such a 'poverty line'. People on supplementary benefit or with incomes below the supplementary benefit level were considered to be in poverty. Although the numbers of people on income support and take-up figures for income support are still published annually by the Department of Social Security, the government no longer recognises any official definition of poverty. Instead, the emphasis has shifted to income distributions, and the publication *Households below average income (HBAI)* contains information about inequalities in income. These statistics show an enormous increase in inequality since 1979.

Compared with income, less information is available about the distribution of wealth among the population, as it is difficult to collect data. How wealth should be defined is a controversial question. Definitions are based on a person's assets. As well as assets like houses or stocks and shares, these can also include the future value of state or occupational pensions. The government attempts to obtain information about an individual's wealth only once. This is at the time of death, when a tax return is completed to assess their eligibility for 'death duty'. The problem is that some people will avoid death duties by transferring their assets to relatives before death. In other cases, the estate will be exempt because it is below the tax threshold.

This means that estimates of wealth derived from these tax returns are based on the wealth of 40 per cent of the population but have been 'adjusted' to make estimates about the whole population. Data published annually in *Inland revenue statistics* estimate the distribution of wealth among rich people but give far less information about assets of the majority and no information at all about the distribution of wealth by age or income.

The final section of the chapter compares the five sources of statistical information about the labour market. Information about employment is derived from three sources: Workforce in Employment (WiE), a survey of employers, National Insurance contributions (NIC) and the Labour Force Survey (LFS), a household survey. The Labour Force Survey is a much better source of information about self-employment and part-time employment than the other two and contains information about employment among specific groups of people, such as minority ethnic groups or people with disabilities.

The two sources of data about unemployment, the count of claimants and the Labour Force Survey, tend to count unemployment among different sections of the population. The count of claimants covers unemployment among middle-aged men well, but the Labour Force Survey provides better information about unemployment among women, young men and older men. Information from any one of these sources on its own can be very misleading, but a more accurate picture of the labour market can be obtained by looking at the relationship between them. Taken together, these data give a considerable amount of information about the national picture, but the information available does not give a complete picture of local employment and unemployment.

Poverty statistics

There are no official poverty statistics published in the UK. The government recognises no official definition of poverty, and there is no agreement among academics and policy analysts about what constitutes poverty.

The reasons for this are not hard to find. There is genuine uncertainty about how poverty might be measured and about whether, indeed, it is possible to measure a single state called poverty. The seemingly never-ending debate about what is meant by poverty and whether it is an absolute or a relative concept is evidence enough of the difficulty of defining, let alone measuring, it. Government nervousness about identifying an official poverty line is unsurprising. Nevertheless, in 2000, the government set targets for child poverty.

Although the concept dates back to the end of the nineteenth century, there has never been agreement about what constitutes a 'poverty line'. It assumes that there is a specific level of resources below which people are excluded from society and disadvantaged in multiple ways, though defining that point is fraught with difficulties. There has also been the long-running disagreement over whether poverty is an absolute or relative concept. Are people who are poor just those without enough physical resources on which to subsist, or are they those who are badly off relative to others in society?

The official statistics that we now have are geared to the concept of relative poverty. The Department of Social Security's annual publication *Households below average income* is the nearest thing we have to a set of official poverty statistics, though in reality it provides more information about low income or inequality. There is other relevant information, in the Department of Social Security's annual publication *Social security statistics*, on the numbers of people on particular social security benefits and on take-up of benefits. This tabulates the numbers of people receiving income support by type, such as whether they are lone parents or pensioners, married or single, disabled or unemployed, and by the amount of money they receive. Both of these sets of figures can be used to tell us something about poverty.

The section which follows describes the *Households below average income* statistics and the information that can and cannot be derived from them. The way the methodology used in their construction affects their interpretation is also discussed.

Households below average income

Households below average income statistics have been produced annually by the Department of Social Security since 1987. The data are derived from a number of primary sources which are described later. Data derived retrospectively on a consistent basis have been published for years back to 1979. As the name suggests, the data relate to households with below average income. In particular, they include analyses of numbers of people in the population with incomes below the contemporary average, and below 40 per cent, 50 per cent, 60 per cent, 70 per cent and 80 per cent of the average. They also include analyses of family and employment status of these groups. Similar analyses are done of households with incomes at various proportions of the 1979 average. Income shares of the poorest 10, 20, 30, 40 and 50 per cent of the population are estimated. This includes analyses of family and employment status of these groups. Detailed analyses are made of the position of children. Receipt of means-tested benefits is analysed according to the household's position in the income distribution. Additional estimates are made showing income dynamics and the ownership of consumer durables.

Evidently this is a rich source of data. To some extent it could be argued that it is too rich. The 1997 edition ran to 260 pages and contained over 50 pages devoted exclusively to tables as well as 56 tables embedded in the text and appendices. Only someone with a great deal of dedication or with years of experience of the publication can find their way around it. Perhaps that is inevitable. There are so many ways of cutting the data and presenting the information that any reduction in the size could well be at the expense of useful analysis.

The data underlying these figures have traditionally come from the Family Expenditure Survey, an annual household level survey undertaken in Great Britain and Northern Ireland. It collects information on income and expenditure from about 7000 households. It was originally started to provide data for the retail price index, but has since been used widely for many other purposes. For further details of the survey, see Chapter 2. The income information is detailed and very suitable for the purpose of creating the *Households below average income* statistics. The Family Expenditure Survey has been undertaken annually since 1961. Analyses, consistent with *Households below average income*, have been carried out for the whole of that period by the Institute for Fiscal Studies.[1]

The Family Expenditure Survey has been superseded for some purposes by the new Family Resources Survey. This survey, first carried out in 1994, is designed by the Department of Social Security specifically to allow work on income distributions, as well as receipt and non-take-up of social security benefits. Its great advantage over the Family Expenditure Survey is its size. It gathers information on people in more than 25 000 households every year. This allows for greater accuracy and, potentially, finer divisions of the population. What it lacks is any information on spending. For income distribution statistics this is not a problem. This means that the Family Resources Survey is better than the Family Expenditure Survey for constructing the *Households below average income* series. The Family Expenditure Survey is still used to look at the distribution of spending and therefore gives useful additional information about living standards.

A BRIEF HISTORY AND INCOME DEFINITIONS

It is instructive to consider the origins of the *Households below average income* series and to compare it with what went before. The previous series of low-income statistics was known as *Low income families (LIF)*. This series had been produced since the start of the 1970s and through to the mid-1980s, though only on a biennial basis by then. It had grown up out of the 'rediscovery' of poverty in the 1960s and was specifically linked to levels of means-tested benefits. What it showed was the number of families in receipt of supplementary benefit (SB), now known as income support (IS), the numbers with incomes below the supplementary benefit level and the numbers with incomes within 10 per cent, 20 per cent and 40 per cent above the supplementary benefit level. The numbers on benefit and with incomes below the benefit level were frequently taken as showing the numbers of people in poverty, while those with incomes within 40 per cent of the line were often referred to as being on the margins of poverty.

These figures had the advantage of linking a measure of 'poverty' to an officially sanctioned minimum benefit level. The whole point of supplementary benefit was that it should provide a floor to living standards. The main reason for dissatisfaction with the figures was that this means of measuring poverty had the perverse effect that raising the level of benefits would appear to increase the numbers in poverty. The numbers were also becoming increasingly difficult to calculate properly, because of the increasing complexity of the supplementary benefit system. It is, of course, still possible to know how many people are in receipt of income support. We also have annually published estimates of the numbers of people who are entitled to receive it but do not do so. What we do not have are estimates of the total numbers of people with incomes below the income support line.

In moving from *Low income families* to *Households below average income*, a number of important methodological changes were made to the definition and calculation of income. The most important is that *Households below average income*, as its name suggests, is based on household incomes. It is assumed that incomes are shared equally within households and so the incomes of all members of a household are added together and assigned to each member of the household. The old *Low income families* data were effectively based on the nuclear family or *benefit unit*. The difference is that where, for example, there are several unrelated people living in one household, or parents living in a household with grown-up children, then these are now treated as single units over which income is shared. Previously, a couple with two grown-up children would have been treated as three separate units. The couple would have been one unit, as would each of their grown-up children.

The effect of this change was to reduce overall recorded inequality since the income is treated as being shared among more people.[2] Neither the household unit nor the benefit unit is unambiguously the right basic unit. The choice depends on how much sharing really takes place. It is at least reasonable to assume that where people live in the same household, they all enjoy access to the same quality of housing, heating and consumer durables, even if they do not explicitly share their income.

In any case, using any unit other than the individual means that some account has to be taken of unit size in calculating living standards. A couple with two children clearly needs more income than a single childless person to achieve the same standard of living. Incomes are therefore rescaled using *equivalence scales*. The particular scale used in *Households below average income* is known as the McClements' Scale, after its originator.[3] This scale gives a weight of 1 to a couple, 0.61 to a single person and a range of weights from 0.09 to 0.36 for children depending on their ages. To bring the income of a single person into equivalence with that of a couple, for example, the single person's income would be divided by 0.61. The income of a couple with an older child would be divided by 1.36, and so on.

The choice of equivalence scale is to some extent arbitrary. The McClements' Scale happened to be devised by an economist at the Department of Social Security in the 1970s. Its main feature is that it gives a low weight to children relative to many other scales.[4,5] Because of the form of the UK income distribution, the lower the weight given to children in an equivalence scale of this sort, the lower the recorded degree of inequality or poverty. On the other hand, using an equivalence scale of this sort leads to a relatively large recorded *growth* in inequality.

Finally, there is the question of whether housing costs should be included. Housing costs are largely made up of the interest component of a mortgage, rent and structural insurance payments. All the tables in *Households below average income* are repeated, once for income 'before housing costs' (BHC), and once for income 'after housing costs' (AHC). The 'before housing costs' measure is the simplest and most obvious. It is just total net income, including housing benefit. The 'after housing costs' measure is this less the housing costs. The reason for having this second measure is partly to take account of the fact that people often have housing costs that are fixed and bear little relation to housing quality. In particular, outright owners of property should be recorded as being better off than people with a mortgage. The 'before housing costs' measure probably understates the relative position of pensioners who own their property outright. The 'after housing costs' measure will understate the position of affluent younger people who have a large mortgage on a nice house.

The 'before housing costs' measure also suffers from a particular problem associated with the treatment of housing benefit. Housing benefit recipients will actually appear to become better off when their rent rises and their housing benefit rises as a consequence. Pensioners who rent their property and receive housing benefit often appear better off than outright owners. There is no simple answer to these dilemmas, but they should be borne in mind when interpreting the figures.

UNDERSTANDING THE FIGURES

The key to understanding the *Households below average income* statistics lies in realising that they are essentially measuring inequality. Like other measures of inequality, they show an enormous increase in inequality since 1979. When they are used to make statements about poverty, this is usually done by stating that the number of people with incomes below half the average is equivalent to the number of poor people. A disadvantage of using this as a measure of poverty is that it is very sensitive to changes in income levels among the richest people. An increase in the average caused by an increase in the incomes of the richest 10 per cent will result in an increase in the number of people recorded as having incomes below half the average. One consequence of this was that measured 'poverty' grew dramatically in the late 1980s, when unemployment was relatively low, but earnings growth at the top end was high.

Estimates based on the half-average income line also turn out to be very sensitive measures, because some of the considerable growth in numbers recorded in the 1980s reflected the fact that some benefit levels had slipped below 50 per cent of average income. As a result, many benefit recipients slipped from not being 'in poverty' to being 'in poverty' according to this measure. As an indicator of poverty, it is purely arbitrary. It can also result in very large numbers of people being recorded as in poverty. In 1991/2 and 1992/3, a quarter of the population had incomes below half average when the 'after housing costs' measure was used.

The *Households below average income* tables can also be used to compare estimates based on contemporary average incomes, with data showing the number of people with incomes below half of the 1979 average. Despite the very rapid growth in average incomes, it is notable that the proportion of the population with incomes below this fixed point has barely changed. It stood at 9 per cent of the population in both 1979 and in 1994/5, on the 'after housing costs' measure. Being constant in real terms, this line can be taken as some measure of absolute poverty.

It is well worth bearing in mind that measures of the numbers of people on income support in conjunction with data on non-take-up of income support are also published annually by the Department of Social Security in *Social security statistics*. These can be very useful, and more easily interpretable, representations of the numbers 'in poverty'. They are not subject to some of the odd features found in the *Households below average income* statistics.

Key official publications

Department of Social Security. *Households below average income: a statistical analysis*. London: TSO, published annually.
Department of Social Security. *Social security statistics*. London: TSO, published annually.

Wealth statistics

What do we mean when we talk about an individual's wealth? Typically, wealth is defined as a stock of assets, net of any debts, but which assets should be included? The choice of some assets such as a house or stocks and shares is fairly uncontroversial. Whether to include non-marketable assets such as the future value of a state pension is more problematic. It is even more difficult to decide whether to include the value of an individual's human capital, in other words, the future value of labour income generated by their skills, as well as their physical assets.

An individual's stock of wealth is different from the current flow of income, but income and wealth are closely related in a number of ways. The current stock of assets will have been accumulated out of past income or, if inherited, out of previous generations' income. Also, the current stock of assets will generate current income flows in the form of dividends or interest income, imputed rent in the case of housing, and earnings in the case of human capital.

Among the questions of interest about the distribution of wealth are:

- How equally or unequally is total wealth distributed in the UK and how has this distribution changed in recent years?
- How does the distribution of wealth compare with the distribution of income?
- What is the typical holding of wealth and how does this vary according to characteristics such as age, income and education?
- What proportion of the population owns particular assets such as a house or stocks and shares?

Official statistics on wealth can answer the first two questions, but tell us far less about the second two.

The main source of official information on personal wealth in the UK comes from the Inland Revenue and the returns people have to make for the purposes of taxing wealth. Unlike income, which is subject to tax every year, and must therefore be revealed to the authorities every year, the only point at which individuals have to reveal their entire wealth to the Inland Revenue is when they die. The returns made for death duties, known as inheritance tax since 1986, form the basis for official estimates of the distribution of wealth in the UK. There are several problems with this methodology, some of which are discussed below. Before doing so, some general issues must be raised about the definition and measurement of personal wealth.

Defining and measuring personal wealth

The official source of information on personal wealth is the annual publication *Inland revenue statistics*. In fact, the official statistics provided by the Inland Revenue offer three alternative measures. The first, narrowest, definition comprises the value of the stock of individuals' marketable assets less any amounts due for debts and mortgages. These assets include land and buildings, stocks and shares, trade assets and shares in partnerships, bank and building society deposits, cash and life assurance policies, and cars and other durable goods. This measure does not include the value of private or state pensions.

This definition measures the current cash value of an individual's stock of assets. In the case of assets with fairly volatile prices, such as stocks and shares, this value may change daily. Fluctuations in house prices will also have a big impact. It should be noted, however, that houses, as well as other durable goods, have a consumption as well as a saving element and may be valued at a constant value for the flow of services they provide as well as being a store of wealth.

There are two further official measures of personal wealth that extend the definition of wealth to include occupational and state pensions respectively. Since saving for retirement is an important economic motivation for wealth accumulation, including the value of pensions is important to gain a more complete picture of personal wealth. Pensions may not have a marketable value today, but they are likely to have an important effect on wealth accumulation in other marketable assets. Including pension wealth is also important because it is such a big part of personal wealth, and often the sole asset, for so many people.

Whether or not the value of private and state pensions is included in the measure of wealth has a considerable impact on the degree of measured inequality in the distribution of wealth. The effect of including the estimated value of occupational and state pensions is illustrated in Table 5.4. It reduces inequality in the distribution of wealth, as measured by the Gini coefficient, by 17 percentage points. Estimating the current value of future state and private pension entitlements is not easy and depends, for example, on estimates of future rates of return.

There may be further items which should be included in a measure of personal wealth. By an analogy with the argument for including pensions, there may be a case for including the value of other contingent state benefits such as unemployment benefit or child benefit. The future value of these benefits does not have any current cash value to the individual, but may reduce the current level of wealth accumulation in other marketable assets. It could even be argued that the value of government-provided services such as health and education should also be taken into account. Since the provision of these goods is universal, it may make little difference to the overall distribution of wealth. On the other hand, in making cross-country comparisons of the levels of saving and wealth, or comparisons over time, it is important to bear different levels of state provision in mind. Finally, it may be argued that the value of human capital, that is, the present value of future skills and education, should be also be included. In practice though, the problems in measuring the returns to human capital are likely to make this a very difficult task.

Limitations of the official wealth statistics

The narrowest definition of personal wealth given in the official statistics is the current value of all marketable assets, net of any debts and mortgages. This is estimated from the returns that have to be filed for the purpose of death duties. There are a number of problems with using this source of information to measure the wealth of the living population. The first is that the sample of those who die in any year is a relatively small and non-random sample. The second problem is that many, smaller, estates are exempt from paying death duties altogether and, therefore, no information is collected on them. Each of these problems is discussed in more detail below and an extended discussion is available elsewhere.[6]

Estimates of personal wealth are constructed using the mortality multiplier method. This means that the estates of people who die are grossed up to form an estimate of the wealth of the total population by multiplying each estate by a factor that is, effectively, the inverse of the mortality rate. Since death is non-random, conditional mortality rates that vary by age, gender and marital status are chosen. Different grossing factors are also used for people with estates above and below a certain threshold to reflect the fact that death rates are also correlated with wealth itself.

The main problem with this method is that the number of young people who die each year is relatively small and hence the grossing factors are correspondingly very large. This will tend to reduce the reliability of the estimates of personal wealth for these groups, since they will be based on a small number of estates that may not be representative of the population as a whole. For the same reason, very wealthy people, currently defined as those with estates worth more than £10 million, are excluded from the calculations, because otherwise their wealth would tend to dominate the total. Detailed information on the methodology used to estimate personal wealth is published in an article in the government publication *Economic trends*.[7] To illustrate the size of the grossing factors that are used, a table from that article is reproduced as Table 5.1.

A second problem with the mortality multiplier method is that not all estates are liable for death duty. Estates that are too small in total value, currently less than £215 000, are excluded, or are exempted because wealth is held in certain assets. The most important of these is housing that passes directly to the spouse of the deceased person. The problem is compounded by the fact that many individuals transfer their wealth before they die in order to reduce their tax liabilities. This practice is so widespread that death duties have been referred to as a 'voluntary tax'. Of course, such transfers reduce the size of the tax burden, not the amount of total wealth. This wealth will be picked up in the official estimates as the recipients of transfers themselves die.

Table 5.1 Mortality multipliers used in estimates of personal wealth, England and Wales only, 1985

Age (years)	Married men	Single men	Married women	Single women
18–24	2132	1229	5477	3112
25–34	1730	816	2914	1598
35–44	778	324	1040	510
45–54	236	130	356	228
55–64	70	47	125	115
65–74	27	23	55	43
75–84	11	11	21	16
85+	5	6	9	6

Source: Economic trends, No. 444, October 1990.

It means that estimates of total wealth may depend on a very small number of estates of people who die without making transfers, making the estimates of total wealth more unreliable.

The estates that exceed the minimum threshold in size and that require returns to be filed make up the 'identified population'. When grossed up, the 'identified population' comprises around 40 per cent of the total adult population, although this varies from year to year, not least because the threshold at which death duty becomes liable changes over time. The total wealth of the 'identified population' is known as 'identified wealth'. Adjustments are made to the estates of the 'identified population' to correct for under-recording and non-recording of small assets. These include national savings, cash, bank and building society accounts and consumer durables that can be transferred without a grant of representation, in other words without returns needing to be made. Adjustments are also made to correct for the valuation of life insurance policies. Table 5.2 shows the effect of these adjustments for official wealth statistics for 1996.

To estimate total personal wealth, a further adjustment is made to take account of the wealth of the rest of the population, known as the excluded population. Estimates of the total wealth of the excluded population are

Table 5.2 Estimates of total personal wealth, UK, 1996

	Net wealth (£ billion)
Total wealth of identified population	1398
Adjustment for:	
under-recording	+351
valuation	−181
adjusted wealth	1568
Excluded property:	536
Total marketable wealth	2103

Source: Inland revenue statistics, 1999.

obtained from a number of independent sources, including personal sector balance sheets and, indirectly, from financial institutions. Information from government surveys such as the Family Expenditure Survey and the General Household Survey is also used. The effects of these adjustments on the estimate of total personal wealth are also shown in Table 5.2.

The distribution of excluded wealth between adults is determined according to known information about its distribution among the 'identified population'. This reflects a general problem with the official estimates of wealth. They are much better at estimating the wealth of the top of the distribution than the bottom. This is a problem largely caused by estimating the total wealth of the adult population using tax returns for a tax which the overwhelming majority of the population, people still alive, does not have to pay at all, and from which a majority of estates that are potentially eligible are exempt.

Table 5.3 uses the official estimates to show the distribution of wealth across the population. It shows that the distribution is very concentrated, with the top 1 per cent of the population owning nearly one-fifth of all wealth, and that this distribution changed very little between 1980 and 1996. In contrast, the distribution of income became more concentrated over the same period. An article in the *Oxford Review of Economic Policy* used official statistics for a detailed discussion of the main trends in the distribution of wealth since before the Second World War.[8] The author concluded that there has been a fairly dramatic equalisation of wealth over this period. This conclusion is based on an analysis of changes at the top of the wealth distribution, and in the proportion of total wealth held by the top 5 per cent in particular. The main problem is that the official statistics tell us something about the way the majority of wealth is distributed, but almost nothing about the distribution of wealth among the majority of the population.

A further limitation with the published official statistics is that they contain no information on how the distribution of wealth varies according to characteristics

Table 5.3 Distribution of marketable wealth among the adult population in the UK

	Percentage of total wealth held	
	1980	**1996**
Most wealthy 1 per cent	19	19
Most wealthy 5 per cent	36	39
Most wealthy 10 per cent	50	52
Most wealthy 25 per cent	73	74
Most wealthy 50 per cent	91	93
Gini coefficient	65	67

Source: Inland revenue statistics, 1999.
The Gini coefficient measures the degree of inequality in the distribution of income or wealth among the population, on a scale from 0 to 100. A Gini of 0 represents perfect equality, with 20 per cent of the population owning 20 per cent of the wealth, 50 per cent owning 50 per cent, and so on. A Gini of 100 represents perfect inequality, with one person owning all of the wealth.

such as age or income. They also contain no information on the levels of owner-ship of or the distribution of particular assets such as housing or stocks and shares. For answers to these questions, there is some information from other gov-ernment household surveys. For example, the Family Expenditure Survey con-tains reliable information on interest and dividend income that can be used to impute ownership of different financial assets over a reasonably long time period. A descriptive analysis of this information was published by the Institute for Fiscal Studies.[9] Also, Wave 5 of the British Household Panel Survey, collected in 1995, contains information about financial assets. One of the most detailed sources of information on financial wealth is data collected privately by National Opinion Polls. A detailed analysis of one wave of the National Opinion Polls Financial Resources Survey can be found in a publication by the Institute for Fiscal Studies.[10]

A further problem with the official statistics on the distribution of wealth is that the distribution is measured across the adult population. In fact, the household may be a more appropriate unit for analysing the distribution of wealth if the whole household benefits from assets held by individual mem-bers. Looking at the distribution of wealth between individual adults rather than between households may overstate the degree of inequality by increas-ing the number of units with zero or very little wealth.

The degree of inequality in the distribution of wealth is also overstated if the value of state and private pensions is excluded. As has already been argued, the value of pensions should be included since they are substitutes for other forms of wealth. They are also, for many people, their only, or at least their most important, asset. The official statistics have two further estimates of personal wealth that add up to total marketable wealth. These are Series D, the value of occupational pension rights, and Series E, the value of occupa-tional plus state pension rights.

The effect of including pension rights is to reduce the degree of inequality measured by the Gini coefficient by around 17 percentage points, as Table 5.4 shows. The estimate of the value of occupational pension rights combines infor-

Table 5.4 Distribution of marketable wealth and pension wealth among the adult poulation in the UK, 1994

	Percentage of total wealth held		
	Marketable wealth only	Including occupational pensions	Including state pensions
Most wealthy 1 per cent	19	14	11
Most wealthy 5 per cent	39	31	25
Most wealthy 10 per cent	52	43	36
Most wealthy 25 per cent	74	66	58
Most wealthy 50 per cent	93	89	83
Gini coefficient	67	59	49

Source: Inland revenue statistics, 1998.
For an explanation of the Gini coefiicient, see Table 5.3.

mation on pension rights in self-administered funds and group pension business in insurance companies. Until recently, the methodology for estimating pension rights assumed long-term membership of final salary pension schemes. Given the growing importance of personal pension schemes, particularly among younger workers, this assumption has become less valid. Estimates of the value of money purchase schemes, which are typical personal pension schemes, are very sensitive to differences in estimates of future rates of return.

To summarise, the official wealth statistics provide information on the broad distribution of wealth across the population. They show very well the concentration of the majority of wealth at the top of the distribution, but provide far less information on the wealth holdings of the majority of the population. This stems largely from the less than ideal way in which the official wealth statistics are compiled from information contained in the returns filed for the purposes of inheritance tax. To address policy issues such as the current concern about the level of individual saving, more detailed information is needed on the wealth of people in the bottom half, or even lower, in the wealth distribution. Information is also needed on the distribution of wealth according to key characteristics such as age and income.

Key official publication

Inland Revenue. *Inland revenue statistics*. London: TSO, published annually.

Employment and unemployment

Original and published sources

Whether men and women work, and what sort of work they do, can have a direct influence on their health. Earnings from work can influence health, and this extends beyond the period of working life. Employment, for most of the population, provides the capital necessary for house purchase and for investment in pension funds. These should provide for the years of retirement, which can be longer than the years spent in employment. If people are unemployed, that too can influence their health, and that of their family, often beyond the loss of earnings.

The mass media often give the impression that public interest in labour market statistics reflects their importance as indicators of the current condition of the labour market. This section takes a longer-term view, focusing on trends in employment and unemployment since the late 1970s. What is known about the trends in the labour market, and what is not known, help to reveal the strengths and limitations of the currently available statistics.

The Office for National Statistics (ONS), under the Labour government elected in 1997, promised substantial expansion in the availability of labour market statistics,[11] but there is no commitment by the Office for National

Statistics to developments in the original data sources from which the statistics are produced. Some emphasis has therefore been given in this section to the distinction between the published statistics and the surveys and administrative data that constitute their original sources. The distinction between the published statistics and the original sources is of particular importance at a local level, where there is considerable scope for development, leading to fuller publication. In the case of unemployment, there is also scope for correcting misleading forms of publication.

The next section examines the original sources of employment and unemployment statistics as measured by the count of claimants and by the Labour Force Survey. This is followed by a summary account of published statistics and the use of information technology to make data available in other ways. The final section discusses problems in getting statistics of employment and unemployment at a local level.

Data sources and how they measure the growth of part-time employment

The UK has three series of data relating to the level of employment. The ONS uses surveys of employers to produce the Workforce in Employment series, and the European Union Labour Force Survey, a survey of households (described in Chapter 2), to produce the Labour Force Survey series. The Department of Social Security counts the number of people who paid National Insurance contributions (NIC) at any time during the financial year. Figure 5.1 indicates the ups and downs in the labour market over the period 1978 to 1997, but also shows that each of these series gives a different picture of changes over time.

The Workforce in Employment and Labour Force Survey series move fairly closely together, although there are differences in conception and coverage. The Workforce in Employment series measures jobs, but the Labour Force Survey series estimates numbers of people. The Workforce in Employment series is based on surveys of employers. It excludes most self-employed people, many home workers, domestic servants, and people in part-time and low-paid jobs, but counts some people twice because they have two jobs. The Labour Force Survey series follows the International Labour Office definition and counts everyone who does more than one hour's paid work a week as in employment and thus has a wider coverage than Workforce in Employment surveys. The differences between the trends shown by the two series are difficult to explain,[12] but reconciliation of the totals for the 1990s have been described in detail by the ONS.[13-17]

The big difference, shown in Fig. 5.1, is between the estimates based on the count of National Insurance contributors and the Labour Force Survey series. The numbers in employment according to the National Insurance contribution series fell by a million between 1979/80 and 1994/5. The Labour Force Survey series shows an increase of more than a million between the spring of 1979 and the spring of 1995. The ONS has not published any attempt to reconcile this difference. The National Insurance contribution series (shown in

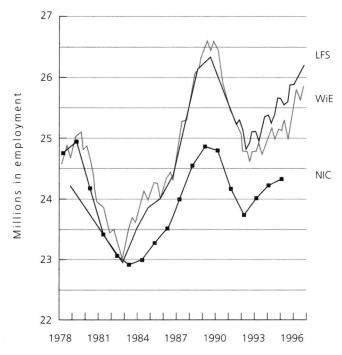

Fig. 5.1 Employment in Britain, 1978–97. The ONS produces WiE series from postal surveys of employees that ask about the numbers employed on a particular day in each quarter. The WiE series counts jobs rather than people, so counts people with two jobs twice, but misses about a million jobs which are not covered by the PAYE sampling frame used. The Labour Force Survey Employment series is based on surveys of households carried out over a quarterly period. It covers all people working more than 1 hour a week, but nearly a million in 1997 had two or more jobs. The National Insurance Contributors series covers employees and self-employed contributing at any time during the financial year ending in April, is published only about 18 months after the end of the financial year, and is subject to retrospective revision. The National Insurance Contributors figures in this chart are based upon the most recently published figure for each year, and are centred on the previous September. (Sources: Historical supplement No. 5 – *Workforce data back series*, ONS disk; *Labour Force Survey Historical supplement 1997*, ONS, 1997. Social Security Statistics.)

Fig. 5.1) comes from returns made retrospectively by employers to the Department of Social Security. Neither the Workforce in Employment nor the Labour Force Survey collects information on National Insurance contributions, so that it is impossible to be precise about the discrepancy of about two million. The difference can be attributed largely to the growth of employment that falls below the National Insurance exemption limit, which was £64 per week in 1997.

Both the Labour Force Survey and the Workforce in Employment distinguish between full and part-time work. The Workforce in Employment questionnaires invite employers to classify jobs with less than 30 hours a week as part-time. Data from this source tell us that the numbers of part-time jobs increased by about three million over the period 1971 to 1997, and the increase in part-time workers was mostly among women. Figure 5.2 illustrates this

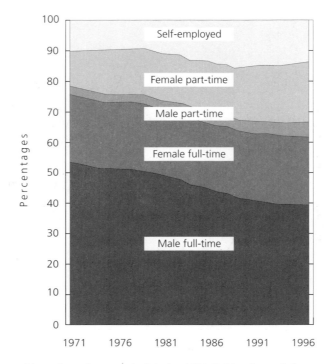

Fig. 5.2 Composition of employment in Britain, 1971–7. Members of the armed forces and of government training schemes have been included in the self-employment category. (Source: Historical supplement No. 5 – *Workforce data back series*, ONS disc.)

trend by showing the changing pattern in the composition of employment. Over the period 1971 to 1997, the proportion of full-time jobs among men fell from 53 per cent to 38 per cent. The proportion of full-time jobs for women did not change. There were small increases in the proportion of part-time jobs taken by men. The other major change was that part-time jobs done by women increased as a proportion of total employment from 12 to 20 per cent.

According to the Labour Force Survey estimates, there were 5.4 million part-time women employees in 1993. This is close to the estimate of 5.2 millions in the Workforce in Employment series in the same year. Differences in coverage and definition make the extent to which these estimates cover the same population unclear. According to the Labour Force Survey, nearly all of the part-time jobs were for less than 30 hours per week, with about two-thirds being for less than 20 hours.[18] The number of part-time jobs has increased substantially in recent decades in most other advanced industrial countries, not just in the UK. The use of the International Labour Organisation one-hour rule means that the aggregate statistics for employment may not give an accurate picture of employment growth, and may be misleading in concealing the extent of unemployment and under-employment.

The number of National Insurance contributors can be estimated from the Labour Force Survey on the basis of earnings data. In 1997, 2.5 million people in employment did not earn enough to pay National Insurance contributions and four-fifths of these were women.[19]

The differences between what is available from the Workforce in Employment and Labour Force Survey on women's part-time work typify other differences. The Workforce in Employment censuses and surveys are the prime source of data about employment by industry and by location, and about labour turnover, in spite of the limitations in coverage. The detailed character of the Labour Force Survey questionnaire, with 386 questions in 1996, makes it the prime source of a wide variety of data about the personal characteristics of the employed and unemployed populations. These include occupation, ethnic group[20] and disability.[21] The Labour Force Survey is also the main source of statistics on self-employment, on the numbers of people who have more than one job, and on people such as home workers who are not covered in the Workforce in Employment series.

'On the dole' and 'on the sick'

The UK has two series of data about unemployment. The Labour Force Survey unemployment series, following International Labour Organisation criteria, estimates the numbers of people seeking work. The monthly count of claimants, based on administrative data about claims for benefits, gives the numbers of people who successfully claim Unemployment Benefit or Job Seekers Allowance.

For a wide variety of purposes, the count of claimants is a more useful statistic. The series has been in its present form since 1983, and has antecedents going back to the nineteenth century.[22,23] The administratively based count has 100 per cent coverage, and data are available for areas as small as individual postcode areas. The count is also up to date, being published 5 weeks after the day to which it relates. It is also definite and unambiguous. The introduction of the Job Seekers Allowance in October 1996 symbolises the tightening up of the rules for entitlement. Since the 1980s, it has become increasingly difficult for anyone to be counted unless they are fairly desperately seeking work and are able to cope with the negotiation processes involved in making a successful claim. On the other hand, people entitled to receive Unemployment Benefit, Job Seekers Allowance or National Insurance contribution credits have a financial incentive to claim, simply because those who do not claim do not get benefit.

Figure 5.3 compares trends in the count of claimants with those of the Workforce in Employment series for the period 1971 to 1997. Despite many changes in the regulations affecting entitlement to unemployment pay, the count of claimants consistently mirrors trends in employment.

The sensitivity of the count to year-to-year changes in the level of employment does not make it a good measure of unemployment over a longer period. Figure 5.3 shows the long-term growth of unemployment up to the early 1980s. Since the early 1980s, some thirty changes in the regulations affecting entitlement to unemployment benefit have reduced the numbers of

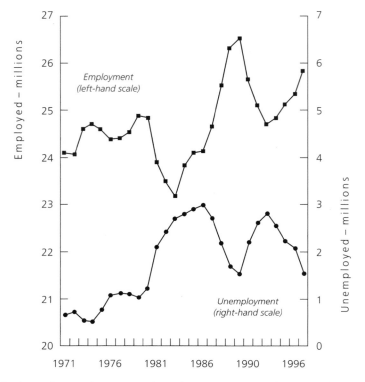

Fig. 5.3 Registered unemployment and employment, 1971–97. (Sources: Historical supplement No. 5 – *Workforce data back series*, ONS disc.)

people claiming[24] and led to charges that the statistics were being 'fiddled'. The experience of trying unsuccessfully to defend this appears to have soured the ONS against the claimant series,[25] but changes in the formal regulations governing entitlement to unemployment benefit have not been the main factor in reducing the numbers of claimants counted.

Since the early 1980s, and perhaps up to 1998, Employment Offices have been encouraged to transfer claimants to Incapacity Benefit in order to reduce the count of claimants. In some parts of the country, like Merthyr Tydfil, Liverpool and Tyneside, more than 20 per cent of men of working age are classified as incapacitated. It was estimated that in January 1997 the national 'excess' of permanently sick people was 1.3 million.[26]

Table 5.5 shows that the number of people of working age receiving sickness-related benefit for a period of 6 months or more increased by 1.3 millions over the period 1971 to 1997, reaching nearly 2 million in 1997. This was substantially greater than the numbers receiving Unemployment Benefit at that time. Rather less than half of the growth occurred in the over-50 age group. The greatest proportionate increase has been in the younger age groups. The number of people in their thirties receiving long-term sickness benefits increased more than fivefold over the period. By 1997, it had reached just under 230 000. The persistence of high levels of employment at a national

Table 5.5 Claimants of sickness, invalidity and incapacity benefit for more than 6 months in Great Britain, 1981 and 1997

Age (years)	Number of claimants (thousands)			1997 as a percentage of 1981
	1981	1997	Increase 1981–97	
Under 30	33	158	125	479
30–39	55	284	229	516
40–49	95	412	317	434
50–59	214	697	483	326
60–64, men only	176	331	155	188
All of working age	573	1882	1309	328

Source: Department of Social Security. *Social security statistics.*

level has sent out a message that labour is not needed. In the coalfields and centres of heavy industry, where the job losses have been greatest, this message has encouraged acceptance of incapacity.[26,27]

The statisticians who worked in the former Department of Employment do not seem to have been aware of the magnitude of the flow from the count of claimants. Although the Department co-operated with the Royal Statistical Society's study of unemployment statistics in 1995, the resulting report shows no evidence of this movement to sickness benefits,[28] nor did the report published by the House of Commons Select Committee on Employment in the following year.[29]

An ONS study, based on record linkage, showed large flows of people in both directions between the count of claimants and Incapacity Benefit over the period March 1995 to August 1997.[30] The average annual flow from Incapacity Benefit to the count of claimants was 15 000 a month, compared to a flow of 21 000 a month in the other direction. There is promise that integration of records held by the Department of Social Security would routinely provide such statistics.[31]

Unemployment according to the Labour Force Survey and the International Labour Organisation

The major strength of the Labour Force Survey is that it aims to cover the whole population of working age. It uses criteria established by the International Labour Organisation to divide the population into three conceptual categories: employment, unemployment, and economic inactivity. As was mentioned earlier, the International Labour Organisation defines employment as paid work of more than 1 hour a week. Unemployment is defined as having taken steps to seek employment within the previous 4 weeks, and by being available to start a job within 2 weeks.

The Labour Force Survey does not directly ask respondents if they are unemployed, but does ask if they are claimants. The inclusion of this question makes it possible to compare directly the International Labour Organisation/Labour Force Survey measure of unemployment with the count of claimants. Figure 5.4 shows that the proportion of unemployed people classified as 'inactive claimants', who are included in the count but not in the Labour Force Survey unemployment series, fell substantially over the period 1984 to 1997. The numbers counted in both series, 'Labour Force Survey claimants', accounting for less than half of the total covered by either series, also fell. By contrast, the proportion of 'Labour Force Survey non-claimants' included in the Labour Force Survey series but not in the count has generally increased. The proportion of 'employed claimants', included in the count but classified as in employment by the International Labour Organisation 1-hour rule, was fairly constant.[32]

In the mid-1980s, the grossed up estimates of the number of claimants derived from the Labour Force Survey were higher than those given by the count of claimants itself. In the 1990s, the Labour Force Survey estimates were consistently about 20 per cent below the count. Attempts to explain these discrepancies are not wholly convincing.[33] The ONS calls the statistics shown in

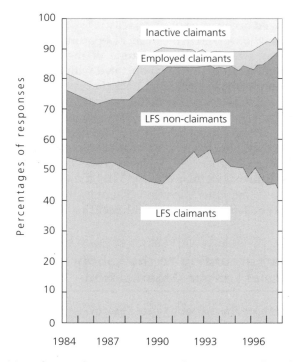

Fig. 5.4 Composition of unemployment, 1984–97. The statistics are based on responses to the Labour Force Survey. It is known that these statistics are subject to error because they do not correspond to the Count of Claimants itself. For the period 1984 to 1988, the Labour Force Survey overestimated the Count of Claimants. Then, with a change in the Labour Force Survey questionnaire in 1989, the Labour Force Survey underestimated the Count of Claimants. By 1997, the shortfall had increased to 20 per cent. Figure 5.3 gives 'unscaled' estimates based upon the number of responses given in the Labour Force Survey without any attempt at adjustment for consistency with Count of Claimants. The figures for Labour Force Survey non-claimants were obtained by deduction from the total number of Labour Force Survey unemployed. (Source: *Labour Market Trends*.[15])

Fig. 5.4 'unscaled', because they are based directly upon responses given to the Labour Force Survey and are not adjusted to correspond with the count. The unscaled statistics treat the responses to the Labour Force Survey questionnaire as valid, but are not consistent with the count of claimants itself.

The ONS is attempting to model the relationship between the statistics from the Labour Force Survey and the count of claimants,[34] but it is doubtful whether this is appropriate. The straightforward solution would be to use claimant records as a sampling frame for part of the Labour Force Survey, enabling comparable statistics to be produced for claimants and non-claimants.[32,35]

The count of claimants and the Labour Force Survey unemployment series cover rather different populations, as Fig. 5.4 shows. The count covers unemployment among the middle-aged male population fairly well, but the Labour Force Survey has better coverage of women, young men and older men who do not easily achieve claimant status.[29] The populations covered also differ in their behaviour. Charts published by the ONS indicate that the two series run more broadly in parallel, but the Labour Force Survey series is less responsive to changes in the level of employment than the count. The relative insensitivity of the Labour Force Survey series is attributable to the constant size of the 'Labour Force Survey non-claimants' group. This contains people counted as unemployed according to the International Labour Organisation criteria but who are not claimants and are therefore excluded from the count.

These differences are likely to be of growing importance. The tightening of the regulations affecting entitlement to Job Seekers Allowance reduces the proportion of 'Labour Force Survey claimants'. A continuation of this trend would increase the proportion of people who are neither claiming benefit nor in employment and who can be considered as hidden unemployment.[36] It is argued that the 'Labour Force Survey non-claimants' group constitutes the top layer of a reserve army of labour, and that its constant size through the trade cycle conceals substantial changes in its composition.[35]

The main publications

The ONS's free introductory booklets *How exactly is unemployment measured?*[37] and *How exactly is employment measured?*[17] are good starting points, but both are limited to a discussion of the statistics at a national level. They give the greatest emphasis to the series derived from the Labour Force Survey, on the grounds that it is produced in accordance with International Labour Organisation definitions.

The monthly *Labour market trends,* formerly the *Employment gazette,* covers most of the published series, and includes many articles giving commentary or more detailed information on the regularly published series. It is the most likely source of information about future developments in these statistics.

Data about unemployment benefits are also published in the annual *Social security statistics.* This includes the eligibility criteria, benefit rates, and data about numbers of claimants by age, dependency and region. For interpretation of the trends in the claimant statistics it is useful to examine the *Annual report and accounts* of the Employment Service, its *Operational plan*, and its *Annual performance agreement*. These publications contain information on performance targets related to the count of claimants.

Apart from the series published in *Labour market trends*, the main publication containing statistics from the Labour Force Survey is the *Labour Force Survey, quarterly supplement*, formerly called the *Quarterly bulletin*. The first *Labour Force Survey, historical supplement*, published in 1997, covers Britain and includes some statistics going back to 1979. The ONS published a further historical supplement in 1999, covering the whole of the UK. Eurostat's annual *Labour Force Survey, results* includes comparative statistics for the UK going back to the 1980s.

The main publications containing Workforce in Employment statistics are in the *Annual employment survey* series. These have been published from 1995 onwards and include subnational statistics. Earlier volumes, entitled *Census of employment*, were published in 1991 and 1993. Historical data at a national level were formerly published as *Historical supplements* and distributed with *Labour market trends*. The version which was used to construct Figs. 5.1 and 5.2 was published on disc as *Historical supplement No. 5, Workforce data back series*.

The decennial census of population is the major source of employment and unemployment statistics at a local level. One of the most useful volumes from the 1991 census was *Key statistics for local authorities*, published by the Office of Population Censuses and Surveys (OPCS) and the General Register Office, Scotland (GRO), Scotland. It included tables on activity rates, occupation and means of transport for the journey to work. The census included questions on the location of people's workplaces and these were used to derive statistics on journeys to work. These journey to work statistics are used to define 'Travel to work areas' and provide background data which influence many other labour market statistics.

Other published and available information

The available data are much more extensive than is indicated by this summary. For example, since April 1998, the *First release* series has been published monthly for each of the standard regions. These press releases, each with about forty pages, are themselves statistical publications, and contain core data which are later published in *Labour market trends* and the *Quarterly supplement* of the Labour Force Survey. These press releases give the greatest emphasis to statistics from the Labour Force Survey.

Statistics are also made available through three organisations that store databases of labour market statistics. These are the Data Archive at Essex University, SPSS MR in London, and Nomis at the University of Durham.

The Data Archive gives access to the Labour Force Survey microdata and the six volumes of the *User guide*. The archive also provide access to two Joint Unemployment and Vacancies Operating System (JUVOS) databases. These are derived from count of claimants records, which include details of claimants' occupations and basic socio-demographic information. The main Joint Unemployment and Vacancies Operating System database is a full count of all claimants. The Joint Unemployment and Vacancies Operating System cohort longitudinal database is a 5 per cent sample of all claims selected by National Insurance number. The use of the insurance number makes it possible to do analyses related to individuals' experience of unemployment, including the length, number and location of unemployment spells. It is thus a source of data about the characteristics and frequency of spells of unemployment and rates of long-term unemployment.[38]

SPSS MR, formerly Quantime Ltd, is a commercial organisation that provides a range of data and services, including Labour Force Survey data, going back to 1979. It also has databases for individual surveys, time series databases, and databases giving basic data by local authority. Users can specify and buy tables to meet their requirements, or access the data online, or they can purchase Quanvert software and access CD-ROMs on a personal computer.

The National Online Manpower Information System (NOMIS) is a service provided by the University of Durham under contract with the Office for National Statistics. Nowadays, the National Online Manpower Information Service provides a wide range of statistics from sources which include the Census of Population, the New Earnings Survey, job vacancies as well as statistics of employment and unemployment. Nomis supplies Joint Unemployment and Vacancies Operating System data and Workforce in Employment statistics for local areas, including historical series.

Problems with data at a local level

Relatively little attention is given to data on employment and unemployment at a local scale. They are not mentioned in the *Guide to official statistics*, for example. Statistics on employment from the Annual Employment Survey, including a breakdown by local authority, have been published, but Workforce in Employment statistics for local authority areas are not included in *Labour Market Trends*, or in any other serial publication.

The major advantage of the Labour Force Survey, for producing compatible statistics for employment, unemployment and economic inactivity, is largely lost at the local scale. This is because it is a sample survey and there is wide sampling variability in the less populous areas. The ONS believes that reliable estimates of the size of economically active populations can be produced for most local authority areas,[24] but depend upon population data from other administrative sources. Labour Force Survey estimates of employment for local authority areas are less reliable. The ONS says that reliable quarterly estimates of employment can be derived from the Labour Force Survey for only about 40 of the 400 or so local authorities, and reliable annual estimates for only about 110 local authorities. Reliable estimates of unemployment and the size of the economically inactive population can be made for even fewer local authority areas.

By contrast, statistics for the count of claimants have been available down to the level of postcode areas since the count was computerised in 1982. *Labour Market Trends* publishes these statistics for 'Travel to work' areas, counties, local authority areas, and parliamentary constituencies.

The value of these local statistics is severely limited by the lack of a suitable denominator to facilitate comparison of unemployment rates in different areas. The traditional solution was to use statistics for the numbers in employment in an area as the main item in the denominator. This was a reasonable solution in an era of full employment, but has become irrelevant and misleading in an era in which unemployment is not just fractional, in other words comprising of just short-term unemployment between jobs, and where the 'daytime' and 'nightime' populations have become increasingly differentiated. Where there is an inflow of commuters into the area, the unemployment rate is understated, and where there is a net commuting flow from an area, the unemployment rate is exaggerated.

The official response to this problem has been to produce census statistics for 'Travel to work' areas, defined in terms of patterns of commuting. This facilitates broad-brush comparisons that are used for European Social Fund allocations, but systematically conceals the growth of concentrations of unemployment in inner city areas.[39–41]

Reforms instituted by the ONS since the Labour government was elected in 1997 have, ironically, made this problem worse. The same workforce ratios, as they should be called, are now published for local authority areas. This is systematically misleading, because most urban authorities are net daily importers of workers, and most rural authorities are net daily exporters of labour. The workforce-based ratios therefore generally understate unemployment rates for urban areas and overstate unemployment ratios in suburban and rural districts.[42] Estimates of true local unemployment rates for local authorities, taking into account commuting patterns, have been posted to the mailbase unemployment-research home page, whose address is given at the end of the chapter.

For many purposes, the most useful data on local unemployment are those of parliamentary constituencies, and perhaps those for wards. The populations of constituencies, averaging 69 000 in 1996, do not vary as much as those for local authority areas. Direct comparisons can therefore be made between constituencies, without the need to use a denominator. Figure 5.5 shows that twenty-two constituencies shown in Inner London each had more than 5000 claimants. There were only ten constituencies with more than 5000 claimants in other parts of England, but analysis in terms of population units smaller than constituencies is necessary to delineate concentrations of unemployment with a comparable degree of accuracy in other smaller cities. A study of the English coalfield communities demonstrates the value of detailed examination of unemployment at a local scale.[43]

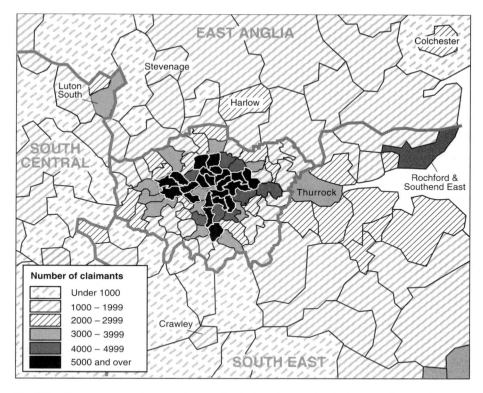

Fig. 5.5   Unemployment by constituency in the London region in June 1997.
(Source: *Labour market trends*. Map produced by John Hunt, Open University.)

Key official publications

Office for National Statistics. *Labour market trends*. London: TSO, published
  monthly.
Office for National Statistics. *Labour Force Survey quarterly supplement*. London:
  TSO, published quarterly.
Office for National Statistics. *Annual employment survey*. London: Office for
  National Statistics, published annually.
Department of Social Security. *Social security statistics*. London: TSO, published
  annually.

Contact addresses and web sites

Contact addresses and web sites

Labour Market Statistics
Office for National Statistics
1 Drummond Gate
London SW1V 2QQ
Telephone:
Labour market statistics helpline
020 7533 6094
Web site: http://www.statistics.gov.uk/

Statistics Research Branch
Department of Economic Development
Netherleigh
Massey Avenue
Belfast BT4 6JP
Telephone: 028 9052 9900
Web site: http://www.nisra.gov.uk/dept/ded.htm

Nomis online statistics database
Telephone: 0191 374 2468

Department of Social Security
Analytical Services Division
The Adelphi
1-11 John Adam Street
London WC2N 6HT
Telephone 020 7962 8000
Web site: http://www.dss.gov.uk/asd/

Statistics and Economics Division
Inland Revenue
West Wing
Somerset House
Strand
London WC2R 1LB
Telephone: 020 7438 6267
Web site:
http://www.inlandrevenue.gov.uk/

References

1. Goodman A, Johnson P, Webb S. *Inequality in the UK*. Oxford: Oxford University Press, 1997.
2. Johnson P, Webb S. Counting people with low incomes: the impact of recent changes in official statistics. *Fiscal Studies* 1989; **10**(4): 66–82.
3. McClements L. Equivalence scales for children. *Journal of Public Economics* 1977; **8**: 191–210.
4. Coulter F, Cowell F, Jenkins S. Equivalence scale relativities and the extent of inequality and poverty. *Economic Journal* 1992; **102**: 1067–82.
5. Banks J, Johnson P. Equivalence scale relativities revisited. *Economic Journal* 1994; **104**: 883–90.
6. Atkinson A, Harrison A. *Distribution of personal wealth in Britain*. Cambridge: Cambridge University Press, 1978.
7. Good F. Estimates of the distribution of personal wealth. *Economic Trends*. London: HMSO, November 1990.
8. Feinstein C. The equalising of wealth in Britain since the Second World War. *Oxford Review of Economic Policy* 1996; **12**(1): 96–105.
9. Banks J, Tanner S. *Household saving in the UK*. London: Institute for Fiscal Studies, 1999.
10. Banks J, Dilnot A, Low H. *The distribution of wealth in the UK*. Commentary No. 45. London: Institute for Fiscal Studies, 1995.
11. Labour Market Division. Improved Office for National Statistics Labour Market Statistics. *Labour Market Trends* 1998; **106**: 55–8.

12. Thomas R. The Labour Force Survey in the dock. *Radical Statistics* 1997; **65**: 4–16.
13. Spence A, Watson M. Estimating employment: a comparison of household and employer-based surveys. *Employment Gazette* 1993; **101**: 465–70.
14. Perry K. Measuring employment: comparison of official sources, *Labour Market Trends* 1996; **104**: 19–27.
15. Pease P. Comparisons of sources of employment data. *Labour Market Trends* 1997; **105**: 511–16.
16. Pease P. The Labour Force Survey in the Dock. *Radical Statistics* 1998; **67**: 62–4.
17. Office for National Statistics. *How exactly is employment measured?* London: Office for National Statistics, 1998.
18. Naylor K. Part-time working in Great Britain – an historical analysis. *Employment Gazette* 1994; **104**: 473–84.
19. MacLennan E. *Low paid and excluded – the effect of the National Insurance threshold on the rights and benefits of low paid workers.* London: Trade Union Congress, 1998.
20. Sly F. Ethnic groups and the labour market: analyses from the Spring 1994 Labour Force Survey. *Employment Gazette* 1995; **103**: 251–62.
21. Sly F, Duxbury R. Disability and the labour market: findings from the Labour Force Survey. *Labour Market Trends* 1995: **103**: 439–59.
22. Denman J, McDonald P. Unemployment statistics from 1881 to the present day. *Labour Market Trends* 1996; **104**: 5–18.
23. Southall H. Working with historical statistics on poverty and economic distress. In: Dorling D, Simpson S, eds. *Statistics in society.* London: Arnold, 1999, pp. 350–8.
24. Fenwick D, Denman J. The monthly employment count: change and consistency. *Labour Market Trends* 1995; **103**: 397–400.
25. Thomas R. Integrity of statistics or integrity of statisticians: a critique of the Green Paper Statistics – a matter of trust. *Radical Statistics* 1998; **68**: 60–71.
26. Beatty C, Fothergill S, Gore T, Herrington A. *The real level of unemployment.* Sheffield: Centre for Regional Economic and Social Research, Sheffield Hallam University, 1997.
27. Davies R. Unemployment and permanent sickness in Mid-Glamorgan. In: Dorling D, Simpson S, eds. *Statistics in society.* London: Arnold, 1998, pp. 335–9.
28. Working Party on the Measurement of Unemployment in the UK The measurement of unemployment in the UK (with discussion). *Journal of the Royal Statistical Society Series A* 1995; **158(3)**: 363–418.
29. Office for National Statistics. Employment and unemployment statistics: response to the Employment Select Committee's Report. *Labour Market Trends* 1996; **104**: 463–66.
30. Edgeley J, Sweeney K. Characteristics of JSA claimants who have joined the claimant count from Incapacity Benefit. *Labour Market Trends* 1998; **106**: 79–83.
31. Stanton D. Developments in social security statistics. In: *Official statistics beyond the year 2000.* Esher, Surrey: Statistics Users Council, IMAC Research, 1997: 54–5.
32. Thomas R. International Labour Organisation unemployment and registered unemployment – a case study. *Bulletin Methodologique de Sociologie* 1998; **59**: 5–26.
33. Pease P. Labour Force Survey estimates of unemployment-related benefits: the results of an Office for National Statistics record linkage study. *Labour Market Trends* 1997; **105**: 455–60.
34. Haworth M, Bowman L. Improved labour market statistics. *British Urban and Regional Information Systems Association*, 1998; **134**: 1–4.
35. Thomas R. The politics and reform of unemployment and employment statistics. In: Dorling D, Simpson S, eds. *Statistics in Society.* London: Arnold, 1999, pp. 324–34.

36. Green A. Problems in measuring participation in the labour market. In: Dorling D, Simpson S, eds. *Statistics in society*. London: Arnold, 1998, 312–23.
37. Office for National Statistics. *How exactly is unemployment measured?*, 3rd edition. London: Office for National Statistics, 1998.
38. Ward H, Bird D. The JUVOS cohort: a longitudinal database of the claimant unemployed. *Employment Gazette* 1995; **103**: 345–50.
39. Webster D, Turok I. The future of local unemployment statistics: the case for replacing TTWAs. *Quarterly Economic Commentary* 1997; **22**(2): 36–40.
40. Turok I, ed. *Travel to Work Areas and the measurement of unemployment*, Conference Proceedings. Glasgow: Centre for Housing Research and Urban Studies, University of Glasgow, 1997.
41. Thomas R, Coombes M. How enlarged Travel to Work Areas conceal inner city employment. *Radical Statistics* 1998; **67**: 35–49, 62–4.
42. Webster D. Local unemployment statistics and the diagnosis of Britain's unemployment problem. *British Urban and Regional Information Systems Association* September; **134**: 5–10.
43. Coal Fields Task Force. *Making the difference – A new start for England's coalfield communities*. Wetherby: DETR free literature, 1998.

Health at work and home

6

OCCUPATIONAL ILL-HEALTH, HOUSING AND DIET

Ben Armstrong, Rebekah Widdowfield,
Yoav Ben Shlomo, Eric Brunner and Annette Boaz

Occupational ill-health and injury

Housing statistics: a shaky foundation for monitoring the
causes of ill-health?

Diet: how the state watches what we eat

This chapter describes data about three areas of life which can profoundly
affect people's health. These are their environment at work, their housing conditions and their diet. As the first section outlines, no single source of official
data can give an accurate assessment of the burden of occupational ill-health
and industrial injury. A rather patchy picture has to be built up from many
different sources, all of which have significant limitations.

The main source of official statistics is the count of people who qualify for
benefits under the government's Industrial Injuries Scheme (IIS). This compensates not only people suffering from an industrial injury, but also those
suffering from 'prescribed' industrial diseases. There are many barriers to
claiming under the scheme. Therefore, the figures provide no more than an
indicator of the absolute lower limit of the number of more serious cases of
industrial disease. The second main source is the Reporting of Injuries,
Diseases and Dangerous Occurrences Regulations 1985 (RIDDOR). This
requires employers to report injuries, fatalities and absence from work of
more than 3 days which are thought to be related to industrial disease. There
are few incentives and many disincentives for employers to report such incidents and it is estimated that at least half of the occurrences are not reported.

Data from these two sources give a very different picture of occupational
disease from those collected in the Labour Force Survey (LFS). This assesses
people's own perception about the cause of their poor health by asking them
whether they suffer from any illness or disability which is caused or made
worse by their work. Reports of deafness due to work are about a hundred
times more common in the Labour Force Survey than in the Reporting of
Injuries, Diseases and Dangerous Occurrences Regulations and Industrial

Injuries Scheme, for example. The current set of prescribed diseases is associated with effects of working in heavy industry, now in decline. Many legal battles will have to be fought by workers before the occupational effects of work in new industries become officially recognised. Meanwhile, a fourth source of data relates people's deaths to their occupations. The Registrar General's decennial supplements on occupational mortality compare death rates around the time of each census of people in particular occupations with those in other occupations and those of people of the same age in the general population.

While a few people may be compensated for the effects of work on their health, no-one is compensated for the effects of poor housing, despite the considerable evidence which suggests that bad housing is associated with poor health. As the second section of this chapter shows, a wealth of information is collected about condition of the housing stock, tenure, renovations and rents.

In contrast, it is difficult to quantify 'poor housing' and homelessness, both of which have major effects on health. Traditionally, overcrowding, lack of amenities such as central heating and unfitness for habitation have been used as indicators of 'poor housing'. With the exception of unfit accommodation, their relevance as measures is now questionable. Instead, other problems such as rent or mortgage arrears, eviction and repossession may be better indicators.

Defining homelessness is notoriously difficult. It is generally accepted that government statistics grossly underestimate the number of homeless people. 'Official' figures record the numbers of people accepted as eligible for rehousing by local authorities, but they are allowed considerable discretion about whether to accept people as homeless. Recent attempts to estimate the numbers of people sleeping rough are also likely to produce underestimates, mainly because of the practical difficulties involved in locating people sleeping out in the open.

The final section describes the information the government collects about what people eat. Because diet has been implicated as a factor in many common diseases, there is increasing official interest in what is consumed by the population as a whole and by people in high-risk groups. Two major types of survey are undertaken. The long-standing National Food Survey provides information about household food purchases. This survey has been undertaken continuously since 1940 and has therefore charted the changes in food purchases. What it does not tell us is what individual people eat. The second is the series of National Diet and Nutrition surveys. They collect information about individual dietary intakes of people in different age groups, including children and elderly people. The main problem with these surveys is that some people, particularly those who are excessively overweight, under-report their food intake. To complement these surveys, the McCance and Widdowson's *The composition of foods* tables estimate the nutritional value of food purchased in the National Food Survey and eaten in the National Diet and Nutrition Surveys.

Occupational ill-health and injury

Two main sources of statistics on officially recognised occupational diseases and injuries count the numbers of people who have been compensated, or whose conditions have been reported by their employees. First, the Department of Social Security publishes data from administrative returns from the Industrial Injuries Scheme. These give information about people who qualify for and claim benefits under the scheme. Under the Reporting of Injuries, Diseases and Dangerous Occurrences Regulations, employers should report occupational disease and injury among their staff.

In addition, for respiratory disease and dermatitis, specialist doctors contribute to special reporting systems. For reasons which are described below, the official counts and special reporting systems underestimate the numbers of people with conditions caused by their work. Surveys of people's own experience of ill-health caused or made worse by their work give much higher estimates. In 1990 and 1995, the Labour Force Survey (described in Chapter 2), collected information about whether respondents attributed a period of ill-health to their work.

Another important source of data is the *Registrar General's* decennial supplements on *Occupational mortality*. These show overall rates of mortality according to the occupation recorded at death registration and data collected in the census. The decennial supplement for 1991 also includes data about cancer incidence and a summary of information from all the statistical systems mentioned above.

Statistics from all except the last of these are published in the Health and Safety Commission's annual *Health and safety statistics*.[1] In what follows, we give an overview of some general issues in interpreting these statistics, then we describe each data source and outline its strengths and limitations.

Interpreting statistics about occupational health

Agreeing that a person is suffering from a disease caused by work is far from simple, and the process is somewhat arbitrary. A few diseases such as lead poisoning and asbestosis are very clearly occupational, since the exposures needed to cause them are highly unlikely to be found outside of workplaces. Many other diseases have multiple causes, only some of which are occupational in origin. Conditions in this second category range from those with a well-established occupational link, such as lung cancer in asbestos workers, to the more speculative, such as 'sick building syndrome'.

For cases of 'very clearly occupational' disease, data collection can in theory be almost complete, but for conditions with multiple causes, even those with 'well-established links' to occupations, it is not possible to know with certainty whether an individual case of disease was due to occupational exposure. Thus, it is unclear which cases should be counted as 'occupational'. Recognition and attribution of disease to work by individuals and their doctors and subsequent reporting are further hurdles to providing a complete picture.

Official recognition of disease: prescribed diseases

The official recognition of a disease as occupational for compensation and statistical purposes is called 'prescription'. Diseases are prescribed by the Industrial Injuries Advisory Council (IIAC). A prescribed disease is both a specification of a disease and a list of occupations or occupational conditions under which the disease is classified as occupational. For example, the cancer angiosarcoma of the liver is a prescribed disease, but only for workers manufacturing vinyl chloride.

To place a disease–occupation combination on the list, the Industrial Injuries Advisory Council requires clear evidence that working in the occupational conditions specified doubles risk of the disease. This criterion is used to select easily identified groups of workers in which the disease is 'more likely than not' to have been caused by work. Groups of workers for whom the risk is raised but less than doubled will experience occupationally caused disease, but they will not be compensated or counted in official statistics. For example, suppose that a work exposure does not double the risk of cancer but increases it by a factor of 1.5. Then, if a group of exposed workers had 150 cancers, fifty of these are probably attributable to their work, but none will be compensated or appear on Industrial Injuries Scheme statistics. Workers with disease which has an established link to their occupation, but who are not proven to the Industrial Injuries Advisory Council's satisfaction to have a doubled risk include people who have lung cancer and are exposed to environmental tobacco smoke at work and foundry workers exposed to the vapour from coal tar.

The sources of data on occupational disease

THE INDUSTRIAL INJURIES SCHEME

This compensates workers injured or killed by an accident at work, or their dependants, and workers suffering from a prescribed disease. The diseases for which there were more than 200 compensated cases in 1996[1] are shown in Table 6.1.

In the past, it was possible to claim three benefits under this scheme: injury benefit, industrial death and disablement benefit. The first two have been abolished. The disablement benefit remains, but the rules have been tightened considerably since 1 October 1986, generally requiring proof of at least 14 per cent disablement. These changes, and changes in the list of prescribed diseases, make the interpretation of trends difficult.

One lung disease, coal workers' pneumoconiosis, has long been a prescribed disease for underground coal miners. Another, chronic bronchitis or emphysema, was not prescribed until 1993. This resulted in the appearance in the Industrial Injuries Scheme statistics of 1560 new cases of disabling disease in 1993, 2594 in 1994, followed by 268 in 1995 and 269 in 1996. This reflected a change in the rules, not an increase in occupational disease. The high numbers in 1993 and 1994, which accounted for almost half the overall total number compensated, were due to the processing of a backlog of cases. Once this

Table 6.1 Diseases with more than 200 cases compensated under the Industrial Injuries Scheme, 1996

	Compensated cases, 1996
Pneumoconiosis	841
Mesothelioma	642
Deafness	531
Vibration white finger	411
Asthma	410
Chronic bronchitis or emphysema	269
Tenosynovitis or repetitive strain syndrome	223

Source: Health and Safety Commission, *Health and safety statistics, 1996/97.*[1]

backlog was cleared, there was a big drop from 1994 to 1996. Actual trends in the incidence of disabling emphysema or bronchitis in coal miners are impossible to determine from these data.

The rules for eligibility for benefit are very restrictive, and benefit will be granted only if an application is made. Therefore, data from the Industrial Injuries Scheme provide a reliable indicator only of the absolute lower limit of the number of more serious cases of industrial disease.[2]

REPORTING OF INJURIES, DISEASES AND DANGEROUS OCCURRENCES REGULATIONS 1985

There are similar problems with the data from this system. In this case, designation and recognition may be less important than both the employers' and individuals' willingness to report. The regulations require employers to report injuries, fatalities and absence from work of more than 3 days if they are thought to be related to industrial disease. Employers should report all cases of occupational disease where they receive a doctor's written diagnosis and the affected employee's current job involves the work activity specifically associated with the disease. With some exceptions, the diseases that employers should report are based on the Department of Social Security's Prescribed Diseases List, used in the assessment of claims under the Industrial Injuries Scheme. There is no requirement for the employers to report occupational deafness, which is one of the most common of the prescribed diseases. Dermatitis and musculoskeletal disease, such as tenosynovitis or repetitive strain syndrome, became reportable only in 1995. Studies have confirmed that there is substantial under-reporting in the Reporting of Injuries, Diseases and Dangerous Occurrences Regulations, even in relation to its own very restrictive rules, when compared to the already restrictive Industrial Injuries Scheme.[1,2] This is illustrated below.

SPECIAL REPORTING SYSTEMS: SWORD AND EPIDERM

Since 1989, the Epidemiology Research Unit at the London Chest Hospital, in collaboration with the British Thoracic Society and the Society of Occupational Medicine, has been funded by the Health and Safety Executive to operate the SWORD reporting system.[3] Occupational and chest physicians report new cases which they recognise as occupationally related respiratory disease. Since 1992, some chest physicians have sent in reports for only 1 month each year and the figures are grossed up, while the remainder of chest physicians and all occupational health physicians report all cases. EPIDERM, which came into operation in 1992, is a similar system for work-related skin disease.[4] It is based at the University of Manchester.

These systems provide useful information to complement the administrative counts from the Industrial Injuries Scheme and Reporting of Injuries, Diseases and Dangerous Occurrences Regulations, but they too have limitations. Like all voluntary reporting systems, accuracy and completeness are hard to ensure. Furthermore, only cases that come to the attention of a specialist doctor can be reported, and their designation as occupational depends on the specialist's judgement. For example, not all cases of asthma which may be occupationally related will be seen by specialist chest or occupational physicians; many will be seen only by a general practitioner. Also, not all specialists will agree on whether a case of asthma is occupationally related. Finally, these special systems exist only for respiratory disease and dermatitis.

THE LABOUR FORCE SURVEY

This general questionnaire survey about employment, administered to 60 000 private households every year, is described in Chapter 2. In 1990, this survey included a supplementary questionnaire which asked respondents to assess whether, in the last 12 months, they had 'suffered from any illness, disability or other physical problem that was caused or made worse by (their) work'.[5] Follow-up questions were asked about the nature of the illness and whether work was thought to have caused the condition or made it worse. The nature of the work and the number of days sick leave taken due to the complaint were also noted. Therefore, the replies are based on the individual's own perception of the link between occupation and ill-health. Similar questions were asked in the 1995 Labour Force Survey, but methods changed, so that comparison of results from the two surveys are problematic. Preliminary tables were given in *Health and safety statistics 1996/97*, and fuller tables will appear in subsequent volumes. These surveys have shown that many more people are suffering from occupational ill-health than is suggested by the counts of people with officially recognised diseases.

DECENNIAL SUPPLEMENT ON OCCUPATIONAL HEALTH

The most recent of these was published by the Office of Population Censuses and Surveys (OPCS) and Health and Safety Executive. Since 1881, the General Register Office has published statistical tables comparing occupations of people dying around the time of each census with the occupations of the population recorded in the census. This is one of the series of 'decennial supplements' described in Chapter 3. It differs from the other statistical systems discussed in this section in that it does not count individual deaths recognised as being caused by occupational conditions. Instead, it looks at all deaths according to the occupation stated on the death certificate, regardless of whether the doctor certifying death recognised an occupational cause. Death rates classified by the immediate 'underlying cause' such as heart disease or cancer are tabulated by occupation. For example, the *Occupational health* decennial supplement for 1991 reported mortality rates for bronchitis and emphysema in coal miners as being 167 per cent of the overall rate in men of working age.[2] Similar data for the previous decades were probably part of the evidence which led the Industrial Injuries Advisory Council to accept the association as causal and to prescribe this disease.

The analyses made in the decennial supplements, together with data from other sources, can identify and quantify occupational disease risks. Because of the various biases, discussed in some detail in the supplements, their results should be interpreted with caution. All elevated rates are not necessarily due to direct occupational hazards. Some are thought to reflect people's 'way of life'. For example, occupations with higher than average rates of smoking would be expected to have higher than average mortality from lung cancer. Conversely, normal or depressed rates cannot always be taken to imply the absence of a hazard. A major deficiency is that information about many women's occupations is not recorded on their death certificates. As a consequence, many tabulations analyse married women's mortality according to their husband's occupations. This reduces their usefulness as a source of data about the hazards in occupations in which women predominate.

Occupational health was broader in scope than previous decennial supplements. In addition to the traditional analysis of mortality, it included similar analyses of cancer incidence by occupation and summarised information from other sources of data about recognised occupational disease. In particular, it included an excellent chapter on 'Monitoring occupational diseases', which brought together and compared information from the various sources.

OTHER SOURCES

Copies of death certificates mentioning certain known occupational diseases, such as mesothelioma, are sent by the Office for National Statistics (ONS) to the Health and Safety Executive, the government body responsible for policing health and safety at work. The 10-yearly Morbidity Statistics from General Practice described in Chapter 8 recorded illnesses which led to consultations with a general practitioner. The Communicable Disease Surveillance Centre receives and collates reports on work-related infections, as Chapter 3 describes.

Comparing sources of data

The systems described above produce very different pictures of the extent of occupational disease. Some examples are shown in Table 6.2, which shows estimates and counts of occupational disease from the various sources for

Table 6.2 Comparison of estimates of numbers of people with selected occupational diseases in 1990

Condition	Labour Force Survey Caused or made worse	Caused	Industrial Injuries Scheme	RIDDOR
Asthma	68 100	19 700	476	70
Back problem	460 400	297 200	–	–
Deafness	121 400	103 100	1041	–
Dermatitis	84 600	54 200	583	–
Lung cancer	–	–	63	–
Mesothelioma	–	–	476	13
Stress or depression	182 700	104 900	–	–
Vibration white finger	7300	7300	5444	120
All conditions	2 240 200	1 302 200	9463	309

Source: Occupational health, decennial supplement. [2]
Labour Force Survey: estimated numbers of persons reporting that their work caused or made worse disease in the last 12 months.
Industrial Injuries Scheme: new cases of assessed disablement due to prescribed diseases.
Reporting of Injuries Diseases and Dangerous Occurrences Regulations – (RIDDOR): reports by employers of absences for more than 3 days due to prescribed diseases.

1990. Comparison between figures from the various sources should take into account that the Labour Force Survey and the Reporting of Injuries, Diseases and Dangerous Occurrences Regulations report both new diseases and their recurrence, whereas the Industrial Injuries Scheme reports new cases only. It is nevertheless clear that, compared to people's own views of the extent to which illness is caused by work, official figures count only a tiny proportion of overall occupational disease. Even if we allow for some incorrect attribution of disease to work in the Labour Force Survey, there is no doubt that neither the Industrial Injuries Scheme nor the Reporting of Injuries, Diseases and Dangerous Occurrences Regulations can be used to estimate the total burden of occupational disease. This is obvious both for conditions not prescribed for any occupation, such as stress or depression, and also for diseases with well-established occupational causes, such as asthma or deafness. The Reporting of Injuries, Diseases and Dangerous Occurrences Regulations are particularly unhelpful.

A survey such as the Labour Force Survey cannot estimate numbers of people with diseases such as mesothelioma and lung cancer, which are rapidly fatal. For mesothelioma, which is recognised as unequivocally occupational, the Industrial Injuries Scheme figures are relatively good. Even here, however, there is under-counting. In 1990 there were 880 deaths from mesothelioma, all but a handful likely to have been caused by occupational exposure to asbestos, yet only 476 cases were reported. This suggests that the Industrial Injuries Scheme covers only about a half of occupationally caused mesothelioma. There is no direct way to count occupationally caused lung cancers, because lung cancer has multiple causes and these are impossible to distinguish from the nature of the cancer. We can be certain that the sixty-three cases included in the Industrial Injuries Scheme are a gross underestimate of the total. Most studies of workers exposed to asbestos find that the excess of lung cancers is as great as or greater than the number of mesotheliomas. Thus, we would expect at least 880 cases of lung cancer due to asbestos alone.

More generally, several reviews have made estimates of total numbers of cancers caused by occupation, by piecing together information on relative risks from epidemiological studies, and separate information on the extent of exposure. An estimate towards the bottom of the range was made by Richard Doll and Richard Peto in 1981.[6] They estimated that 4 per cent of cancer deaths were due to known occupational risks. Although that estimate was made for the USA in 1980, it is reasonable to expect a similar proportion in Britain in the 1990s. Given about 150 000 deaths due to cancer annually, this would imply 6000 annually due to occupational exposures. In 1996, the Industrial Injuries Scheme reported just 889 cases of occupational cancer, all but 28 due to asbestos.

Although the substantial disagreement between published statistics illustrates their weakness, a consensus does not necessarily mean that the agreed figure is correct. For example, in 1990, neither the Industrial Injuries Scheme nor the Reporting of Injuries, Diseases and Dangerous Occurrences Regulations reported any cases of occupational bronchitis and emphysema. In the reports from the Labour Force Survey, chronic bronchitis and emphysema cannot be distinguished from other types of 'lower respiratory disease' as the survey did not involve an examination by a health professional.[7] After the Industrial Injuries Advisory Council prescribed this disease for coal miners in 1992, 1560 new cases appeared for the first time in the 1993 Industrial Injuries Scheme statistics. After a judge ruled in 1998 that coal dust was the cause of disabling bronchitis and emphysema in six miners seeking damages from British Coal, it was estimated that 100 000 similar cases met the same criteria.[8] Thus, a disease that appeared in the statistics up to 1990 to have no occupational causes appears in 1998 to be one of the major occupational diseases.

Finally, until an association between occupation and a disease is identified, no statistics can reflect its impact on health. In the 1950s, counts or estimates of occupational disease could not include cancers caused by asbestos, as it was not yet known that asbestos could cause cancer. Unless other associations are known or even suspected, their impact cannot be measured.

Occupational injuries

Occupational injury statistics are published annually by the Health and Safety Commission in the same volume as occupational disease statistics.[1] The main source is the Reporting of Injuries, Diseases and Dangerous Occurrences Regulations system, to which employers should report injuries resulting in 3 or more days' absence from work. As for occupational disease, questions in the Labour Force Survey have been used to supplement information obtained from the Reporting of Injuries, Diseases and Dangerous Occurrences Regulations. For injuries, it is the employers' willingness to report, rather than difficulties of definition, that is the main problem. The Labour Force Survey returns suggest that in 1996/7, the Reporting of Injuries, Diseases and Dangerous Occurrences Regulations data include less than half of the reportable injuries to employees, and only 10 per cent of injuries to self-employed people.

Injury rates from the two systems are shown by industry in Table 6.3. Reporting rates vary from 11 per cent in finance and business to 86 per cent in extraction and utility supply. Agriculture appears to have quite low injury rates according to the Reporting of Injuries, Diseases and Dangerous Occurrences Regulations, but high rates according to the Labour Force Survey. As a general rule, the likelihood of reporting depends on the severity of the injury. There is evidence, however, that even major injuries are under-reported.[9] For fatal injuries, the Reporting of Injuries, Diseases and Dangerous Occurrences Regulations data are supplemented by data from other sources, notably death certificates, so that the data are likely to be very nearly complete. Useful reviews by Theo Nichols of the Health and Safety Executive's industrial injury statistics were published in 1996[9] and 1998.[10]

Key publications

Since 1992/3, statistics relating to occupational death, injury and diseases in Great Britain have been published annually by the Health and Safety Commission[1] in *Health and safety statistics*. In Northern Ireland, accidents statistics reported by the Reporting of Injuries, Diseases and Dangerous Occurrences Regulations are published biannually by the Health and Safety Executive for Northern Ireland. The Health and Safety Commission publication

Table 6.3 Rates of reportable injury by industry from workers' self-report from the Labour Force Survey and employers' reports from the RIDDOR

Industry	Injury rate per 100 000		Percentage reported under RIDDOR*
	Labour Force Survey	RIDDOR	
Agriculture	2180	656	30
Extraction and utility supply	1910	1637	86
Manufacturing	2130	1198	56
Construction	2890	1254	43
Distribution and repair	1450	477	33
Hotels and restaurants	1450	244	17
Transport and communication	2440	1398	57
Finance and business	760	81	11
Public administration and defence	1870	1151	62
Education	740	325	44
Health and social work	1830	579	33
Consumer/leisure services	1350	450	33
All industries	1640	684	42

Source: Health and safety statistics 1996/97.[1] Rates per 100 000.
*Percentage of reportable injuries estimated from the Labour Force Survey reported to RIDDOR system

includes very clear notes on the sources of data. It is forthright about their limitations, but others citing them are not always so careful. It also contains statistics and commentary on dangerous occurrences, gas safety and enforcement. A statistical summary is published with the Health and Safety Executive's *Annual report*. Before 1992, health and safety statistics were published in the *Employment Gazette*, now called *Labour Market Trends*[11-13] The most recent decennial supplement, *Occupational health*,[2] was produced jointly by the Health and Safety Executive and the OPCS, now part of the ONS. It includes an excellent summary of sources of statistics on occupational disease.

Key official publications

Health and Safety Commission. *Health and safety statistics*. London: HSE books, published annually from 1992/3 onwards.

Health and Safety Commission. *Annual statistical supplement*. London: HSE books, published annually.

Office of Population Censuses and Surveys, Health and Safety Executive. *Occupational health*. Series DS, No. 10. London: HMSO, 1995.

Health and Safety Executive for Northern Ireland. *Biannual report*. Department of Enterprise, Trade and Development Northern Ireland. Belfast: TSO.

Contact addresses and web sites

Great Britain
Health and Safety Executive
Health Directorate: Epidemiology and
Medical Statistics Unit (EMSU)
Magdalen House
Stanley Precinct
Merseyside L20 3QY
Telephone: 0151 951 4000
Web site: http://www.open.gov.uk/hse/
hsehome.htm

Health and Safety Executive Automatic fax system
Information about publications and facts sheets
Telephone: 0839 060606

OHSRom – Silver
Health and Safety Executive database
on CD ROM – includes regulations,
legislation and publications on nuclear
energy, hazardous substances, health
and safety and occupational hygiene.

Northern Ireland
Health and Safety Executive for
Northern Ireland
83 Ladas Drive
Belfast BT6 9FR
Telephone: 028 9024 3249
Web site: http://www.hse-ni.org.uk

Housing statistics: a shaky foundation for monitoring the causes of ill-health?

There is now a wealth of research showing links between poor housing and ill-health.[14-16] For example, the Standing Conference on Public Health has estimated that people in poor housing use the National Health Service 50 per cent more than average and that poor living conditions cost the service some £2 billion a year.[17] Other epidemiological research confirms this association. For example, overcrowding, poor amenities and dampness have been linked to reduced life expectancy,[18] increased risk of infectious diseases and accidental death,[19,20] mental health problems,[21] respiratory conditions[22] and other complaints, compared with people who are better housed. In addition, numerous studies have demonstrated that, for a whole host of ailments, homeless people are considerably less healthy than the general 'homed' population. [23-5]

Despite this long-standing recognition of the links between housing and health, there is a surprising lack of statistical information. Difficulties involved in both defining and measuring poor housing and homelessness cast doubt upon the extent to which these problems can be quantified, while the tendency for national statistics to relate predominantly to *either* housing *or* to health makes it hard to establish empirically the associations between the two. These difficulties notwithstanding, there is a wealth of statistical information which can inform debates about housing and health.

This section describes the information that is available. It begins with an overview of the principal sources of housing statistics before turning its attention to housing conditions and homelessness, two particular aspects of housing which are more directly associated with well-being. It describes in each instance the data available, where they can be found, and their usefulness and limitations. Table 6.4 summarises the sources of housing statistics for each of the topics discussed, as well as a number of other aspects of housing less directly associated with health, including, for example, house-building, renovations and housing costs.

Housing statistics in general

The main publications containing official data on housing and homelessness in England are compiled by the Department of the Environment, Transport and the Regions (DETR) from statistical returns completed by local authorities and from continuous or *ad hoc* surveys organised centrally.

Housing and construction statistics draws together information from local authority returns, along with that from other sources such as the census, Council of Mortgage Lenders[26] and the Family Resources Survey.[27] Its aim is 'to provide a broad perspective on developments in housing and construction over the past decade'. As well as the annual publication, which details changes over the preceding 10 years, *Housing and construction statistics* is also published quarterly as a two-part report giving the latest figures on a range of

Table 6.4 Sources of official housing statistics

Topic	Sources
Housing conditions/unfitness	Census, *English house condition survey, Housing and construction statistics*, Survey of English housing
Homelessness	*Local housing statistics*, Survey of English housing, *Homelessness actuals*[33]
Housing stock: size, type, tenure	*Housing and construction statistics, Local housing statistics*
House-building	*Housing and construction statistics, House-building information bulletin, Local housing statistics*
Renovations/slum clearance	*Housing and construction statistics, Local housing statistics, House renovations information bulletin*
Housing costs: rents, prices, rent/mortgage arrears, repossessions, evictions	*Housing rent actuals,*[34] *Family resources survey,*[27] *Family expenditure survey,*[35] *Housing and construction statistics, Rent officer statistics*, Survey of English housing, *Housing finance quarterly*[26]
Allocations	Survey of English housing

housing topics, including housing stock, tenure, new build, renovations, council house sales, rents and mortgage repayments.

While *Housing and construction statistics* contains data for England and the regions as a whole, the quarterly *Local housing statistics* (LHS), provides regular statistics on house-building, renovations, slum clearance, council house sales and the provision of specially designed accommodation for elderly or disabled people for individual local authorities in England. These statistics are consequently useful sources of data for researchers seeking to identify differences between areas or requiring information for a particular authority. *Local housing statistics* also records the number of households accepted for rehousing under the homelessness provisions of the 1996 Housing Act, as reported by local authorities in their homelessness returns to the Department of Environment, Transport and the Regions. Figures for acceptances nationally are provided in the quarterly *Homelessness information bulletin*, which also provides further information, including reasons for homelessness and local authority use of temporary accommodation.

Similar information can be found for Wales in the annual *Welsh housing statistics*, for Scotland in the quarterly *Housing trends in Scotland*, and for Northern Ireland in the annual *Northern Ireland housing statistics*. Details of these publications are given at the end of this section.

As well as these regular sets of official statistics, there are two major continuous surveys in England devoted to housing alone: the Survey of English Housing and the English House Condition Survey. The annual

Survey of English Housing, published as *Housing in England*, involves face-to-face interviews in 20 000 private households. First introduced in 1993, the survey updates information formerly collected in the Labour Force Survey's 'housing trailers'. These surveys give a comprehensive range of basic information at both national and regional level on households and their housing circumstances, including, for example, type of accommodation, tenure, housing costs, and repossessions. Since 1994, they have also asked people's views about their housing and the area in which they live. The survey has also provided a basis for reports examining the characteristics, circumstances and attitudes of particular groups such as private tenants[28,29] and households living in shared accommodation.[30]

While the Survey of English Housing provides a general overview of housing, the English House Condition Survey focuses specifically on housing conditions. Undertaken every 5 years since its introduction in 1966, the survey collects information through a four-stage process involving interviews with householders, a physical survey of dwellings, a postal survey of local authorities and housing associations, and a survey of current market values of the property assessed. The information collected includes property and household characteristics, tenancy, levels of occupancy, stock condition, repair and improvement. While most of the tables in the published report relate to England as a whole, some provide a breakdown by region or for groups of local authorities.

Although both the Survey of English Housing and the English House Condition Survey ask questions about the ethnic group of occupants, the small sample size makes analysis difficult and only a few tables are published. The *English house condition survey 1991* included tables showing the distribution of unfit, poor and the worst 10 per cent of housing by ethnic minority status. More detailed data examining the links between housing circumstances, conditions and ethnicity can be found in the London Research Centre's regular publication, *London housing statistics*,[31] but there is a paucity of such information for the country as a whole.

Similar, but less detailed, information to that contained in the English House Condition Survey is available from housing condition surveys conducted in Scotland, Wales and Northern Ireland, while a useful overview of poor housing across the UK can be found in *The state of UK housing*.[32] This report draws together information from the four national housing condition surveys and other sources to provide a comprehensive body of information on housing conditions, detailing both the latest information and trends over time.

Two general surveys described in Chapter 2, the 10-yearly census and the General Household Survey, are further sources of data about housing. The main census volume on housing, *Housing and car availability*, contains information on housing tenure, density and household amenities, but housing data are also cross-tabulated with other variables in other volumes. The General Household Survey contains similar information to the census, but on an annual basis, along with additional information on a range of housing topics including housing costs, age of building and number of bedrooms.

A general overview of housing and the statistics available can be found in

Social trends, which draws together data from all the various sources detailed above 'to paint a broad picture of British society today'. Published annually, *Social trends* devotes a whole chapter to housing. In 1998, this included information on characteristics of households living in different types of tenure, home ownership, rented housing, experience of homelessness, types and conditions of housing, house-building, and housing costs and expenditure. Although figures are usually only given at a national level and the accompanying text is predominantly descriptive, *Social trends* is a useful starting point for conducting housing research. The source of data is given below each table, and chapters conclude with a list of other relevant published information and contacts for further details.

A further source of information worth consulting is the *Housing digest*. First produced in 1997 and updated twice a year, the digest, available on CD-ROM or disk, collates much of the housing data from the official sources referred to above to provide detailed information on some ninety housing topics. Details are given in the contact list at the end of this section.

Housing conditions

Overcrowding, lack of amenities or central heating and unfitness for habitation are the data items used most frequently as indicators of 'poor housing'. Their relationship with health has been extensively explored,[17-21] but they apply to a very small proportion of the population. Changing standards and expectations, along with a general improvement in housing conditions in the post-war period, cast doubt upon the usefulness of overcrowding and lack of amenities as a measure of poor housing in the twenty-first century.

OVERCROWDING

Information about overcrowding can be gleaned from the census, the General Household Survey and the English House Condition Survey. The census does not actually define overcrowding, but simply records the number of rooms the household has for its own use. Used in conjunction with the number of persons in the household, this can provide a measure of overcrowding or, alternatively, under-occupancy. Published data cross-tabulate the number of persons per room by shared accommodation, household composition, dependent children, households with pensioners, households with dependants and ethnic group. Although, as noted above, there is no explicit definition of overcrowding, publications based on census output, such as the county reports, tend to refer to overcrowding as levels of occupancy of greater than one person per room.

This seems an inadequate measure of overcrowding and one which is increasingly out of line with contemporary standards and expectations. In particular, the census does not record the *different uses* of rooms and the only rooms excluded from the count are bathrooms, toilets and kitchens under 2 metres wide. Under such a definition, a household comprising five people living in a property with three bedrooms, a living room and a medium-sized kitchen would not be considered to be overcrowded, even if one of its members was having to sleep in the living room. The Scottish censuses use an indicator of overcrowding more appropriate to contemporary society, the 'occupancy norm', shown in Table 6.5. This relates the number of rooms available to a household to its need, on the basis of age, sex and marital status.

A similar definition is used for England in the General Household Survey and the English House Condition Survey. The 'bedroom standard' variable relates the number of rooms a household is deemed to need with the number of bedrooms available, again on the basis of household composition. The English House Condition Survey is the more useful of the two surveys, relating overcrowding, defined as a dwelling which is below the bedroom standard, to tenure, ethnic identity, age of household head, household type and type of area.

AMENITIES AND CENTRAL HEATING

The census tabulates the number of households lacking or sharing use of a bath or shower and/or inside toilet. In the past, sharing or lacking amenities was a useful indicator of poor housing, but its relevance to contemporary society is questionable, given that in 1991 only 1.3 per cent of households fell into this category. More useful information is available in the English House Condition Survey. This records not just the provision of amenities but also the age and condition of major internal services and facilities. The English House Condition Survey data are available only at national or regional level, however, so the census remains the principal source of data about amenities for areas below regional level.

As the number of households lacking or sharing amenities has fallen, researchers have increasingly looked for alternative indicators of poor housing. To this end, the availability of central heating was recorded for the first time in the 1991 census. Although adopted in a number of deprivation indices as a measure of housing quality, possession of central heating is of limited value. It gives no indication of the efficiency of the heating system or, more importantly, how often it is used. A number of studies have highlighted what has become known as 'fuel poverty', whereby households are unable to afford to heat their homes adequately. This problem is likely to have been exacerbated following the imposition of Value Added Tax (VAT) on fuel at a rate of 8 per cent in April 1994.

Table 6.5 Definition of 'occupancy norm' used in Scotland

Room entitlement is calculated on the basis of household composition. A one-person household is assumed to require only one room. Where there are two or more residents, it is assumed that they require one room, as a common room, and one additional room, as a bedroom, for each of the following:

- married couple
- any other person aged 21 or over
- each pair of adolescents of the same sex aged 10–20
- each pair of children under 10
- each pair formed from an adolescent aged 10–20 with a child under 10 of the same sex
- each child unable to form a pair

The English House Condition Survey goes some way towards addressing these limitations, recording both the existence and type of heating in a property by room. It also records a variety of other information, including times the heating is on, heating regimes and use of additional heating. Together, these give a comprehensive picture of heating provision, efficiency and use, but once again only for England as a whole.

UNFIT HOUSING

Of course, the ultimate in poor housing conditions is property which is unfit for human habitation. In 1996, some 1.47 million dwellings, 90 per cent of which were inhabited, fell into this category,[18] having failed to meet the new fitness standard set out in Section 604 of the Local Government and Housing Act 1989, shown in Table 6.6.

Determining unfitness is a subjective process, resting as it does upon the interpretation of such ambiguous terms as 'serious', 'adequate' and 'satisfactory'. Local authorities are statutorily obliged to take action on any property identified as unfit, whether by serving notice, making a closing or demolition order, or including the property in a clearance area. In addition, the standard of fitness determines eligibility for mandatory renovation grants. As a result, authorities may be reluctant to declare a property unfit in situations which are not clear-cut and there may be a number of unfit properties which fail to be officially defined as such.

Statistics on dwellings which are declared unfit for human habitation and action taken by local authorities in response can be found in Part 2 of the quarterly *Housing and construction statistics*. Although the published data are broken down only into England and the regions, information at county and local authority level is available on request. In Scotland, similar data can be found in the annual publication *Dwellings below the tolerable standard*, which contains statistics for Scotland as a whole and for each of the individual local authority districts. More detailed information on unfit properties in England is available from the English House Condition Survey. It gives a more

Table 6.6 Dwellings defined as fit for human habitation

Under the fitness standard set out in Section 604 of the Local Government and Housing Act 1989, a property is deemed fit for human habitation unless it fails to meet any of the following requirements in the opinion of the local authority:

- it is structurally stable
- it is free from serious disrepair
- it is free from dampness prejudicial to the health of any occupants
- it has adequate provision for lighting, heating and ventilation
- it has adequate supply of wholesome piped water
- it has satisfactory facilities for preparing and cooking food, including a sink with supplies of hot and cold water
- it has a suitably located toilet
- it has a bath or shower and basin, each with supplies of hot and cold water
- it has an effective system for draining foul, waste and surface water.

comprehensive breakdown of poor housing conditions than the *Housing and construction statistics*, considering not just dwellings which are statutorily unfit but also those in substantial disrepair or requiring essential modernisation. In addition, the English House Condition Survey relates these to other variables. For example, the survey tabulates reasons for unfitness by tenure and dwelling age as well as giving detailed information on the households living in poor or unfit accommodation, including the type of household and the age, economic status and ethnic group of household members.

Homelessness

As mentioned earlier, there is widespread recognition that homeless people experience a range of health problems and are considerably less healthy than the population as a whole. Although the definition of homelessness is subject to much debate,[36-9] there is a general acceptance that homelessness encompasses not only roofless people, but also people living in various other forms of inadequate or insecure housing situations, including hostels, bed and breakfast hotels or sharing accommodation with another household.

'OFFICIAL' HOMELESSNESS STATISTICS

Published official homelessness statistics simply record the number of households statutorily accepted as homeless and eligible for rehousing under the provisions of the 1985 and, latterly, the 1996 Housing Acts. This information is published both nationally and for individual local authorities in *Local housing statistics*. The *Homelessness information bulletin*, published quarterly by the Department of the Environment, Transport and the Regions, gives further details, recording not only the number of homeless acceptances but also the numbers of applications, numbers of households in priority need, reasons for homelessness, and local authority use of temporary accommodation. The figures in the bulletin refer to England as a whole, but it may be possible to obtain more detailed data for individual authorities from the Department of the Environment, Transport and the Regions or from the relevant local housing departments. Local departments often include these statistics in their annual housing reports and housing investment programme strategies or make them available on request. Similar data for Scotland, provided both at national and district level, can be found in *Operation of homeless persons legislation in Scotland*.

Official statistics on the numbers of homeless households are widely considered to grossly underestimate the extent of the problem. Many people who live in unsatisfactory situations or who are roofless are deterred from seeking help because of the stigma and humiliation attached to being classified as homeless. Other groups of homeless individuals, such as young single people, may not approach their local authority for assistance in the belief that the council is unable, or unwilling, to help.

Furthermore, for those households who do approach their local authority for assistance and complete the application process, being accepted for rehousing is far from guaranteed. Even if accepted as homeless, other conditions then apply. Applicants have to be in 'priority need', a category defined as including families with children, pregnant women, or 'vulnerable' individuals/households unintentionally homeless, and to have a local connection before they are eligible for rehousing and thus appear in the official statistics. Although legislation lays down criteria about the circumstances in which a household is considered homeless and the nature of the local authority's duty towards them, determining homelessness and the duty owed is far from being a straightforward objective process and authorities have a considerable degree of flexibility.

As a result, the number and proportion of homeless applications and acceptances vary considerably between authorities. Whether or not a household is accepted as homeless would seem to depend as much on the way in which individual local authorities interpret the homelessness legislation as on a household's housing circumstances. The number of homelessness acceptances is also affected by the way in which authorities deal with homeless households. In particular, many local authorities altered their allocation policies following the 1996 Housing Act to enable homeless households to be rehoused directly from the waiting list rather than via the homelessness route, which, under the new legislation, restricted homeless households to temporary rehousing in the first instance. With this change in local authority rehousing practice, many homeless households effectively disappear from the official homelessness statistics. As a result, the official figures now represent an even less accurate reflection than before of the extent of homelessness.[40]

Quite clearly, then, the official homelessness statistics represent only a proportion of the total homeless population. For a variety of reasons, large numbers of homeless people, including people sleeping rough, living in hostels, bed and breakfast accommodation or squatting, are not included in these figures.

ROUGH SLEEPERS

In recent years, the most frequent and co-ordinated attempts to quantify the extent of this 'unofficial' homelessness have consisted of an assessment of the numbers of people sleeping rough. Although the association between all forms of homelessness and poor health is widely recognised, the link between rough sleeping and ill-health has been particularly well documented. Research shows that the street homeless are less healthy than both the homed population and other homeless people.[23] People sleeping rough are more likely to catch tuberculosis,[41] more likely to have a mental health problem[42,43] and often face difficulties gaining access to primary health care.[44,45] Knowing the number of rough sleepers, therefore, has important implications for health service provision. Practical difficulties in establishing the extent of such homelessness suggest, however, that, as with the official homelessness figures, rough sleeper counts severely underestimate the scale of the problem. In particular, rough sleeping is often hidden from view and the number of rough sleepers identified depends on the enumerator's knowledge of where and when people are sleeping rough.

Statistics are also affected by the time period over which rough sleeping is assessed. Research suggests that, for many homeless people, rough sleeping is a temporary or periodic experience. It can be interspersed by periods of time in various forms of temporary accommodation, such as staying with friends, in a hostel or in bed and breakfast accommodation. Not surprisingly, therefore, studies which record the incidence of rough sleeping over a period of time identify a greater number of rough sleepers than head counts taken on a single night.[46]

In terms of available figures, information about the number of rough sleepers is somewhat patchy. The 1991 census included a count of rough sleepers but has been widely criticised for severely underestimating the extent of the problem.[47] In the late 1990s, a large number of local authorities undertook such counts in a bid to obtain money under the Government's Rough Sleepers' Initiative. Many more authorities made no assessment, and there is no specific publication which details numbers of rough sleepers by area. Researchers seeking details of rough sleeping should therefore approach the Department of the Environment, Transport and the Regions or individual authorities for the latest figures.

'OTHER' HOMELESSNESS

Of course, rough sleeping represents just one, and the most extreme, dimension of homelessness. As Shelter points out on its web site, 'for every person literally without a roof over their head there are hundreds of thousands more who may be less visible but just as much in need of a proper home'. Yet, with no single organisation charged with responsibility for the task, there has been no concerted attempt to establish the extent and nature of such unofficial homelessness. Various organisations have attempted at different times to establish the numbers of people living in hostels and bed and breakfast establishments, and the numbers squatting or staying with friends or relatives. Many of these estimates are quite dated and, although they are sometimes extrapolated to provide national estimates, they are predominantly London based. The figures vary according to which groups are considered, the area covered and the time period over which an assessment is made. Given the ad-hoc and inconsistent nature of these assessments, there is no regular publication of the resulting information. The best point of contact for the latest estimates of the number and circumstances of homeless people who are not included within the official homelessness statistics is therefore probably Shelter, or one of the other main homelessness charities, such as Centrepoint or Crisis.

Although published statistical data tend not to establish explicitly the widely recognised connections between housing and well-being, there is a wealth of housing statistics which can inform debates about the impact of housing circumstances on the nation's health. While statistics on housing conditions and homelessness are most obviously relevant to these debates, further research suggests that other, perhaps less immediately apparent, aspects of a person's housing circumstances also have important implications for their health and well-being. For example, there are now a growing number of studies which point to the detrimental impact on health experienced by house-holds with rent or mortgage arrears or facing eviction or repossession.[48,49]

At the end of the day, statistical information is limited, although such data undoubtedly have an important contribution to make. Difficulties in both defining and measuring poor housing and homelessness suggest that only by using statistical data in conjunction with other, more qualitative, forms of information will it be possible to obtain a comprehensive understanding of the relationship between housing and health.

Key official publications

Statistics about housing in general
Department of the Environment, Transport and the Regions. *Housing and construction statistics Part 1*. London: TSO, published annually.
Department of the Environment, Transport and the Regions. *Housing and construction statistics Part 2*. London: TSO, published quarterly.
Department of the Environment, Transport and the Regions. *Local housing statistics*. London: Department of the Environment, Transport and the Regions, published quarterly.
The Welsh Office. *Welsh housing statistics*. Cardiff: TSO, published annually.
The Scottish Office Development Department. *Housing trends in Scotland*. Edinburgh: TSO, published quarterly.
Department of the Environment (Northern Ireland). *Northern Ireland housing statistics*. Belfast: TSO, published annually.

Survey of English Housing
Office for National Statistics. *Housing in England*. London: TSO, published annually.

House condition surveys
Department of the Environment, Transport and the Regions. *English house condition survey*. London: TSO; published every 5 years.
Scottish Homes. *Scottish house condition survey 1991*. Edinburgh: HMSO, 1993.
Welsh Office. *Welsh house condition survey 1993*. Cardiff: HMSO, 1995.
Department of the Environment (Northern Ireland). *Northern Ireland house condition survey 1991*. Belfast: HMSO, 1993.

Homelessness statistics
Department of the Environment, Transport and the Regions. *Homelessness information bulletin*. London: Department of the Environment, Transport and the Regions, published quarterly.
The Scottish Office Development Department. *Operation of homeless persons legislation in Scotland*. Edinburgh: TSO, published annually.

Contact addresses and web sites

Department of the Environment, Transport and the Regions
Housing Data and Statistics Division
Eland House

Bressenden Place
London SW1E 5DU
Telephone: 020 7890 3303
Web site: http://www.detr.gov.uk

Housing digest is available from:
Crown Business Communications
United House
9 Pembridge Road
London W11 3JY
Telephone: 020 7727 7272

Housing Resource Guide – a guide to
housing sites on the internet
Web site: http://www.housinguk.org

Shelter
Web site: http://www.shelter.org.uk

Joseph Rowntree Foundation
Web site: http://www.jrf.org.uk

Diet: how the state watches what we eat

Since the Second World War, public policy on food has changed its emphasis. In the early part of the century, the focus was on ensuring the adequacy of the food supply, on identifying malnutrition among poor people and, because of novel discoveries in the vitamins' field, on intakes of 'protective foods'. Now, because diet has been implicated as a factor in common diseases such as cardiovascular disease, diabetes and cancers of the digestive system, the emphasis is on the types and quantities of food consumed by the population as a whole, as well as by particular high-risk groups. Further modern concerns include public perception of and the potential risks from food additives, contaminants and food-borne diseases such as bovine spongiform encephalopathy. As in the UK, European countries, Japan and the USA all collect dietary information for public health and commercial purposes.[50]

There are three major sources of dietary data. The long-established National Food Survey (NFS),[51] originally set up in 1940 to monitor the adequacy of the wartime diet, collects data on household food purchases. Since 1994, information has been collected about food eaten outside the home, thereby correcting a long-standing gap in the data. The survey is useful in analysing changes in food purchases at household level. Using the National Food Survey to estimate individual intake is problematic, because food may be distributed unequally between members of the household, and information on food wasted or thrown away is not collected. A general review of the problems with the National Food Survey was published in *Statistics in society.*[52]

The second source is a programme of nutrition surveys of different age groups initiated in the early 1990s following the success of the survey of adults.[53] The National Diet and Nutrition Surveys (NDNS)[53–7] collect information about individual dietary intakes. These include detailed information at an individual level, which is unavailable from the National Food Survey.

In order to estimate the nutritional value of the food purchases in the National Food Survey and individual diets in the National Diet and Nutrition Surveys, the composition of the foods bought or eaten must be known. This information can be found in *McCance and Widdowson's The composition of food and its supplements.*[58]

These three major sources of information are described in detail below. In addition, the Family Expenditure Survey and the Family Resources Survey (described in Chapter 2) collect information about household expenditure on food and drink. Several ad-hoc surveys, not described in detail here, provide population-based dietary data. They include the British arm of the European Prospective Investigation into Cancer and Nutrition (EPIC) study,[59] the Medical Research Council's National Survey of Health and Development[60] and the 'Whitehall II' study of civil servants.[61]

National Food Survey

Since the Second World War, the National Food Survey[51] has documented food purchases, expenditure and nutrient intakes at household level. Initially, the wartime Ministry of Food used the survey to monitor consumption amongst the urban working classes, the most vulnerable group under rationing. Now the survey is commissioned by the Ministry of Agriculture, Fisheries and Food (MAFF). Since 1950, samples of households in Great Britain have been randomly selected from the Post Office address file, which later became its postcode file. Results are published in summary form on a quarterly basis.

More detailed annual reports, including a commentary, appear in November of the year following data collection. Tabulations according to the income group of the head of household are a standard feature of the reports. In 1985, the annual reports switched to a glossy format with selective presentation of results and a section of special analyses. For example, the report for 1992 looked at cooking and spreading-fat purchases over the years 1975–92. Additional detailed data can be found in the *Compendium of results of the National Food Survey*. The 1996 compendium costs £177.00, with a discounted price of £43.00 to academics, but is available for public inspection free of charge at the Ministry of Agriculture, Fisheries and Food library. Anyone wishing to inspect one should ring 020 7270 8000 and give 24 hours' notice. National Food Survey datasets for 1974 onwards are available from the Data Archive at the University of Essex.

The ONS has conducted the National Food Survey since 1996. Fieldwork is conducted throughout the year, thus capturing seasonal effects in food purchases. Interviewers contact selected households, with some 65 per cent agreeing to keep a 7-day diary of all food and drink purchases, home-grown produce and gifts of food and drink coming into the home. The participating household member, who is the person doing most of the food shopping, is also asked to record details of each meal and snack, and who was present or absent for each meal.

In 1992, two important improvements were made to the National Food Survey protocol. Recording was extended to include confectionery and soft and alcoholic drinks. In half of the sample, each member of the household over the age of 11 is now asked to keep an individual diary of food and drink eaten outside the home. Data on eating out were released for publication from 1994, following 2 years of development.

The National Food Survey data series allows examination of food consumption and nutrient intake trends. Longitudinal analyses suggest, for example, that household food energy and fat intake decreased by some 15 per cent between 1980 and 1990. A likely explanation is that there was an increase in sedentary habits over this period, as well as some reductions in high-fat food purchases. A time bias may also contribute to the apparent trends, since food prepared at home tended to form a decreasing proportion of the diet during the 1980s.

Analysis of trends using National Food Survey data has been taken a step further with the use of statistical modelling. This allows the estimation of nutrient intake for different types of individuals, despite the fact that the unit of observation in the National Food Survey is the household. The effect on food purchases of variations in household composition, according to age, sex and occupation, permits the estimation of average nutrient intakes for children, men and women. Trends have been examined in this way in a secondary analysis of the data series from 1979,[62] with the latest being published in 1997.[63] Because data about eating out, confectionery and alcoholic drinks were not collected before 1992, the contributions these items make to the diet are consequently discounted. In 1996, the National Food Survey was extended to include Northern Ireland.

National Diet and Nutritional surveys

The National Diet and Nutrition Survey programme was set up following on from the Dietary and Nutritional Survey of British Adults.[53] Fieldwork for this survey, of 2197 adults aged 16–64, was carried out in 1986/7 under the supervision of the OPCS, and the main report appeared in 1990.[53]

The National Diet and Nutrition surveys programme is jointly funded and directed by the Department of Health and the Ministry of Agriculture, Fisheries and Food. Its purpose is to monitor food consumption patterns, nutrient intake and related physiological factors in various age groups. The surveys are undertaken in England, Wales and Scotland but not in Northern Ireland. The first survey in this programme, conducted by the OPCS, was of young children and its reports were published in 1995.[54,55] An informed source indicates that the commentaries on these tables were closely scrutinised by government officials and, to accommodate government ideology at that time, the authors were not permitted to use the terms 'poverty' or 'social deprivation'.

Subsequent surveys have gone out to tender, in line with national and European Union requirements. Accordingly, the survey of people aged 65 years and over, which included a sample of men and women living in institutions, was contracted to Social and Community Planning Research, now known as the National Centre for Social Research, and the Department of Epidemiology and Public Health at University College London. Fieldwork for this survey was completed in September 1995 and the main report was published in 1998.[56] Fieldwork for a survey covering 4–18 year olds was undertaken during 1997, with publication expected in 2000. A further study of adults aged 19–64 years is expected to start in 2000.

In all surveys of diet, it is difficult to achieve an accurate picture. The first survey of adults, carried out in 1986/7 by the OPCS, is probably the largest survey to date to utilise the 7-day weighed intake method.[53] This method is widely regarded as one of the most precise techniques for assessing diet. Yet, because of the complexity of contemporary eating patterns, the many factors which influence dietary behaviour and the unavoidable intrusiveness of any attempt to measure diet, the adults' survey data are not free of bias. This is a universal problem with dietary surveys, making interpretation of their results a difficult task.

The most important source of measurement error in the survey of adults is probably reporting bias. Many participants apparently under-recorded food intake, consciously or unconsciously, during the period of the survey. This is evident because the dietary energy intakes calculated for some individuals from food tables were implausibly low when compared with the basal metabolic rates. This measure of minimal energy requirements can be calculated with some confidence for a group of people with a set of simple formulae involving the sex, age and weight of the subject. Bearing in mind the imprecision of this measure for individuals, 'energy under-reporters' can be defined as people reporting energy intakes of less than 1.2 times the calculated basal metabolic rate, providing barely enough energy to watch TV, let alone to fuel an active life. Thus defined, 30 per cent of men and 47 per cent of women in the survey of adults appear to have under-reported food intake.[64]

Widespread under-reporting has ramifications for the interpretation of many of the survey's results. For instance, the observed relationships between nutrient intakes and obesity will tend to be distorted by this reporting bias. Obese people are more likely to be energy under-reporters,[61] and the Medical Research Council Dunn Nutrition Laboratory has shown that obese people may selectively under-report consumption of fat and sugar-rich foods. These and related problems can, to an extent, be compensated for by the collection of samples which yield 'objective' diet-related measurements or biomarkers such as urinary sodium, serum ferritin and plasma vitamin E concentration. Biomarkers are not available for many nutrients, however.

Despite the difficulties outlined above, the survey of adults and the later surveys of elderly people and children are a large step forward in the monitoring of the nation's diet. These surveys provide information on variations in intakes of some fifty food groups, dietary fatty acids, protein, carbohydrates, sugars, vitamins and minerals. They are analysed by Registrar General's social class and region, employment status and other demographic variables. The surveys of children and people aged over 65 also included an examination of oral health.[55,57] In addition to the substantial official report, the adults and pre-school children survey datasets are available to academic and other researchers from the Data Archive. Subsequent surveys will also be available from the same source.

McCance and Widdowson's *The composition of foods*

Publication of food composition tables began at least as long ago as 1921. *McCance and Widdowson's The composition of foods* is in its fifth edition, and nine supplements have appeared at intervals since 1988. These publications contain the composition of some 3000 food items analysed for over 100 nutrients and fatty acids. This represents a substantial proportion of the 10 000 or so foods and food products available in the UK, but it is difficult to keep it up to date, with about 200 new products being added every month.[51] Most of the data are derived from chemical analysis, though some table entries are estimated from analyses of similar food items. The tables have a number of uses, including providing estimates of nutrient intake from dietary surveys. Exact nutrient content will depend on how the food is stored and cooked.

In 1987, the Ministry of Agriculture, Fisheries and Food, which previously had sole responsibility for the food tables, made an agreement with the Royal Society of Chemistry for the publication of tables, amounting to a semi-privatisation. Copyright of this public asset has now been returned to the Crown. An electronic version of each supplement is available. These are difficult to use as they require considerable additional checking and editing in order to produce an integrated table. The contract for the compilation of the sixth edition was awarded to the Institute of Food Research, Norwich. When completed, the paper version of the sixth edition will be published by the Royal Society of Chemistry. The electronic versions of all supplements and the fifth edition are available from The Stationery Office.

Reports of surveys of diet and nutrition

National Food Survey
Ministry of Agriculture, Fisheries and Food. *National Food Survey.* London: TSO, published annually.

National Diet and Nutrition Survey Programme
Gregory J, Foster K, Tyler H, Wiseman M. *The Dietary and Nutritional Survey of British Adults.* London: HMSO, 1990.

Gregory J, Collins DL, Davies PSW, Hughes JM, Clarke PC. *National Diet and Nutrition Survey: children aged 1.5 to 4.5 years. Vol. I Report of Diet and Nutrition Survey.* London: HMSO, 1995.

Gregory J, Hinds K. *National Diet and Nutrition Survey: children aged 1.5 to 4.5 years. Vol. II Report of the Dental Survey.* London: HMSO, 1995.

Finch S, Doyle W, Lowe C, Bates CJ, Prentice A, Smithers G, Clarke PC. *National Diet and Nutrition Survey: people aged 65 years and over, Vol. I.* London: TSO, 1998.

Steele JG, Sheiham A, Marcenez W, Walls AWG. *National Diet and Nutrition Surveys: people aged 65 years and over. Report of the oral health survey.* London: TSO, 1998.

McCance and Widdowson's *The composition of foods*
Holland B, Welch AA, Unwin D, Buss D, Paul AA, Southgate DAT. *McCance and Widdowson's The composition of foods,* 5th edition. Cambridge: Ministry of Agriculture, Fisheries and Food and Royal Society of Chemistry, 1991.

Contact address and web site

Ministry of Agriculture, Fisheries and Food
Whitehall Place (West Block)
London SW1E 6QW
Telephone: 020 7270 3000
Food helpline: 0645 335577
Web site: http://www.maff.gov.uk

References

1. Health and Safety Commission. *Health and safety statistics 1996/97*. London: HSE Books, 1997, published annually from 1992/3.
2. Office of Population Censuses and Surveys Health and Safety Executive. *Occupational health*. Decennial Supplement. Series DS No. 10. London: HMSO, 1995.
3. Meredith SK, Taylor VM, McDonald JC. Occupational respiratory disease in the UK 1989: a report to the British Thoracic Society and the Society of Occupational Medicine by the SWORD project group. *British Journal of Industrial Medicine* 1991; **48**: 292–8.
4. Cherry NM, Beck M, Owen-Smith V. Surveillance of occupational skin diseases in the United Kingdom. In: *Proceedings of the* 9th *International Symposium on Epidemiology in Occupational Health*. US Department of Health and Human Services, Cincinatti: NIDSH, 1994: 608–10.
5. Health and Safety Executive. *Self reported work related illness survey*. Research Paper 33. London: HSE, 1993.
6. Doll R, Peto R. Quantitative estimates of avoidable risks of cancer in the US today. *Journal of the National Cancer Institute* 1981; **66**: 1191–308.
7. Stevens G. Workplace injury: a view from Health and Safety Executive trailer to the 1990 Labour Force Survey. *Employment Gazette* 1992; **100**(12).
8. Miners win historic claim. *Guardian*, Saturday, January 24, 1998.
9. Nichols T. Problems in monitoring safety in British manufacturing at the end of the twentieth century. In: Williams R, Guy W, eds. *Interpreting official statistics*. London: Routledge, 1996: 115–20.
10. Nichols T. Industrial injury statistics. In: Dorling D, Simpson S, eds. *Statistics in society*. London: Arnold, 1998, pp. 263–70.
11. Health and Safety Statistics 1988–1989. Employment Gazette Occasional Supplement No. 1. *Employment Gazette* 1990; **98**(11).
12. Health and Safety Statistics 1989–1990. Employment Gazette Occasional Supplement No. 2. *Employment Gazette* 1991; **99**(9).
13. Health and Safety Statistics 1990–1991. Employment Gazette Occasional Supplement No. 3. *Employment Gazette* 1992; **100**(9).
14. Burridge R, Ormandy D, eds. *Unhealthy housing: research, remedies and reform*. London: E & FN Spon, 1993.
15. Ineichen G. *Homes and health: how housing and health interact*. London: E & FN Spon, 1993.
16. Leather P, Mackintosh S, Rolfe S. *Papering over the cracks – housing conditions and the nation's health*. London: National Housing Forum, 1994.

17. Standing Conference on Public Health. *Housing, homelessness and health.* London: Nuffield Provincial Hospitals Trust, 1994.
18. Shelter. *Behind closed doors.* London: Shelter, 1998.
19. Barker D, Osmond C. Inequalities in health in Britain. *British Medical Journal* 1987; **294**: 749–52.
20. Kellett J. Health and housing. *Journal of Psychosomatic Research* 1989; **33**: 255–68.
21. Pleace N, Quilgars D. Health, housing and access to health care services in London. In: Burrows R, Pleace N, Quilgars D. *Homelessness and social policy.* London: Routledge, 1997; pp. 149–58.
22. McCarthy P, Byrne D, Harrison S, Keithley J. Respiratory conditions: effect of housing and other factors. *Journal of Epidemiological Community Health* 1985; **39**: 15–19.
23. Bines W. The health of single people. In: Burrows R, Pleace N, Quilgars D. *Homelessness and social policy.* London: Routledge, 1997; pp. 132–48.
24. Kearns R, Smith C. Homelessness and mental health. *Professional Geographer* 1994; **46**(4): 418–42.
25. Wright JD, Weber E. *Homelessness and health.* Washington DC: McGraw-Hill, 1987.
26. Council of Mortgage Lenders. *Housing Finance Quarterly.* Published quarterly.
27. Department of Social Security. *Family Resources Survey.* London: TSO, published annually.
28. Green H. *Private renting in five localities.* London: HMSO, 1994.
29. Carey S. *Private renting in England.* London: HMSO, 1995.
30. Green H. *Shared accommodation in five localities.* London: HMSO, 1994.
31. London Research Centre. *London housing statistics.* London: London Research Centre, 1994.
32. Leather P, Morrison T. *The state of UK housing.* Bristol: Policy Press, 1998.
33. Chartered Institute of Public Finance and Accountancy. *Homelessness Actuals.* London: CIPFA, published annually.
34. Chartered Institute of Public Finance and Accountancy. *Housing Rent Actuals.* London: CIPFA, published annually.
35. Office for National Statistics. *Family spending.* London: TSO, published annually.
36. Watson S, Austerberry H. *Housing and homelessness: a feminist perspective.* London: Routledge & Kegan Paul, 1986.
37. Watson S. Definitions of homelessness: a feminist perspective. *Critical Social Policy* 1984; **11**(4): 60–73.
38. Greve J, Currie E. *Homelessness in Britain.* York: Joseph Rowntree Foundation, 1990.
39. Hutson S, Liddiard M. *Youth homelessness: the construction of a social issue.* Basingstoke: Macmillan Press, 1994.
40. Widdowfield R. The limitations of official homelessness statistics. In: Dorling D, Simpson L, eds. *Statistics in society.* London: Arnold, 1999, pp. 181–8.
41. Citron K, Southern A, Dixon M. *Out of the shadows: detecting and treating tuberculosis among single homeless people.* London: Crisis, 1995.
42. Cohen C, Thompson K. Homeless mentally ill or mentally ill homeless. *American Journal of Psychiatry* 1992; **149**(6): 816–21.
43. Geddes J, Newton R, Young G, Bailey S, Freeman C, Priest R. Comparison of the prevalence of schizophrenia among residents of hostels for homeless people in 1966 and 1992. *British Medical Journal* 1994; **308**: 1125–7.
44. Anderson I, Kemp P, Quilgars D. *Single homeless people.* London: HMSO, 1993.
45. Stern R, Stilwell B, Heuston J. *From the margins to the mainstream: collaboration in planning services with single homeless people.* London: Church Action with the Unemployed and West Lambeth Health Authority, 1989.
46. Fisher N, Turner S, Pugh R, Taylor C. Estimating the number of homeless and

homeless mentally ill in North Westminster by using capture–recapture analysis. *British Medical Journal* 1994; **308**: 27–30.

47. Wright J, Everitt R. *Homelessness in Boston.* Sleaford: Shelter Lincolnshire, 1994.
48. Davis R, Dhooge Y. *Living with mortgage arrears.* London: HMSO, 1993.
49. Nettleton S, Burrows N. Home ownership, insecurity and health in the United Kingdom. In: Peterson A, Waddell C, eds. *Health matters.* Hemel Hempstead: Allen and Unwin, 1998.
50. Schmitt A, Chambolle M, Millstone E, Brunner E, Lobstein T. Nutritional surveillance in Europe. IPTS/ESTO Task C Project No. 10 1998. See web site http://esto.jrc.es/cg-ga/exsumm97.html
51. Ministry of Agriculture, Fisheries and Food. *National Food Survey 1996.* London: TSO, 1997.
52. Shaw M. *Measuring eating habits: some problems with the National Food Survey.* In: Dorling D, Simpson S, eds. *Statistics in society.* London: Arnold, 1999, pp. 140–7.
53. Gregory J, Foster K, Tyler H, Wiseman M. *The Dietary and Nutritional Survey of British Adults.* London: HMSO, 1990.
54. Gregory J, Collins DL, Davies PSW, Hughes JM, Clarke PC. *National Diet and Nutrition Survey: children aged 1.5 to 4.5 years.* Vol. I, *Report of Diet and Nutrition Survey.* London: HMSO, 1995.
55. Gregory J, Hinds K. *National Diet and Nutrition survey: children aged 1.5 to 4.5 years.* Vol. II, *Report of the Dental Survey.* London: HMSO, 1995.
56. Finch S, Doyle W, Lowe C, Bates CJ, Prentice A, Smithers G, Clarke P. *National Diet and Nutrition Survey: people aged 65 years and over,* Vol. I, London: TSO, 1998.
57. Steele JG, Sheiham A, Marcenez W, Walls AWG. *National Diet and Nutrition surveys: people aged 65 years and over. Report of the Oral Health Survey.* London: TSO, 1998.
58. Holland B, Welch AA, Unwin D, Buss D, Paul AA, Southgate DAT. *McCance and Widdowson's The composition of foods, 5th edition.* Cambridge: Ministry of Agriculture, Fisheries and Food and Royal Society of Chemistry, 1991.
59. Riboli E, Kaaks R. The EPIC Project: rationale and study design. *International Journal of Epidemiology* 1997; **26** (Suppl. 1): S6–14.
60. Braddon FEM, Wadsworth MEJ, Davies JMC, Cripps HA. Social and regional differences in food and alcohol consumption and their measurement in a national birth cohort. *Journal of Epidemiology and Community Health* 1988; **42**: 341–9.
61. Stallone DD, Brunner EJ, Bingham SA, Marmot MG. Dietary assessment in Whitehall II. The influence of reporting bias on apparent socioeconomic variation in nutrient intakes. *European Journal of Clinical Nutrition* 1997; **51**: 815–25.
62. Chesher A. Changes in the nutritional content of British household food supplies during the 1980s. In: *Household food consumption and expenditure 1989: annual report of the National Food Survey Committee.* London: HMSO, 1990; pp. 24–39.
63. Chesher A. Semi parametric estimation of nutrient intake–age relationships. *Journal of the Royal Statistical Society, Series A.* 1997; **160**: 389–428.
64. Pryer JA, Brunner EJ, Elliott P, Nichols R, Dimond H, Marmot MG. Who complied with COMA 1984 dietary fat recommendations among a nationally representative sample of British adults in 1986–7 and what do they eat? *European Journal of Clinical Nutrition* 1995; **49**: 718–28.

7 Environment matters

INDUSTRIAL POLLUTION, AIR POLLUTION AND TRANSPORT

Mary Taylor, Susan Kerrison, Sue Hare,
Stephen Potter, Adrian Davis and Ben Lane

Industrial pollution: a limited right to know
Air pollution
Transport and health

Industrial pollution, air pollution and transport are highly interrelated. The data collected about them are continually changing, driven by European Union legislation, public concern and increases in scientific knowledge. The first section of this chapter describes the limited data that are available on emissions of pollutants to the environment from industrial processes and the problems members of the public encounter in gaining access to them. Until recently, the data have been held on a number of separate public registers in different geographical locations. The new Chemical Release Inventory is an attempt to provide a central register of all releases from the more polluting industries, but the data held on this register are difficult to interpret because of the lack of standardisation.

The statistics available on air pollution present different problems. Data are collected from numerous different monitoring sites and made publicly available almost instantaneously on the worldwide web. Despite this, it is unclear whether the most damaging pollutants are being monitored and whether other pollutants are monitored in the most useful way. The primary source of the major air pollutants is now road transport, but transport statistics provide little information to further understanding of how road use may be controlled. The section concludes by considering the other impacts transport has on health. Reduction in road accidents was set as a target in the green paper *Our healthier nation*, but the road accidents statistics are notoriously unreliable, so it will be difficult to know whether the targets have been achieved.

The Department of the Environment, Transport and the Regions (DETR) and the Environment Agency, which is responsible for enforcing the environmental legislation, are the main government bodies responsible for pollution and transport. The contact details and web sites for each are shown later in this chapter.

Industrial pollution: a limited right to know

Every day, thousands of industries produce waste streams containing a myriad of different substances, which are released into the environment or transferred to disposal facilities, such as landfills, incinerators or sewage treatment works. These facilities are themselves further sources of environmental pollution. The majority of these 'transactions' are covered by legal rules of one sort or another, so it might be presumed that they would generate data to allow the impact of these activities to be assessed. The reverse is true. Relatively little information is collected about substances released from industrial sources, and the few data collected are often inconsistent and difficult to collate.

It may seem surprising that monitoring of releases can be rather haphazard, but access to information about industrial pollution is a battleground where public and private interests clash. On the one side industry argues that increased costs of monitoring and reporting emissions would be burdensome and result in insignificant or uncertain gains in environmental protection. On the other side lie arguments for the public's right to know about releases of chemicals and concerns about their environmental impacts. Companies are likely to regard their data about the chemical composition of the substances they release as private unless there is legislation to the contrary. Historically, the presumption is of secrecy rather than disclosure.

Another factor which limits the availability of information is our vast ignorance and uncertainty about the toxicological and ecotoxicological effects of the majority of substances in use. Some 100 000 different chemical substances have been catalogued in commercial use,[1] but there are national air quality standards for only eight of them.[2] If there are no benchmarks or acceptable levels, then it can be difficult for a regulator to insist on particular controls or monitoring, even assuming that some concern has been identified. This leads to considerable gaps in our knowledge of emissions. For example, hormone-mimicking 'gender bender' chemicals have caused alarm, but there are virtually no data on emissions. These substances affect the development of reproductive systems. They are suspected to decrease sperm counts and to increase the incidence of certain cancers and other reproductive abnormalities. Although they are active in minute quantities, a special investigation in 1998 revealed that one ICI plant alone is discharging tens of tonnes of them into the Tees estuary.[3] This information was not available from the routine monitoring data.

The regulatory system

Legislation to control industrial pollution developed considerably during the nineteenth and twentieth centuries and there are now a large number of laws on the subject. The historical development led to a patchwork of bodies having different responsibilities for pollution control, and identifying which of them regulates what can be confusing at first. Regulation has also developed separately in Scotland and Northern Ireland, although membership of the European Union now means that many national environmental laws have a common origin as a European Directive.

The formation of the Environment Agency in England and Wales and the Scottish Environmental Protection Agency (SEPA) brought some functions together. These bodies have major responsibilities for protecting the environment, extending well beyond controlling polluting processes. They are government-funded quangos and have brought together the former waste regulators, water pollution regulators and industrial inspectorates. So far, there is no such quango in Northern Ireland, and sections of the Department of the Environment still have responsibilities there. Local authorities also have some responsibilities, particularly for smaller industrial sites. Water companies with sewage treatment works connected to industrial sites via sewers are also involved. Tables 7.1 and 7.2 summarise the functions of the regulatory agencies, their areas of responsibility and how to access the information they collect. Table 7.1 summarises the sources of data about major industrial processes covered by 'Integrated pollution

Table 7.1 Sources of information on industrial emissions covered by 'Integrated pollution control' processes

Country	Regulator	Release inventory	Other release data available?	Location of registers
England and Wales	Environment Agency	Chemical Release Inventory (CRI)	Yes	Regional offices of Environment Agency, plus copies at local authority
Scotland	Scottish Environmental Protection Agency (SEPA)	–	Yes	Regional offices of Scottish Environmental Protection Agency, plus copies at local authority
Northern Ireland	Industrial Pollution Inspectorate, Environment and Heritage Service of Department of the Environment, Northern Ireland	–	Registers being established; some data may be available on request	Inquire with the Industrial Pollution Inspectorate

Table 7.2 Sources of information on industrial emissions from processes not covered by 'Integrated pollution control'

Medium	Country	Regulator	Annual release inventory?	Other release data available?	Location of registers
Air	England and Wales	Local authority	–	Yes	Local authority
Air	Scotland	Scottish Environmental Protection Agency	–	Yes	Regional offices of Scottish Environmental Protection Agency, plus copies at local authority
Air	Northern Ireland	Local authority or Industrial Pollution Inspectorate	–	System being established	
Water	England/Wales/ Scotland	Environment Agency/ Scottish Environmental Protection Agency	–	Yes	Regional offices of Environment Agency/Scottish Environmental Protection Agency

Table 7.2 Continued

Medium	Country	Regulator	Annual release inventory?	Other release data available?	Location of registers
Water	Northern Ireland	Environment and Heritage Service	–	Yes	Environment and Heritage Service
Sewer discharges	England and Wales	The water service company responsible for sewerage	–	Confidential	Permits available at offices of sewerage service provider
Sewer discharges	Scotland	Water authority	–	On request	Inquire with water authority
Sewer discharges	Northern Ireland	Water Service of Department of the Environment Northern Ireland	–	No (but change afoot)	Inquire with Water Service

control' (IPC), while table 7.2 summarises sources of data about processes which are not covered. 'Integrated pollution control' is described below.

Industrial pollution control is usually exercised through issuing a legal permit to a company. The permit will set out various conditions of operation, often including specified limits on release of pollutants into the environment, along with monitoring and reporting requirements. Much of the monitoring is done by companies themselves, but the regulatory bodies also have powers to take samples. The permits and conditions are usually, but not always, regarded as public information, as are the monitoring data. How to access this information is explained below, in the section on public registers.

Most of the monitoring data on emissions are presented as the concentration of a substance in a waste stream. Further information is therefore required on the volume released in order to calculate how much of a substance is actually entering the environment. This information is often not readily available. The Chemical Release Inventory is of particular interest, because it attempts to quantify total quantities of a substance released on an annual basis, making comparisons between sites possible.

The Chemical Release Inventory and 'Integrated pollution control' of major industrial processes

Around 2000 industrial sites are regulated through 'Integrated pollution control', which was established under the Environmental Protection Act 1990. They are regulated by the Environment Agency in England and Wales, the Scottish Environmental Protection Agency in Scotland and, more recently, the Industrial Pollution Inspectorate of the Environment and Heritage Service in Northern Ireland.

'Integrated pollution control' processes are those regarded as the more polluting or complex industrial processes. These are controlled with a view to preventing or minimising pollution of air, land and water. Sometimes, reducing pollution of one medium leads to increasing pollution of another medium. 'Integrated pollution control' also tries to find the best practicable environmental option, bearing in mind the possible trade-offs between media. This is why it is called 'integrated'. Since the regulators have to consider all three media, at least some data are available for emissions to air, land and water.

One industrial site might be operating several different types of processes and each process will receive a separate permit, legally termed an 'authorisation'. Each permit has various conditions for operation, usually including requirements to monitor for specified substances in waste streams at specified frequencies. Substances are usually reported as a concentration, for example milligrammes per litre. The monitoring data are used, in the first instance, to judge performance of the plant against the imposed emission limits. The applications for permits, the permits themselves and monitoring reports are available in public registers in England, Wales and Scotland. In Northern Ireland, public registers were not set up until the late 1990s, although any monitoring data should be available under the environmental information law described below.

In 1991, it was proposed to produce an annual inventory of emissions from the 'Integrated pollution control' processes in England and Wales. Unfortunately, Scotland and Northern Ireland were not included in this plan. Industrial operators usually report data showing the concentration of each chemical in a waste stream during the year, but at the end of each year they must report the total quantities released. These reports are filed on public registers. An example, the report for 1996 for Britannia Zinc Limited, a smelting company operating at Avonmouth, Bristol, under authorization AS7396, is shown in Table 7.3.

The Environment Agency also combines the data into a centrally held database, which forms the Chemical Release Inventory (CRI). This consists of nearly 10 000 records for approximately 2000 processes and over 400 different substances. On the face of it, this sounds like a useful resource. Unfortunately, the Chemical Release Inventory has fundamental flaws which have seriously limited its use so far.

The main problem is that reporting requirements have not been applied consistently. The Chemical Release Inventory is based on permit data rather than being constructed from, say, a standard list of pollutants. This has led to inconsistencies in reporting and a lack of reporting requirements for many substances. It was set up at a time when the government did not want to impose any extra monitoring costs on industry, so the Environment Agency could require only reports on chemicals already mentioned in the existing permits.[4] Pollution inspectors from the Environment Agency had varied in their monitoring requirements, even when writing permits for similar processes. For example, one incinerator quantified releases of forty-one substances in 1994, while another quantified releases of only four substances. Out of a total of fifteen municipal waste incinerators, ten reported dioxin releases, but five did not, even though all incineration processes will produce some dioxins and all of these incinerators had permits. Although over 400 chemicals are on the list, on average only about five chemicals are reported per process.

It is impossible for the general public to know which substances are released but not reported by any particular industrial process. Easy compar-

Table 7.3 Chemical release data for Britannia Zinc Limited, Avonmouth, Bristol, during 1996

Medium	Substance	Actual release	Annual limit
Air	Sulphur dioxide	3316 tonnes	None
	Sulphur trioxide	8.7 tonnes	None
	Particulates	191 tonnes	None
	Lead	19.5 tonnes	47.3 tonnes
	Zinc	49.6 tonnes	96.4 tonnes
	Cadmium	1.6 tonnes	6.1 tonnes
	Arsenic	661 kilograms	None

Note: some releases may be indirectly controlled through other conditions of operation.
Source: adapted from Environment Agency public register information.

isons of emissions are impossible because so much of the information is inconsistent or missing. Emission inventories should be simple tools enabling the public to get some measure of pollution by comparing emissions between companies or from year to year. In the USA, such a public database, the Toxics Release Inventory (TRI), was begun in 1987. By 1995, it had a standard list of some 600 chemicals and its existence has led to considerable reduction in pollution.[5] Considerable efforts have been made to inform the public and to capture people's attention. For example, the inventory has been used as a basis to compile lists of 'top ten' polluters. The public then demanded improvements, and embarrassed companies set about removing themselves from leading positions in the league tables. In England and Wales, the whole spirit of the idea has been lost through compromises made in the way data are collected.

Another disadvantage of linking the Chemical Release Inventory to the permits is that the system is being phased in over several years, so not all industries have reported annual releases from the beginning. Industrial processes are divided into the six major sectors shown in Table 7.4, with further subdivisions. Processes in existence when the 'Integrated pollution control' system began have been brought under control in phases, beginning with the fuel and power sector in 1991/2, and ending with 'other' industries in 1995/6. New processes in any sector have had to seek immediate 'Integrated pollution control' authorisation before coming into operation.[6] This means that data for a full set of 'Integrated pollution control' processes were not available at the end of the 1990s, even though the first entries in the database date back to 1992. Given political will, an inventory could have applied to all sectors immediately, regardless of the rate of 'Integrated pollution control' authorisation.

Another shortcoming is that, in the database, environmental media are divided into only three classes: air, land and water. More useful analysis could occur if further distinctions were made. For example, to group releases to a sewer and sewage treatment works with releases direct to a river or coastal water makes no sense, environmentally speaking. Sewage treatment may result in transformation of the substance. Alternatively, it may be released to land in sewage sludge or to water in the liquid effluent from the works, or both. These are quite different environmental fates, but all are covered by the term 'releases to water'. The US Toxics Release Inventory distinguishes between many different fates, including waste destined for off-site recycling,

Table 7.4 The major industrial sectors of 'Integrated pollution control'

Sector	Processes included
Fuel and power	Power stations, petroleum sector
Waste disposal	Incineration, chemical recovery and production of waste-derived fuel
Mineral industry	Production of cement, glass, ceramics
Chemical industry	Production of pesticides, pharmaceuticals, organics and inorganic chemicals
Metal industry	Iron and steel, smelting and non-ferrous sectors
'Other'	Paper manufacturing, timber preparation, uranium processing

energy recovery, fugitive or non-point emissions, sewage treatment and underground injection. Information at this level of detail can lead to a much deeper understanding of trends in waste management.

Further information is masked by the way that the chemicals are reported as a group, even though their chemical or toxicological properties may vary. For instance, some reports refer to 'heavy metals'. Others specify groups of named metals or name individual metals or their compounds. 'Volatile organic compounds' have varying potential for causing photochemical smog. Over 95 per cent of solid waste releases have been called 'non-prescribed solids not otherwise specified', a particularly unhelpful description.

Even identification of a particular site can be a problem. Postcodes and addresses of 'Integrated pollution control' sites have to be obtained from a separate database and no unique identifying code is used for each industrial site. If a common identifier was used for each site, it could help link the Chemical Release Inventory database to other databases of information. For example, linkage could be made with water discharge data, also held by the Environment Agency, but under different legislation, described below. This would greatly increase the usefulness of the various sets of information.

Ironically, the best of industry's voluntary reports on environmental releases are more comprehensive, in at least some respects, than the Chemical Release Inventory. Some even show production data, giving an idea of the underlying reasons for increases or decreases in amounts reported. It may be worth approaching a particular industry to request further detail. For example, British Petroleum publishes annual reports, with data on a diskette relating to its individual sites.

To add further to the confusion, industrial sites which do not fall within the net of 'Integrated pollution control' do not report to the Chemical Release Inventory, even though they may have significant emissions. This includes sectors such as mining, gas drilling and exploration, sewage treatment, and landfill of waste, and smaller industries which do not meet the relevant threshold for 'Integrated pollution control' regulation. Industrial sites may even have a mixture of 'Integrated pollution control' processes and processes which are not covered, yet only emissions from the 'Integrated pollution control' processes will appear in the Chemical Release Inventory.

Some of the shortcomings of the Chemical Release Inventory database have been recognised, and moves to make the data more consistent began in 1997.[7] It is still likely to fall far short of a thoroughly comprehensive inventory. A new European law, not yet in force, on 'Integrated pollution prevention and control' (IPPC) will possibly increase the scope of data available to include information on resource consumption, energy and water use. Unfortunately, it will be some years before this system is fully in place.

Sites and processes not covered by 'Integrated pollution control'

AIR POLLUTION CONTROL

Smaller or less complex industrial processes which do not meet the criteria for 'Integrated pollution control' regulation but which still have potential for air pollution are also regulated. In England and Wales, the job falls to local authorities, which have responsibility for about 12 000 smaller industries. Paint sprayers, waste oil burners and small-scale incinerators are typical processes. Only air pollutants are regulated. Data are not held centrally, but local authorities hold public registers which show the permit details and any monitoring data required to be reported.

In Scotland, these processes are regulated by the Scottish Environmental Protection Agency. In Northern Ireland, where new legislation came into force only at the end of the 1990s, some processes are controlled by the Industrial Pollution Inspectorate, while others are controlled by the local authorities.

This system of local authority air pollution control was also established under the Environmental Protection Act 1990. These smaller industrial processes are often referred to as 'Part B' processes, as opposed to the 'Part A' processes regulated under 'Integrated pollution control'.

DISCHARGES TO WATER

Many industrial sites may also have water pollution permits, known as 'discharge consents'. These apply where an industry is discharging waste liquids directly into a river, estuary or coastal water. Sewage treatment works have such permits and can be a considerable source of water pollution, even when operating within permit limits. Permits are issued by the Environment Agency, the Scottish Environmental Protection Agency, and the Environment and Heritage Service in Northern Ireland. These bodies also monitor discharges and the results are kept in public registers, along with the permits.

The monitoring data show the concentrations of substances in the discharge. Total amounts of substances released are impossible to quantify without further information on the volumes discharged. Typical indicators of water pollution include ammonia, suspended solids and a measure of the oxygen demand of the effluent, but other substances will be measured, depending on the nature of the particular industry and its discharge.

TRADE EFFLUENT

Unless authorised under 'Integrated pollution control', permits to release liquid wastes to sewers are obtained from the water company that operates the sewerage service. In Scotland, the public water authorities fulfil this function, and in Northern Ireland it is exercised by the Water Service of the Department of the Environment, Northern Ireland. Many small and large businesses have such permits.

In England and Wales, the permits are public documents, and can be seen by contacting the relevant water company, but legislation explicitly forbids the release of any monitoring data. An individual industry might not mind disclosing the information, so it is worth contacting individual dischargers.

In Northern Ireland and Scotland, there is no public register of trade effluent permits as such at the time of writing, although the Scottish water authorities and the Water Service envisage improved public access in the future. Some information, including monitoring data in Scotland, may be obtained in response to a specific inquiry. The Environmental Information Regulations ought to be relevant here too, although arguments might arise about what should be 'commercially confidential'.

The permits contain information such as maximum permissible volumes and concentrations of various substances. These limits may bear little or no relationship to what actually goes into the sewer, so beware of assuming that the permits convey information about any quantities, or even types, of chemicals released.

RADIOACTIVE SUBSTANCES

The Environment Agency and Scottish Environmental Protection Agency also have responsibilities for registering users of radioactive materials. They maintain public registers of specified information, which includes the permits and any monitoring data relating to disposal of radioactive substances. At one time, the Environment Agency was considering producing an inventory of annual releases of radioactive substances. This inventory has received even less commitment within the agency than the Chemical Release Inventory and the idea appears to have fallen by the wayside. In Northern Ireland, local authorities maintain registers of the user registrations, but no monitoring data are available.

ATMOSPHERIC EMISSIONS INVENTORIES

Now that there are national air quality targets, there is considerable interest in better documentation of sources of air pollutants. Both national and local atmospheric emissions inventories are being compiled. These are described in the section on air pollution.

Public registers

It has been recognised, if not fully practised, that polluters and regulators should become more accountable to the public. Laws and systems have gradually allowed access to information about the regulation and performance of a polluter. Public registers, essentially sets of documents and/or computer files in a publicly accessible office, have been established by statute. These hold documents and related data specified by the relevant legislation.[8,9] Public registers can be visited, or requests sent to the registrar. A fee may be levied for photocopying and postage. The location of a particular piece of information in a register will depend on who the regulator is, the legislation under which it is available, and the geographic location of an industry. Most public registers are split into regional registers available at offices. Some register information is also sent to the relevant local authority, so it is worth checking with the regulator before travelling to find information.

For industrial pollution control, the registers hold items such as applications, permits and any monitoring data required by those permits. The evolution of this public information means that many of the available pollution data depend on the nature of the permits, which, in turn, depend on the scale and type of the industrial activity. If a sewage treatment works has a permit for certain water pollutants, but air pollutants are not specifically controlled, they are not monitored. Under different legislation, a power station may have a permit covering pollution of air, land and water. In this case, some air pollutants will be included in the monitoring programme. Other smaller industries are controlled with respect to air pollutants only.

The Environmental Information regulations

A further general right to environmental information, including pollution data but by no means limited to this, has been established by law. The Environmental Information regulations (SI 1992/3240) confer significant rights of access to information held by a public authority on the state of the environment or on matters which may affect the environment.[10-12] The regulations do not cover information which is privately held. If the data required are not available through public registers but are held by a public body, then it is worth requesting the information through these regulations. The type of information could include the results of a one-off survey or data which pre-date the establishment of a public register.

The regulations have undoubtedly improved rights to information, but the law contains grounds for refusing a request for information. In practice, public bodies reluctant to part with information have made considerable use of the clauses allowing these exceptions.[13] It can be all too easy to claim that work is 'still in the course of completion' or that it is 'commercially confidential'. Similarly, although 'reasonable' charges are permitted, there is scope for over-charging. The view that charges should extend only to the costs of copying the information and no attempt should be made to recoup costs of collection of the data or retrieval from filing systems or archives is supported by the Minister for Agriculture, Fisheries and Food.[14] Currently, such decisions can be difficult to challenge if the information holder is stubborn. It is to be hoped that future 'freedom of information' legislation will provide an effective and affordable appeal system.[15]

The way forward

When arguing for increased information, or better ways of presenting information, it is often claimed that 'the public' is not interested. 'Only consultants and pressure groups look at these data' is a typical comment, as if to justify lack of information or difficulties of access. Data are patchy, inconsistent and not easy to track down. Third parties, including pressure groups, researchers, the press, all of whom may represent the public interest, play a vital role in converting data into information with meaning for the public. Not only should all emissions be quantified or estimated and catalogued, but also active efforts should be made to pro-actively disseminate information and explain it to the public and polluters. Increasing availability of data via the internet has also greatly increased the potential for public access to information. Interactive facilities mean that a member of the public can be provided with local, relevant information without having to 'buy the whole book'.

Two examples of industrial pollution data which use the internet may be of interest to readers. The US Environmental Defense Fund uses data from the Toxics Release Inventory, while the Friends of the Earth site uses Chemical Release Inventory data. Details are given below. Both sites have been produced by environmental campaign groups, and show how quite detailed information can be put to use. In the USA, the proximity of schools to industrial sources of pollutants has been mapped by the Environmental Defense Fund, and the site links particular chemical names to databases of toxicology information. Armed with such information, citizens can begin to question industrial waste and demand cleaner environments. The site is a fine example of the 'right to know' developing into the right to understand and the right to act.

Key official publications

Department of the Environment, Transport and the Regions. *Digest of environmental statistics.* London: TSO, published annually.
Department of the Environment. *Environment facts: a guide to using public registers of environmental information.* London: TSO, 1996.
Environment Agency. *Improved consistency of reporting in the Chemical Release Inventory: a consultation document.* Bristol: Environment Agency, 1997.

Contact addresses and web sites

Friends of the Earth
26–28 Underwood Street
London N1 7JQ
Friends of the Earth's Chemical Release
Inventory
Web site: http://www.foe.co.uk/
factorywatch

Scottish Environmental Protection
Agency
Web site: http://www.sepa.org.uk/
index.htm

Environment and Heritage Service of
the Department of the Environment for

Northern Ireland
Web site: http://www.ehsni.gov.uk:
8080/enviprot/enviprot.htm

Information about the Atmospheric
Emissions Inventory
Web site: http://www.aeat.co.uk/
netcen/airqual/emissions/welcome.html
http://www.london-research.gov.uk/
emission/main.htm

Environmental Defense Fund's Toxics
Release Inventory
Web site: http://www.scorecard.org

Air pollution

A change of air? Current sources of air pollution

Road transport has now replaced fossil fuels as the major source of many air pollutants in the UK. Emissions of pollutants from this (shown in Table 7.5) now match or exceed emissions from other sources for all the most important pollutants except sulphur dioxide. In some cities, the contribution of road transport to pollution is even greater. For example, it is estimated that in London road transport is the source of over 75 per cent of emissions of nitrogen dioxide.[16]

The pollutants in Table 7.5 are called primary pollutants as they are emitted directly into the atmosphere. Ozone is an important secondary pollutant. Instead of being released directly, it is formed from the interaction between oxides of nitrogen and volatile organic compounds. The next section gives a brief overview of standards for air quality, monitoring networks and the data publicly available.

Table 7.5   Emissions of air pollutants in the UK by source, 1994

Air pollutant	Percentage of emission from each source			
	Road transport	Power stations	Industrial	Other, including domestic, other transport
Benzene	68	–	27	5
1,3 Butadiene	77	–	18	5
Carbon monoxide	90	1	3	6
Lead	65	2	33	10
Oxides of nitrogen	49	24	16	11
Volatile organic compounds	37	–	30	33
Particulates <10 microns (PM10)	26	15	42	17
Sulphur dioxide	2	65	24	9

Source: National Air Quality Strategy Consultation Draft.[17]

The health effects of poor air quality

Considerable evidence has now accumulated about the health effects of air pollution.[18–20] In the early 1990s, the Department of Health set up two committees to advise on this subject, the Advisory Group on the Medical Aspects of Air Pollution Episodes, and the Committee on the Medical Effects of Air Pollutants (COMEAP). They have produced reports on individual pollutants[21–4] and exposure to mixtures of pollutants.[18] Some individual pollutants such as ozone, sulphur dioxide, oxides of nitrogen and carbon monoxide are known to exacerbate the problems of people with lung disease and asthma. In high concentrations, they cause breathing problems in healthy people. Others, such as benzene and 1,3 butadiene, are known to cause cancer. The Committee on the Medical Effects of Air Pollutants attributed 12 500 premature deaths to ground-level ozone from all sources, 8100 to all particulate emissions, and 3500 to all sulphur dioxide emissions. It has been estimated that in the UK the additional hospital admissions account for 2.7 per cent of all hospital admissions for respiratory diseases in urban areas.[24]

Of particular concern are links between lung function impairments and motor traffic emissions. There is a growing consensus that the rise in childhood asthma is related to the ability of emissions to lower tolerance thresholds.[25] Small particles less than 10 microns in diameter (PM_{10}) associated with diesel emissions are increasingly believed to be associated with cancer and premature deaths. In a number of studies, correlations between neighbourhood traffic volumes and respiratory symptoms in children and hospital admissions for asthma have also been reported.[26,27] One report stated that 'recent evidence has convincingly shown that death rates from heart and lung disease are up to 37 per cent higher in cities with high levels of fine particulates'.[27]

As well as the effects of individual pollutants, there are concerns about 'pollution episodes', more commonly known as smogs. The Advisory Group on the Medical Aspects of Air Pollution Episodes identified three common types of episode[18] which occur under particular metereological conditions. These are summer smog, where the main pollutant is ozone, vehicle smog, where the main pollutants are oxides of nitrogen, and winter smog, where the main pollutants are sulphur dioxide and oxides of nitrogen. Under these conditions, concentration of pollutants, for example oxides of nitrogen, particulates or benzene, can build up over several days, causing high levels of pollution.

During these episodes of air pollution, there are increases in numbers of hospital admissions and of deaths of people who are already in poor health, such as those with chronic respiratory disease and elderly people with heart and lung diseases. For example, in December 1991, London experienced levels of nitrogen dioxide in excess of the World Health Organisation (WHO) guidelines for 4 days. At that time, the peak hourly concentration of oxides of nitrogen reached 423 parts per billion, exceeding the World Health Organisation guideline of 105 parts per billion by a factor of four.[17] During that week, numbers of deaths from respiratory diseases were over 20 per cent more than expected, and admissions to hospital for people aged 75 and over for obstructive lung disease were 55 per cent higher than expected.[20]

Using such studies, the Committee on the Medical Effects of Air Pollution estimated that air pollution is responsible for the premature deaths of between 12 000 and 24 000 people each year in the UK.[19] This is likely to be a low estimate, as little evidence is available about the damaging long-term effects of pollution incidents.

Setting standards and objectives for the National Air Quality Strategy

The National Air Quality Strategy (NAQS), first published in 1997,[2] received its first review in 1999.[28] A continuous programme of further reviews and revision has been promised and a new version was published in January 2000. The strategy aims to ensure that air quality throughout the country does not cause significant harm to human health or the environment. The Expert Panel on Air Quality Standards (EPAQS) was set up to advise on standards. These standards are similar to both the World Health Organisation guidelines and European Union standards, and have been adopted for eight pollutants which are widespread and known to affect human health. They are sulphur dioxide,[29] oxides of nitrogen,[30] black smoke or particulate matter which includes PM_{10},[31] benzene,[32] 1,3 butadiene,[33] carbon monoxide[34] and ozone.[35] In addition, the WHO standard has been adopted for lead. Other pollutants, such as $PM_{2.5}$ (particles less than 2.5 microns in size) and polycyclic aromatic hydrocarbons, may be considered for inclusion at a later date. Less information is available for these, but they are nevertheless causing increasing concern.

The National Air Quality Strategy standards are defined in terms of concentration of the pollutant and duration of the exposure. In other words, they take into account both what is known about the effects of long-term, low-level exposure and the possibility of pollution incidents. Unfortunately, there are gaps in the knowledge about the effects of long-term exposure to low levels of some pollutants and the effects of 'cocktails' of pollutants which city dwellers breathe every day. Therefore, the standards do not necessarily reflect 'safe' levels of exposure, but what is currently known about the risks from particular pollutants.[36]

In setting standards, the panel relied on the known effects of industrial exposure to individual pollutants and experimental evidence. In the case of benzene,[32] for example, there is no completely safe level for exposure, but an exposure of 500 parts per billion over a working lifetime is associated with negligible cancer incidence. The committee divided this level by ten to allow for living all the time in the ambient air, and by ten again for safety. The panel accordingly recommended a 5 parts per billion running annual mean as the immediate target and further recommended that this be reduced to 1 part per billion.[32] There is evidence that other substances, such as carbon monoxide and ozone, damage health in the short term. Therefore, standards measured in terms of 8-hour means have been set to reflect this.

In the strategy, the government also adopted policy targets or objectives for air quality (shown in Table 7.6) to be achieved by the year 2005. For benzene, 1,3 butadiene, carbon monoxide and lead, these are the same as the standards. For oxides of nitrogen, ozone, PM_{10} and sulphur dioxide, they allow for the standard to be exceeded on a number of occasions. For example, the objective for ozone is 50 parts per billion, running 8-hour mean measured as the 97th percentile. This means that the highest 3 per cent of the readings will be discounted or allowed to exceed the standard. In the case of ozone, this means

Table 7.6 Standards and objectives proposed in the National Air Quality Strategy to be achieved by the year 2005

Pollutant	Air quality standard	Measured as	Objective
Benzene	5 parts per billion	Running annual mean	The standard
1,3 butadiene	1 part per billion	Running annual mean	The standard
Carbon monoxide	10 parts per million	Running 8-hour mean	The standard
Lead	$0.5\ \mu g/m^3$	Annual mean	The standard
Nitrogen dioxide	150 parts per billion	1-hour mean	150 parts per billion, measured as the 99.9th percentile
	21 parts per billion	Annual mean	21 parts per billion annual mean
Ozone	50 parts per billion	Running 8-hour mean	50 parts per billion, measured as the 97th percentile
Particles (PM$_{10}$)	$50\ \mu g/m^3$	Running 24-hour mean	$50\ \mu g/m^3$ measured as the 99th percentile
Sulphur dioxide	100 parts per billion	15-minute mean	100 parts per billion measured as the 99th percentile

that the objective will be achieved if the standard is exceeded for less than 11 days or thirty-three 8-hour periods a year.

The analysis in the National Air Quality Strategy[2] suggests that for benzene, 1,3 butadiene and carbon monoxide, current UK concentrations are either close to or already below the standards in all areas, except at kerbside locations with very heavy traffic. The review published in 2000 suggested that these targets should be met by the end of 2003.

For ozone, oxides of nitrogen, PM$_{10}$ and sulphur dioxide, the situation is quite different. In 1994, recommended standards for ozone were exceeded at fifteen out of thirty-three stations for more than 10 days. Annual concentrations of oxides of nitrogen are above the standard in all urban monitoring stations. Hourly standards are exceeded at eighteen out of twenty-three stations on up to 20 days of the year, with some stations recording two or three times the hourly standard. For sulphur dioxide, only two out of twenty-three stations did not report exceeding the standards. In 1994, sites exceeded the standards on from three to forty occasions. The strategy published in 2000 tightened the hourly standard for nitrogen dioxide to 150ppb, allowed more excedances for particles and introduced new 1-and 24-hour mean standards for the ambient concentration of sulpher dioxide.

To achieve the air quality objectives, it is estimated that emissions of these pollutants will have to be reduced by between 60 and 80 per cent. Stricter standards on vehicle emissions and control of the composition of vehicle fuels mean that the objectives will be met for benzene, 1,3 butadiene, carbon dioxide and lead, but only if the growth in road transport is constrained. If the number of vehicles or road journeys increase, then the measures will not be adequate. These measures will have little effect on other pollutants, however.

Ozone is particularly difficult to control, as about half the ozone in southern Britain originates from pollution in continental Europe.

Local authorities have been given responsibility for ensuring that air quality in their area complies with the objectives set in the strategy. The first stage requires the authorities to review and assess local air quality. Where the review reveals areas which do not meet the National Air Quality Strategy's standards and objectives, the authority will be required to set up 'air quality management areas' and design and implement a programme to bring air quality to within the specified limits. It is likely that road transport pollution will be the reason for establishing most of these areas.

Monitoring air pollution

The number of monitoring sites increased significantly throughout the 1990s, with a large number of rural and urban sites currently recording pollutant levels for a wide range of air pollutants, not just those for which there are standards. The monitoring networks are funded by the Department of the Environment, Transport and the Regions and are operated on their behalf. Data from all of the air pollution networks in the UK are available on the National Environment Technology Centre web site, details of which are given below. The sites in the UK are organised in a series of networks, with three automatic networks and six sample-based networks.

THE AUTOMATIC MONITORING NETWORKS

A network of about one hundred automatic air-monitoring stations provides continuous 'real time' measures of ozone, oxides of nitrogen, carbon monoxide, sulphur dioxide, particulate matter (PM_{10}), and twenty-five types of hydrocarbons, including benzene and 1,3 butadiene. Not all of these pollutants are monitored at each site. A second network, based in urban areas, covers the majority of cities and monitors levels of ozone, oxides of nitrogen, carbon monoxide, sulphur dioxide and PM_{10} and provides measurements of background levels and 'hotspots' at the kerbside or in the vicinity of industrial plants. The third network, based in rural areas, concentrates on monitoring ozone, as this is considered to be the main pollutant in rural areas. Many local authorities also undertake significant automatic monitoring and their sites are being brought into national networks.

THE NON-AUTOMATIC MONITORING NETWORKS

There are six non-automatic monitoring networks. A nitrogen dioxide-monitoring network was set up in 1993 and consists of more than a 1000 sites operated by local authorities' monitors. A smoke and sulphur dioxide network, also operated by local authorities and previously known as the National Survey of Air Pollution, has been running since the 1950s. Long-term monitoring through this network has identified the fall in smoke and sulphur dioxide concentrations over this period. The multi-element network monitors eight trace elements – cadmium, chromium, copper, iron, manganese, lead, nickel and zinc – at five urban sites.

Other networks monitor lead and other elements in industrial areas, rural areas and over the North Sea. The acid deposition monitoring network, located at approximately thirty primarily rural sites, monitors rain samples for acidity and other ions, including sodium, sulphate, nitrate, potassium and calcium. Rural sulphur dioxide monitoring is conducted at around thirty sites. The information is used in conjunction with data from the acid deposition network to identify whether excessive quantities of pollution are falling on fresh waters and vegetation. The toxic organic micropollutants network consists of three urban sites in London, Middlesbrough and Manchester, and one rural site in Lancashire. At each site, seventeen species of dioxins are measured and ten species of polycyclic aromatic hydrocarbons.

Estimating emissions

As well as monitoring the quality of air, inventories are compiled of the sources of air pollution. These are used to interpret air quality statistics and to prepare strategies for reducing pollutants. Since 1987, the National Atmospheric Emissions Inventory has mapped estimated emissions of several pollutants on a 10 km^2 basis. This is published as the National Atmospheric Emissions Inventory (NAEI).[37] Data from it are published in the Department of the Environment, Transport and the Regions' *Digest of environmental statistics*.[38] A series of more comprehensive and detailed regional emissions inventories has been specially compiled for the Department of the Environment, Transport and the Regions. These inventories cover Merseyside, Bristol, Southampton/Portsmouth, Swansea/Port Talbot, Manchester, Middlesbrough, West Yorkshire and Glasgow. At the time of writing, the inventories for West Midlands and London had been published.[16,39]

The inventories estimate emissions from point sources such as industrial plants, broad areas sources, such as heating systems, and moving sources, such as roads, railways and livestock. For example, it has been estimated that in the area within the M25 motorway, livestock produce 181 tonnes of methane and other volatile organic carbons per year. The majority of emissions are estimated using local information on consumption of fossil fuels and vehicle kilometres travelled. Eight key pollutants are catalogued: oxides of nitrogen, sulphur dioxide, carbon monoxide, carbon dioxide, non-methane volatile organic compounds, benzene, 1,3 butadiene and PM_{10}. Where there are sufficient data, three additional pollutants – methane, total suspended particulates and black smoke – are included. Notable omissions are the potentially serious air pollutants lead, which is included in the National Air Quality Strategy, and polycyclic aromatic hydrocarbons, which are being considered for inclusion in the strategy. The reports are worth looking at to see what has been feasible and where gaps in the data have caused problems.

Air pollution: access to information

In response to pressure, particularly following the Environment Act of 1995, priority was given in the late 1990s to public access to information on air quality. Data from the UK air pollution monitoring networks are available in annual reports, usually a year or two in arrears. These reports are currently produced by the National Environment Technology Centre for the Department of the Environment, Transport and the Regions.[37] They are currently available in printed format, but the increasing volume of data produced from the expanding network of sites may mean that, in future, printed copies will become less readily available. Data are also accessible via the internet and available in CD-ROM format.

Each year, a *Digest of environmental statistics* is produced by the Department of the Environment, Transport and the Regions.[38] This includes a chapter on air quality and also gives the latest estimates for emissions of pollutants. Reports are also produced at various intervals by the government or its advisory groups. As well as reports on the effects of air pollution on health,[18,19,21–4] reports have covered emissions,[39] air quality,[40,41] critical levels of air pollution,[42] vehicle-related emissions[43] and acid deposition.[44]

Key official publications

Department of the Environment, Transport and the Regions. *Digest of environmental statistics.* London: TSO, published annually.

National Environment Technology Centre. *Air pollution in the UK.* London: DETR, published annually.

Department of Health Advisory Group on the Medical Aspects of Air Pollution Episodes. *Health effects of exposure to mixtures of air pollutants.* London: HMSO, 1995.

Department of Health Committee on the Medical Effects of Air Pollutants (COMEAP). *Quantification of the effects of air pollution on health in the UK.* London: TSO, 1998.

Department of the Environment. *The UK National Air Quality Strategy*, Cmd 3587. London: TSO, 1997.

Department of the Environment, Transport and the Regions. *The air quality strategy.* London: TSO, 2000.

London Research Centre. *London atmospheric emissions inventory.* London: London Research Centre,1997.

London Research Centre. *West Midlands atmospheric emissions inventory.* London: London Research Centre, 1996.

Contact addresses and web sites

Information on air quality can be obtained from local authorities, usually the Environmental Health Department, or from a variety of organisations including the following:

Atmospheric Research and Information Centre (ARIC)
Manchester Metropolitan University
Chester Street
Manchester M1 5GD
Telephone: 0161 247 1590/2/3

Fax: 0161 247 6332
Email: aric@mmu.ac.uk
Factsheets, newsletters, information
Web site: http://www.doc.mmu.ac.uk/aric/arichome.html

National Environment Technology Centre (NETCEN), AEA Technology
Culham
Abingdon
Oxfordshire OX14 3DB
Telephone: 01235 463072
Fax: 01235 463011
Air pollution data, information
Web site: http://www.aeat.co.uk/netcen/airqual/index.html

National Society for Clean Air and Environmental Protection (NSCA)
136 North Street
Brighton BN1 1RG
Telephone: 01273 326313
Fax: 01273 735802
Email: info@nsca.org.uk
Web site: http://www.greenchannel.com/nsca

London Research Centre, now part of Greater London Authority
81 Black Prince Road
London SE1 7SZ
Telephone: 020 7983 4000
Web site: http://www.london.gov.uk

Emissions inventory for several major cities
Web site: http://www.london-research.gov.uk/emission/webhtm.htm

Department of the Environment, Transport and the Regions Information, data
Web site: http://www.environment.detr.gov.uk/airquality/

Environmental Agency
industrial emissions reports
Web site: http://www.environment-agency.gov.uk/epns/isr.html

Air pollution data are available on page 106 of Teletext and pages 410–17 of Ceefax and are updated hourly. A freephone telephone service – 0800 55 66 77 – is also operated by the Department of the Environment, Transport and the Regions.

Environmental Protection Directorate, Environment and Heritage Service of the Department of the Environment for Northern Ireland
Web site: http://www.ehsni:8080/enviprot/ enviprot.htm

Transport and health

Statistics for a new agenda

During the 1990s, the nature of transport policy began to alter radically, giving rise to new information needs. In many cases, the statistics required to serve new transport policies simply do not exist. Furthermore, it has also been realised that the health impacts of transport go well beyond the traditional concerns of road traffic casualties and noise. These other health impacts of transport have only patchy statistical coverage. Added to this, inappropriate measures are used for the traditional concerns of road casualties and noise.

Overall, the impacts of transport on health are being re-evaluated. A new agenda is beginning to emerge, but the information sources needed to service this new agenda are only partially developed. In some cases, it is still unclear what they should be. So, although this section will point the reader to some available statistics, this subject is one in which research studies are likely to yield further information.

Transport policy's changing agenda

Since the Second World War, the traditional approach to transport planning in Britain has been an essentially reactive one of adjusting supply to demand. Predominantly, this has involved building new roads and enlarging old ones, coupled with the trimming of rail and bus services. Some exceptions were made due to 'social need', such as subsidising local bus, rail and ferry services, particularly in rural areas. Only in large cities, particularly London, has further expansion of road transport been rendered impossible by the sheer volume of traffic concentrated into a relatively small area. Even so, the general desire has been to provide as much road capacity as possible.

This traditional 'predict and provide' approach to transport planning has now lost its credibility.[45] Although concerns about the local and global environmental impacts of motor traffic are growing in importance, the major reason for this re-evaluation is the inability of the traditional road building policies to reduce traffic congestion. Forecast growth in traffic of 140 per cent or more simply cannot be accommodated.[46,47] Reports from the Standing Advisory Committee on Trunk Road Assessment[48] and the Royal Commission on Environmental Pollution,[49,50] among others, have shown the futility as well as the environmental and social costs of such an approach. Even British Road Federation research showed that a road-building programme of an uncontemplated vastness, beyond that which Britain's economy could sustain, would fail to stop congestion getting worse. As a policy response, road building will always fail, so policies to manage transport demand are the only option.

The full implications of the shift to demand management transport planning are only beginning to be realised. One important consequence is that the information system designed to service the old approach to transport policy is totally inadequate for the new agenda. Transport is a heavily regulated and taxed area and this provides many opportunities for data collection.

The core data source, the annual *Transport statistics, Great Britain*, published by the Department of the Environment, Transport and the Regions, gathers together statistics from survey and administrative sources. This reports government expenditure on transport, fuel consumption of vehicles, estimates of emissions, vehicle licensing data, traffic speeds, road and public transport accidents, freight transport, air and shipping, the capacity of the bus, coach and railway transport services, and the findings of surveys such as the International Passenger Survey and household travel surveys. The volume also contains some international comparisons and selected time trends.

To support past policies, very detailed information has been collected and reported about travel demand such as traffic levels, passengers carried by bus, rail and air, and transport supply, including roads by type and numbers of railway lines open. With policy shifting to manage the demand for travel, it is vitally important to understand how travel is generated, what elements of the travel-generating system are amenable to policy intervention and what parts are not. For example, the growth of double or triple income households, with members working in widely different locations, is increasing the distances travelled to work. It is difficult to envisage a transport policy approach to address this issue. A policy targeted at the choice of travel method could be more successful, however. When the response was simply to react to the growth in traffic, information on the nature of that traffic and the factors causing its generation was not of particular importance. Demand was taken as given and roads built.

The information needed to explore the nature of travel demand and to design appropriate policy approaches is described in *Vital travel statistics*.[45] Broadly, the old information sources and techniques involved traffic surveys and traffic modelling. To these statistics of measurement need to be added statistics of 'understanding'. These include household travel surveys and qualitative studies of responses to alternative policy scenarios, and 'good practice' case studies. Such information is not readily available. The reports of the National Travel Survey[51] are particularly valuable, but they describe national patterns. Apart from the *London Area Transport Survey*,[52] undertaken every 10 years since 1971, only ad-hoc sources are available at a local level. Local authority planning departments should know if such information has been gathered.

Household travel surveys, such as the National Travel Survey, and Local Area Travel Surveys (LATS) ask people to document their travel behaviour, which allows relationships to their lifestyles to be understood. For example, the National Travel Survey runs continuously, with around 3200 households taking part each year. Information is gathered on personal characteristics such as age, gender, working status, and driving licence holding, and on household characteristics, including numbers of vehicles available, number of people earning and the types of settlements they live in. Details of travel made by individuals over a 7-day period, including purpose, method of travel, time of day and length of journey, are recorded. The annual reports of the National Travel Survey contain a general analysis of travel behaviour, together with specialist reports in each issue. For example, the 1994/6 report examined the travel behaviour of young adults and patterns of company car use. Specialist tables can be ordered from the National Travel Survey to explore specific interests.

The Commission for Integrated Transport, being set up under the 2000 Transport Act,[53] will probably be a core source of information on strategic transport policy issues.

Impacts of transport on health

The trend towards a fundamental change in core transport planning philosophy is strongly reinforced by growing concerns about the environmental impacts of transport, including its health impacts. An environmental view of health is emerging as central to understanding and tackling this issue.

Until the late 1980s, the relationship between transport and health was focused almost entirely on the readily quantifiable effects of transport casualties, which were dominated by road traffic and by noise and air pollution and which were seen largely as a localised city centre issue. While these issues

Table 7.7   Environmental effects of transport

Level	Transport effects	Causes
Local	Noise, smell, air quality, health effects	Particulates, volatile organic compounds, carbon monoxide, ozone, noise
Regional	Waste disposal, land use	Land take of infrastructure
Continental	Acid rain	Nitrogen oxides, sulphur dioxide
Global	Climate change, ozone depletion	Carbon dioxide, ozone, chlorofluorocarbons (CFCs)

continue to be of concern, a more holistic view of transport's health impacts is emerging. This relates not only to emissions from transport sources, but also to the indirect health impacts of a motor transport-oriented lifestyle.

When assessing the direct impacts of the transport system, account should be taken of the detrimental environmental effects at a number of levels. A useful hierarchy of environmental impacts featured in the Dutch National Environmental Policy Plan, upon which Table 7.7 is based.

Transport produces around a quarter of the UK's carbon dioxide emissions, and levels continue to rise. This would make it difficult to achieve the target of a 12.5 per cent reduction in total greenhouse gas emissions from the 1990 level by 2008–12 which was agreed at the 1997 Kyoto Earth Summit, let alone the UK's domestic target to reduce emissions by 20 per cent by 2010.

Transport is thus an important factor in global warming and one of the major impacts of global warming is on health. Some effects would be beneficial, for example a reduction in cold-related disease, but there are real dangers of diseases from warmer climates, particularly malaria, establishing themselves in Britain. Outside the UK, the health effects of global warming could be very substantial.

Air quality

In 1998, the Department of Health Committee on the Medical Effects of Air Pollution estimated that up to 24 000 vulnerable people die prematurely each year, and a similar number are admitted to hospital, because of exposure to air pollution, much of which is due to road traffic.[19] The death toll is over six times the number killed in road accidents. In terms of costs, the best estimate for the cost of impacts of air pollution on mortality and morbidity is £3.9 billion a year, or 0.38 per cent of Gross Domestic Product, with the transport sector responsible for about 60 per cent of this.[54] This figure is confirmed by a European Commission study which estimated that deaths, hospitalisation, work sick leave and other health effects attributable to traffic pollution amount to at least 0.4 per cent of Gross Domestic Product, with estimates as high as 3 per cent being suggested in some cases.[55]

The National Air Quality Strategy set objectives, derived from health-based standards for eight pollutants, to be achieved by 2005. Transport is a major source, and frequently *the* major source, of all pollutants covered in the strategy, except sulphur dioxide. A fuller account of sources of air pollution, the effects on health, the air quality standards and monitoring of air quality can be found earlier in this chapter in the section on air pollution. A comprehensive review of the health effects of car emissions from a transport perspective was published in *Local transport today.*[56]

Noise pollution

Statistics on complaints about traffic noise to environmental health officers and about aircraft noise are found in the annual volumes of *Digest of environmental statistics*, published by the Department of the Environment, Transport and the Regions. Surveys of attitudes to noise, for example two surveys by the Building Research Establishment on noise in the home and noise around dwellings, represent a more realistic assessment of noise impact.[57,58] In such surveys, road traffic noise is noted as the most widespread form of noise disturbance, found at 92 per cent of sites, with aircraft noise found at 62 per cent of sites and noise from railways at only 15 per cent of sites.

Noise from transport sources is unlikely to be sufficiently prolonged and loud to produce tinnitus and hearing loss, but traffic noise does contribute to stress-related problems such as raised blood pressure, minor psychiatric illnesses, and may be an aggravating factor in mental illness.[59] The WHO study sees sleep interference as significant.[58] Up to 63 per cent of dwellings are exposed to a level of night-time noise high enough to interfere with sleep. The main effect of exposure is a reduction of rapid eye movement sleep, which is the deepest stage of sleep, essential for human health. Disturbed sleep can alter mood and the performance of intellectual and mechanical tasks.[60]

As long as flows are not high, traffic management techniques can reduce noise from road vehicles. There are European Union regulations for the maximum sound levels for new vehicles, but these do not currently ensure that exposure is actually reduced to address the concerns described above.

Lifestyle health impacts

In addition to the direct health impacts of pollution and noise, it is now recognised that transport's impact on health also involves subtle and cumulative processes. These include behavioural and lifestyle changes, such as reductions in independent mobility, as traffic levels rise. For elderly people, this may involve withdrawal from street life and loss of social support networks, with the associated increased health risks.[61]

Over several decades, Mayer Hillman's work has charted such effects, particularly with regard to children.[61-4] Loss of independent mobility may damage children's emotional and physical development. This is due to the decline in safe and accessible space for play and exercise, including the school journey. This both reduces children's ability to explore and learn about their environment and contributes to increasingly sedentary lifestyles, with consequent concerns about fitness and heart health.[65] Importantly, it is known that sedentary children are likely to become sedentary adults.[66] Such changes are in part, if not wholly, responses to the noisy and dangerous street environment, of which motor traffic is the prime cause. Thus, the 'systems' health impacts of transport extend well beyond the direct effects of pollutants emitted or casualties inflicted.

Transport casualties and safety

The growing awareness of the direct and indirect health impacts of transport, described above, has been coupled with heightened concerns about the continuing high level of deaths and injuries from road accidents. Road traffic casualties are documented in detail in the Department of the Environment, Transport and the Regions annual *Road accidents, Great Britain*, with information on casualties from all transport methods reported in the annual *Transport statistics, Great Britain*. Information on road traffic accidents is gathered in terms of the severity of the casualties, types of vehicles involved, road classes and results of breath tests. Rail accidents are classified by severity, type of rail activities and whether victims are passengers, staff or others. Air accidents are classified by severity and type of aircraft. Accidents involving public transport by road, rail and air account for 4 per cent of all transport casualties. There are two types of problem with these data: the quality of the data collected, and the ways they are analysed and presented.

Despite the range of data available, the reliability, particularly of road accident data, is questionable. Road accident statistics are compiled from reports of accidents to the police. While fatalities have been found to be recorded and reported accurately, the situation is different for injuries. The uncertainty of the data is greater for less severe injuries. The classification of injuries is not informed by medical assessment, but the police are required to make judgements about whether the injury is slight or serious. These judgements are not reliable and the statistics can be misleading. Furthermore, 30 per cent of traffic accident casualties are not reported to the police, and 70 per cent of cyclist casualties go unrecorded. The recording is also systematically influenced by police numbers. With more police around, it is easier to report an accident, and it is possible to demonstrate a correlation between the number of injuries and the number of tours of duty of uniformed police constables.[67]

Traffic accidents are one of four key action areas proposed in the Department of Health's Green Paper *Our healthier nation*.[68] In 1987, the Department of Transport set a target that, by 2000, road accident casualties would be reduced by one-third compared to a baseline average for the years 1981–5. By 1997, deaths and serious injuries had been reduced by 36 per cent and 42 per cent, respectively, but slight injuries showed no decrease. Indeed, they showed an increase in the previous year. Because slight injuries make up the majority of casualties, this meant that all casualties had dropped only marginally. The difficulties with the reliability of the statistics mean that it is debatable as to whether or not the targets have been achieved at a national level. At a local level, there are many more confounding factors, making geographical comparisons very unreliable. In March 2000, the Road Safety Division of the Department of the Environment, Transport and the Regions published a new road safety strategy with targets to be met by 2010.

Despite the problems, there is general agreement that, although numbers of casualties are decreasing rapidly for some types of road users, they are actually rising for others. For motorists, driving is becoming safer as fatal and serious casualties have been reduced. Accidents which were previously fatal or led to serious injury are increasingly survivable. Changes in road design, general improvements in vehicle collision performance, use of seat belts and air bags and experience in the emergency treatment of injured passengers have all contributed to this general improvement. Despite this, total road casualties rose by 1 per cent in 1997, begging the question as to whether the measures taken have exhausted their potential for reducing casualties.

Vechicle safety features do little to improve the safety of pedestrians and cyclists, who account for 45 per cent of road deaths, a disproportionate percentage, with pedestrians making up 25 per cent of the killed and seriously injured categories. The UK's record for pedestrian and cyclist safety is relatively poor by European standards, particularly among child pedestrians.

Comparisons which relate casualties to a measure of the amount of travel undertaken can be made to produce a rate or frequency of accidents. This raises the question of what measure of travel should be used to generate the casualty rate. Relating casualties to the amount of passenger travel is probably the most satisfactory indicator and preferable to the often-used vehicle-kilometre measure. Whether this is done in terms of distance or journeys can change the appearance of the information significantly, as Table 7.8 shows.[45]

In terms of casualties per billion kilometres, rail emerges as by far the safest transport method, with one-fifth the casualty rate of motorists. The risk of an

Table 7.8 Casualties per billion kilometres travelled

Mode of transport	1994 casualties	Billion km travelled per year	Casualties per billion km	Relative risk (car = 1.0)
Pedestrians	47 354	17.0	2785	6.6
Cyclists	24 149	3.4	7103	16.8
Motorcyclists	24 309	3.4	7149	16.9
Car and lorry drivers and passengers	206 033	487.6	423	1.0
Bus and coach drivers and passengers	10 082	45.3	222	0.5
Rail passengers	2 227	34.0	66	0.2

Source: *Vital travel statistics*,[45] drawing upon information from *Road accidents, Great Britain*, *The National Travel Survey* and *Transport statistics, Great Britain*.

Table 7.9 Casualties per billion journeys

Mode of transport	1994 casualties	Billion journeys in a year	Casualties per billion journeys	Relative risk (car = 1.0)
Pedestrians	47 354	17.0	2 785	0.5
Cyclists	24 149	1.1	21 954	3.8
Motorcyclists	24 309	0.3	81 030	14.0
Car and lorry drivers and passengers	206 033	35.7	5 771	1.0
Bus and coach drivers and passengers	10 082	4.5	2 240	0.4
Rail passengers	2 227	1.1	2 024	0.3

Source: *Vital travel statistics*,[45] drawing upon information from *Road accidents, Great Britain*, *The National Travel Survey* and *Transport statistics, Great Britain*.

accident in a bus is half of that in a car, but pedestrians have nearly seven times more casualties per distance travelled than motorists. Cyclists and motorcyclists have seventeen times the casualty rate of car users.

Relating casualties to journeys, as in Table 7.9, changes the picture. Because pedestrian journeys are very much shorter than car trips, they have a 50 per cent lower casualty rate than car trips rather than being worse than car travel, as the distance rate suggests. For the same reason, cycling drops from having 17 times the risk of driving to under four times. The change in measure slightly improves the relative safety of motorcyclists. The gap narrows a little between car users and public transport, but is still substantial.

Another measure is simply to relate casualties in each group to the number of people in the population, for example child accidents as a rate per 100 000 children. This is often done for international comparisons, where accurate travel data are unavailable or unreliable. One difficulty is that, although demographic groups like children or elderly people are readily identifiable, this measure is very difficult to relate to overlapping groups such as pedestrians, cyclists, motorists or public transport users. Such measures, although useful, are of limited use for informing and developing transport policies, particularly at the local level.

Measuring road safety and danger

One key point is that all the measures mentioned so far are of transport casualties. It is almost taken for granted that a decline in transport casualties represents an increase in 'road safety'. In actual fact, the opposite may well be true. If roads become more dangerous to pedestrians and cyclists, then pedestrians and cyclists may become motorists, car passengers or public transport users. They may even not travel at all. This applies particularly to elderly people and children.[69] As the 1997 transport policy consultation paper noted, 'people are walking and cycling less, so their exposure to danger has reduced. This is because they cannot find safe, unpolluted routes.'[70] *Increased* road danger, perversely, produces fewer road accidents.

Accident statistics and casualty rates, however measured, cannot of themselves provide an adequate measure of road safety. Measuring 'road safety' or 'road danger' is a considerably more difficult task than documenting 'hard' statistics like reported accident casualties.[71,72] It is probably better understood via surveys of perception, or by studies that include a variety of measures of travel and of road casualties in order to obtain a more complete picture. Of the 'hard' indicators, traffic volume and speed are probably most relevant in measuring 'safety'. These figures are gathered by local authority transport departments for other reasons for many roads in their areas.

The possibility exists that, without a road safety perspective, reducing transport casualties could simply involve suppressing travel by those methods perceived as 'dangerous'. Getting people to give up walking and cycling and into cars would leave only other vehicles and their occupants for motorists to hit.

It is possible to explore this safety issue by coupling casualty data with other information. The accident reduction potential of well-designed cycle and pedestrian facilities is demonstrated by the city of York, where a reduction in accidents to pedestrians and cyclists has been combined with a rise in journeys on foot and by bicycle. This achievement is contrary to the experience in other cities and the country in general. The integration of safety for all modes with demand management transport policies has meant that York has easily outperformed the UK average for casualty reduction,[72] as Table 7.10 shows. Robert Davis notes in his report:

> Pedestrian and cyclist levels have held their own while at the same time reported road accident casualties in the City have fallen dramatically. Compared to the government's 1981–85 base level (for the casualty reduction target), overall casualties had fallen by 47 per cent by the end of 1994, with the trend still downwards. Pedal cyclist casualties were reduced 30 per cent and pedestrians 40 per cent.[71]

Table 7.10 Changes in road casualties in York and the UK

Mode of transport	Percentage change in road casualties			
	1988 to 1992		1981–5 base to 1992	
	York average	UK average	York	UK
All casualties	−24	+1	−43	−3
Pedestrians	−18	−8	−41	−18
Pedal cyclists	−18	−8	−33	−13
Car drivers	+9	+35	−3	+40
Car passengers	−7	+16	−12	+14
Motorcycle/mopeds	−44	−42	−67	−57

Source: Davis R. *Is it safe?*[71]

This comparison raises the issue of whether it is possible to achieve a significant cut in all transport casualties outside of an integrated transport planning framework. Within such a framework, reductions approaching a half seem achievable.

Travel demand management is an important element of transport casualty reduction. This indicates that the context in which transport accident statistics are gathered needs to be understood in order to have figures that can be useful in deciding a policy response. Aggregated national data can be misleading. Furthermore, there is a need to use statistics on traffic danger, of which vehicle volumes and speeds are the best readily available indicators, in conjunction with traffic accident statistics.

Developing an environmental perspective on transport statistics

This exploration of the health impacts of transport indicates that this is a subject in transition. There are a number of statistical sources that have built up around the traditional concerns of traffic accidents and serious noise nuisance. These, on their own, are inadequate for an understanding of transport's direct and indirect health impacts. Outside of these traditional areas, sources of information are patchy and questions of interpretation are numerous. Crucially, the health impacts of transport are interwoven with issues of the environmental impacts of our highly transport-dependent lifestyle and need to be viewed and interpreted in this context. Transport is set to become one of the major public health issues of the twenty-first century.

Key official publications

Department of the Environment, Transport and the Regions. *Digest of environmental statistics.* London: TSO, published annually.

Department of the Environment, Transport and the Regions. *Transport statistics, Great Britain.* London: TSO, published annually.

Department of Transport. *London Area Transport Survey.* London: London Research Centre, decennial, 1971,1981, 1991.

Department of the Environment, Transport and the Regions. *Transport statistics report: National Travel Survey.* London: TSO, published annually.

Department of the Environment, Transport and the Regions. *Road accidents, Great Britain.* London: TSO, published annually.

Contact addresses and web sites

Department of the Environment,
Transport and the Regions
Transport Statistics
Zone 1/33
Great Minster House
76 Marsham Street
London SW1P 4DR
Telephone: 020 7944 4847
Web site: http://www.detr.gov.uk/
statistics/transport/index.htm

Department of the Environment for
Northern Ireland
Central Statistics and Research Branch
Clarence Court
Belfast BT2 8GB
Telephone: 028 9054 0808
Transport statistics: 028 9054 0807
Road safety statistics: 028 9054 0877
Web site: http://www.nisra.gov.
uk/dept/doe.htm

London Research Centre
(now part of the Greater London
Authority)
81 Black Road
London SE1 7SZ
Telephone: 020 7983 4000
Web site: http://www.london.gov.uk/

Transport 2000
The Impact Centre
12–18 Hoxton Street
London N1 6NG
Telephone: 020 7613 0743

References

1. Commission of the European Communities. European Inventory of Existing Com
   mercial Chemical Substances (EINECS). *Official Journal of the European Communities*
   1990; C 146 A.
2. Department of the Environment, Transport and the Regions. *The UK National Air
   Quality Strategy.* London: TSO, 1997.
3. ICI (for the Environment Agency). *Review of releases of nonylphenol and nonylphenol
   ethoxylates from Wilton surfactants plants (Authorisation AK6969).* London: ICI, 1998.
4. Her Majesty's Inspectorate of Pollution. *Chemical Release Inventory, Annual report
   1992 & 1993.* London: Department of the Environment, 1994.
5. US Environmental Protection Agency. *1993 Toxics Release Inventory, Public Data
   Release, Executive Summary.* Washington DC: US Environmental Protection Agency,
   1995.
6. Department of the Environment/Welsh Office. *Integrated Pollution Control: a practical guide.* London: Department of the Environment, 1993.
7. Environment Agency. *Improved consistency of reporting in the Chemical Release Inventory: a consultation document.* Bristol: Environment Agency, 1997.
8. Department of the Environment. *Environment facts: a guide to using public registers of
   environmental information.* London: Department of the Environment, 1996.
9. The Scottish Environmental Protection Agency (SEPA). *Guide to environmental information available to the public.* Stirling: Scottish Environmental Protection Agency, 1997.
10. Statutory Instrument 1992/3240 (and amendment). London: HMSO, 1992.

11. Statutory Rules of Northern Ireland No. 45/1993. London: HMSO, 1993.
12. Commission of the European Communities. European Directive, 90/313/EEC, on freedom of access to information on the environment. *Official Journal of the European Communities* 1990; **L 158**: 56–8.
13. Friends of the Earth. *Insisting on our right to know.* London: Friends of the Earth, 1996.
14. Standing Committee C (Pesticides Bill). House of Commons Official Report, 4 March 1998. London: TSO, 1998.
15. Her Majesty's Government. *Your right to know: the Government's proposals for a Freedom of Information Act.* London: TSO, 1997.
16. London Research Centre. *London Atmospheric Emissions Inventory.* London: London Research Centre, 1997.
17. Department of the Environment and the Scottish Office. *The United Kingdom National Air Quality Strategy – consultation draft.* London: Department of the Environment, 1996.
18. Department of Health Advisory Group on the Medical Aspects of Air Pollution Episodes. *Health effects of exposure to mixtures of air pollutant.* London: HMSO, 1995.
19. Department of Health Committee on the Medical Effects of Air Pollutants (COMEAP). *Quantification of the effects of air pollution on health in the UK.* London: TSO, 1998.
20. Macfarlane A, Haines A, Goubet S, Anderson R, Ponce de Leon A, Limb E. Air pollution, climate and health: short term effects and long term prospects. In: Charlton I, Murphy M, eds. *The health of adult Britain 1841–1994.* London: TSO, 1997.
21. Department of Health Advisory Group on the Medical Effects of Air Pollution Episodes. *Ozone.* London: HMSO, 1991.
22. Department of Health Advisory Group on the Medical Effects of Air Pollution Episodes. *Sulphur dioxides, acid aerosols and particulates.* London: HMSO, 1992.
23. Department of Health Advisory Group on the Medical Effects of Air Pollution Episodes. *Oxides of nitrogen.* London: HMSO, 1993.
24. Department of Health Committee on the Medical Effects of Air Pollution. *Non-biological particles and health.* London: HMSO, 1995.
25. Committee on the Medical Effects of Air Pollutants. *Asthma and outdoor pollutants.* London: HMSO, 1995.
26. Wjst M, Reitmeir P, Dold S, Wulff A, Nicolai T, von Loeffelholz-Colberg E, von Matius E. Road traffic and adverse effects on respiratory health in children. *British Medical Journal* 1993; **307**: 596–600.
27. Walters S. What are the respiratory health effects of vehicle pollution? In: Read C, ed. *How vehicle pollution affects our health.* London: Ashden Trust, 1994; 9–11.
28. Department of the Environment, Transport and the Regions. *Report on the Review of the National Air Quality Strategy: proposals to amend the strategy.* London: DETR, 1999.
29. Department of the Environment. *Expert Panel on Air Quality Standards: sulphur dioxide.* London: HMSO, 1995.
30. Department of the Environment. *Expert Panel on Air Quality Standards: nitrogen dioxide.* London: HMSO, 1996.
31. Department of the Environment. *Expert Panel on Air Quality Standards: particles.* London: HMSO, 1995.
32. Department of the Environment. *Expert Panel on Air Quality Standards: benzene.* London: HMSO, 1994.

33. Department of the Environment. *Expert Panel on Air Quality Standards: 1,3-butadiene.* London: HMSO, 1994.
34. Department of the Environment. *Expert Panel on Air Quality Standards: carbon monoxide.* London: HMSO, 1994.
35. Department of the Environment. *Expert Panel on Air Quality Standards: ozone.* London: HMSO, 1994.
36. WHO Regional Office for Europe. *Methodology and format for updating and revising the Air Quality Guidelines for Europe.* Copenhagen: WHO, 1993.
37. Salway AG, Eggleston HS, Goodwin JWL, Murrells TP. *UK emissions of air pollutants 1970–1994.* National Atmospheric Emissions Inventories (NAEI). London: AEA Technology/Department of the Environment, 1996.
38. Department of the Environment Transport, and the Regions. *Digest of environmental statistics.* London: TSO, published annually.
39. London Research Centre. *West Midlands Atmospheric Emissions Inventory.* London: London Research Centre, 1996.
40. Quality of Urban Air Review Group. *Urban air quality in the UK. First report.* London: Department of the Environment, 1993.
41. Quality of Urban Air Review Group. *Airborne particulate matter in the UK. Third report.* London: Department of the Environment, 1996.
42. Critical Loads Advisory Group. *Critical levels of air pollutants for the UK.* London: Department of the Environment, 1996.
43. Quality of Urban Air Review Group. *Diesel vehicle emissions and urban air quality in the UK. Second report.* London: Department of the Environment, 1993.
44. Review Group on Acid Rain. *Acid deposition in the United Kingdom 1992–1994.* London: DETR, 1997.
45. Potter S. *Vital travel statistics.* London: Landor Publishing, 1997.
46. Goodwin PB, Hallet S, Keeny F, Stokes G. *Transport: the new realism.* Oxford: Transport Studies Unit, Oxford University, 1991.
47. Goodwin PB. *Traffic growth and the dynamics of sustainable transport policies.* Oxford: Transport Studies Unit, Oxford University, 1994.
48. Standing Advisory Committee on Trunk Road Assessment (SACTRA). *Trunk roads and the generation of traffic.* London: HMSO, 1994.
49. Royal Commission on Environmental Pollution. *Transport and the environment.* London: HMSO, 1994.
50. Royal Commission on Environmental Pollution. *Transport and the environment – developments since 1994.* Twentieth Report of the Royal Commission on Environmental Pollution. Cm 3752. London: TSO, 1997.
51. Department of the Environment, Transport and the Regions. *Transport Statistics Report: National Travel Survey.* London: TSO, published annually.
52. Department of Transport. *London Area Transport Survey.* London: London Research Centre, decennial, 1971, 1981, 1991.
53. Department of the Environment, Transport and the Regions. *A new deal for transport. The Government's White Paper on the Future of Transport.* London: TSO, 1998.
54. Davis A. Medical thresholds or quality of life assessments? *Clean Air* 1996; **26**: 61–4.
55. Bjerrgaard R, Bangemann M, Papoutis C. *Auto Oil Programme Document, COM 96 248 Final, Sheet 23,* October, European Commission, DGXII, Brussels. On the DGXII web site, 1996.
56. Hughes P. Councils gear up for new air quality standards as national strategy nears completion. *Local Transport Today* 1995; **173**: 13–17.
57. Building Research Establishment. *Information Paper 22/93, Effects of environmental noise on people at home.* London: HMSO, 1993.

58. World Health Organisation Centre for Environment and Health. *Residential noise: concern for Europe's tomorrow.* Wissenschaftliche, Stuttgart: Verlagsgesellschaft mbH, 1995.

59. Jones DM. Noise, stress and human behaviour. *Environmental Health* 1990; **98**(8): 206–8.

60. Berkman L, Syme L. Social networks, host resistance, and mortality: a nine-year follow-up of Alameda County residents. *American Journal of Epidemiology* 1979; **109**: 186–204.

61. Hillman M. Social goals for transport policy. Reproduced in Beattie A, Gott M, Jones L, Sidell M. *Health and wellbeing: a reader.* Basingstoke: Macmillan, 1993.

62. Hillman M. Transport and the healthy city. In: Ashton J, Knight L, eds. *Proceedings of the first United Kingdom Healthy Cities Conference.* Liverpool: University of Liverpool, 1988.

63. Hillman M, Adams J, Whitelegg J. *One false move: a study of children's independent mobility.* London: Policy Studies Institute, 1990.

64. Hillman M, ed. *Children, transport and the quality of life.* London: Policy Studies Institute, 1993.

65. Cale L, Almond L. Physical activity levels in young children: a review of the evidence. *Health Education Journal* 1992; **51**/**2**: 94–9.

66. Health Education Authority/Sports Council. *Allied Dunbar National Fitness Survey, 1992.* London: Health Education Authority/Sports Council, 1992.

67. Adams J. *Risk,* Chapter 5. London: UCL Press Ltd, 1995.

68. Department of Health. *Our healthier nation.* London: TSO, 1998.

69. Adams J, Hillman M, Whitelegg J. *One false move: a study of children's independent mobility.* London: Policy Studies Institute, 1991.

70. Department of the Environment, Transport and the Regions. *The government's consultation on developing an integrated transport policy: a report.* London: TSO, 1997.

71. Davis R. *Is it safe? A guide to road danger safety reduction.* Leeds: The Road Danger Reduction Forum, 1995.

72. West-Oram DF. Measuring danger on the road. *Traffic Engineering and Control* 1989; **30**: 529–32.

8 Health care

MONITORING THE NATIONAL HEALTH SERVICE

Alison Macfarlane, Susan Kerrison, Sylvia
Godden and Declan Gaffney

Development of data collection
How data are collected and published
NHS staff
Clinical activities in hospitals and the community
Diagnostic and therapeutic facilities and activities in hospitals and the community
General medical, dental, optical and pharmaceutical services
Health promotion and contraception
Public expenditure on health care
Monitoring NHS performance

This chapter starts by outlining briefly how the collection of data about health care developed in the wake of the services themselves. It then describes the data collected at the end of the 1990s about staff involved in providing health care, the activities of the services and the finance of health care. This is followed by a discussion of the gaps and deficiencies in the data and of the plans for change which are being published and set in train as this book goes to press.

Development of data collection

The current systems for collecting data about the National Health Service (NHS) have developed as a by-product of the need to monitor how public funds have been spent on health care, public health and health promotion. This process started in the 1890s with notifications of communicable diseases. As publicly funded health services developed in the 1920s and 1930s, the local authorities and voluntary organisations which received central government funds to provide them were required to fill in forms or 'returns' about the services and the numbers of people who had used them.

The establishment of the NHS in 1948 greatly expanded both the range of services funded by the state and the impetus to collect data about how they were used. Aggregated 'returns' were designed to collect information about a range of services, activities and resources. One of the largest and best known was the SH3 hospital return for NHS hospitals in England and Wales. This was used to collect data about the numbers of in-patient stays and the average numbers of beds available and occupied beds in each specialty in each hospital.

More detailed data were collected through systems which recorded individual encounters with the NHS. The Hospital In-patient Enquiry (HIPE) collected data such as age, sex, region of residence, diagnosis and operations performed for a 10 per cent sample of in-patient stays in NHS hospitals in England and Wales. As the data were collected when the person was either discharged or died in hospital, they were counted in terms of 'discharges and deaths'. In Scotland, the SMR1 Scottish Morbidity Record system was set up in 1961 to collect data about all stays in Scottish hospitals. These systems were developed to derive data about the use of hospital services by people of different ages and about operations performed and length of hospital stays.

In 1969, Wales and each English region started to collect and analyse data about all discharges and deaths. As well as being used at regional level, this system, Hospital Activity Analysis (HAA) was used to derive a 10 per cent sample of discharges and deaths to be analysed at national level in the Hospital In-patient Enquiry. Stays in maternity departments were analysed separately as the Maternity Hospital In-patient Enquiry, but because of lack of consensus among the professions concerned, only about a third of districts ever implemented Maternity Hospital Analysis. A system of Hospital Activity Analysis was also implemented in Northern Ireland.

For long-stay hospitals in England and Wales, there was a separate system, the Mental Health Enquiry, which collected data about hospital facilities and basic demographic information about residents and their length of stay and legal status.

In the mid-1950s, the first of four surveys of *Morbidity statistics from general practice* collected data about consultations in a 1-year period from a small set of volunteer practices in England and Wales.[1]

The reorganisation of the NHS and local government in 1974 moved community health services from local authorities, which were also responsible for social services, and placed them under district and area health authorities, which also had responsibility for hospital services. The exception was in Northern Ireland, where all the services were placed together under four health and social services boards. In England, the fourteen pre-existing regional hospital boards were changed into regional health authorities, whose responsibilities included co-ordinating data collection and collating and analysing data for their regions before both passing them on to the Department of Health and Social Security.

As with other aspects of government statistics, the statistics collected by the central government health departments in each of the four countries of the UK were affected by the 25 per cent cut in spending which followed Sir Derek Rayner's review in 1980.[2] In particular, it meant that, for a number of years in the early 1980s, the annual volumes of *Health and personal social services statistics for England* were not published.

The 'Körner' committee

Over the same period, the Steering Group on Health Services Information, which was set up in February 1980, reviewed NHS data collection in England.[3,4] Its recommendations influenced the ways in which data are collected in Wales and Northern Ireland, but had little influence in Scotland, which continued to develop its own system. The Steering Group was chaired by Edith Körner, and her name is usually associated with the system it recommended.

The Steering Group decided that its 'main concern is with information for health service management. Thus we have not tackled specifically the information needed by health professionals to evaluate the results of their care'.[3] It therefore concentrated on data about the use of NHS resources and made recommendations for collecting data about the activities of the NHS, its 'manpower', or 'workforce', as it is now known, and its finances. The activities of the NHS were subdivided into:

Services provided on hospital premises

hospital wards
operating theatres
accident and emergency departments
radiotherapy departments
diagnostic services

Services provided on and off hospital premises

consultant out-patient clinics
day care facilities
paramedical services
family planning services
maternity services

Services provided in or for the community

preventive services
community nursing

The system was based on 'episodes of care'. In particular, a 'finished consultant episode' was an episode of day case or in-patient care under one consultant in a NHS hospital. This means that one in-patient stay or 'hospital spell' could actually consist of more than one episode. For each episode of care, the Steering Group defined a 'minimum dataset' of items to be recorded. Details of these are given later in this chapter.

When implementing the Steering Group's recommendations, the government decided that data should relate to financial years, instead of using calendar years, as had been the practice previously. Most of the recommendations came into operation on 1 April 1987. Some were delayed until April 1988 and those concerning maternity statistics were implemented in September 1988. 'Körner aggregate returns' were also introduced in Northern Ireland on 1 April 1988. Many are also used in Wales.

The majority of statistics published about the NHS in England since the late 1980s are based on the Steering Group's recommendations. Increasingly, the data have been derived from computer systems, rather than from manual form filling. Nevertheless, in some areas, such as maternity and child health surveillance, stand-alone systems had already been developed without linkage to other hospital and community systems, making it difficult to transfer data directly.

Changes in the 1990s

The introduction of the internal market in April 1991 had implications for data collection. Systems had to be adapted because of the split between health authorities, which purchased care, and trusts, which provided it. Minimum datasets were amended to become 'contract minimum datasets', with increasing emphasis on information needed for contracting and decreasing emphasis on the smaller numbers of clinical data items. Systems were set up to collect 'fast track' information to monitor NHS activity and some of these used different definitions from pre-existing activity returns.

In England, the fourteen regional health authorities were reduced to eight in 1994 and abolished in 1996. This meant that their role in data collection disappeared. In addition, most had databases which had been built up over many years, but these were abandoned and the staff who had maintained them left the NHS. Instead of submitting data to be collated by regions before being passed on to the Department of Health, districts and trusts started to submit data directly to the Department of Health. The NHS Clearing Service was set up, so that data could be sent directly via the NHS network, ClearNet, instead of having to be written to magnetic tapes or discs and sent by post.

The change in government in May 1997 led to changes in the NHS which are affecting data collection both directly and indirectly. The establishment in April 1999 of primary care groups to commission services for people in areas smaller than health authorities means that they need data to inform their decisions. At the time of writing, it is not yet clear what these are. At the same time, the four countries of the UK are developing and implementing ambitious information strategies. *Information for health,*[5] the strategy for England, and *A strategic programme for modernising information management and technology in the NHS in Scotland*[6] were published in the second half of 1998. A strategy for Wales, *Better information, better health,* was published early in 1999.[7]

Each strategy is based on setting up an electronic health record for everyone registered with a general practitioner for NHS care. This record will be held on their general practitioner's computer system. It will contain data about the care given by hospitals and other organisations providing care, as well as care given within the practice. Each organisation providing care will have an electronic patient record containing information about the care it gives to each person who uses its services. This information will also be transmitted to their general practice electronically through the NHS network. In the long run, it is envisaged that much of the information needed for statistical returns will be derived from these records. Adequate resources and a number of years' work will be needed to implement these changes.

This chapter describes the data which are currently collected in the four countries of the UK about NHS staff, activities and finance. In doing so, it tries to indicate where readers can find up-to-date information about the changes in data collection as they occur. The chapter concludes by discussing the problems with the data currently collected and whether the proposed changes are likely to solve them.

How data are collected and published

As has already been mentioned, each of the four countries of the UK collects NHS data in a different way. With devolution, these disparities are likely to increase rather than decrease. This section describes the organisations responsible, together with their general statistical publications. Their addresses and other details are given at the end of the chapter. More specialised publications on particular subjects are also described later in this chapter.

In England, the Department of Health's NHS Executive is responsible for collection of data at a national level. Each April, it sends a health service circular, *Central data collection from the NHS*, to health authorities, trusts and regional offices. This sets out details of the central statistical returns that it asks the NHS to provide and describes its process for reviewing its requirements. This circular is available on paper from the Department of Health and also on the internet at http://www.doh.gov.uk/coin.htm. With the introduction of primary care groups in April 1999, the returns are under review, so a detailed list is not given in this chapter.

Data are published annually in *Health and personal social services statistics for England*. The 1998 volume was the first to be made available on the internet. In the late 1990s, the content of the publication was reviewed. As a result, fewer data were published, but each section includes the names and telephone numbers of the statisticians who are responsible for the data and can provide fuller data to people who need them. These include data published in the department's statistical bulletins and booklets, most of which are listed in the back of the publication and on the department's web site. Statistical bulletins are formally published and press released, while booklets are released informally. There is an increasing tendency to convert booklets into bulletins.

National data are also published in the *Annual report of the Department of Health*, which includes the government's spending plans, and in *On the state of the public health: the annual report of the Chief Medical Officer*. Each year, the back bench House of Commons Health Committee sends a detailed questionnaire to the Department of Health asking for financial and other data. The committee publishes the department's replies in its annual reports on *Public expenditure on health and personal social services*.

In Wales, most data are available from the Health Statistics Analysis Unit of the National Assembly for Wales, known as the Welsh Office before July 1999.

As well as collecting data directly itself, it publishes data for Wales obtained from the Office for National Statistics and other agencies. It also publishes some NHS data processed by Health Solutions Wales, formerly known as the Welsh Health Common Services Agency. Up to 1994, data were published in *Health and personal social services statistics for Wales*. In 1995, the publication was split. Since 1995, NHS data have been published in *Health statistics Wales*, with more detailed data on an accompanying diskette. In 1997, the publication became bilingual. Summary data are published in the bulletin *NHS Wales: quarterly statistics*. Data are also published in the *Digest of Welsh statistics* and the *Digest of Welsh local authority statistics*. The Chief Medical Officer's annual report, *Welsh health*, contains some statistical information.

The organisation responsible for data collection in Scotland is the Information and Statistics Division (ISD) of the Common Services Agency for the National Health Service in Scotland. Data are published in *Scottish health statistics*. From 1997 onwards, this has been available on the internet. Health briefings and bulletins on specific subjects and other publications are listed at the back of *Scottish health statistics* and on its web site. Fuller information about data collection and availability is given in the *ISD guide*, which is available free of charge. NHS data are also published in the Chief Medical Officer's annual report *Health in Scotland*, as well as in the *National Health Service in Scotland annual report* and the *Scottish abstract of statistics*. These are published by the Scottish Executive, known as the Scottish Office before July 1999.

In Northern Ireland, many data are collated separately by each of the four health and social services boards before being sent to the Regional Information Branch of the Department of Health, Social Services and Public Safety of the Northern Ireland Executive. Up to 1993/4, data were published in *Health and personal social services statistics for Northern Ireland*. The way NHS data were published was reviewed after the internal market started in Northern Ireland in April 1993. Publications of data about NHS and social services were restructured on the basis of nine programmes of care. These are:

1. Acute services
2. Maternity and child health
3. Family and child care
4. Elderly care
5. Mental health
6. Learning disability
7. Physical and sensory disability
8. Health promotion and disease prevention
9. Primary health and adult community.

The two main annual publications, *Hospital statistics* and *Community statistics*, are available on paper or on disc, with the tables as Excel spreadsheets. Some data are also available on the Regional Information Branch's web site. *Hospital statistics* contains data about programmes of care 1,2 and 4–6, while *Community statistics* contains data about programmes of care 3–9.

Key official publications

Department of Health. *Health and personal social services statistics for England*. London: TSO, published annually.

Welsh Office. *Health statistics Wales*. Cardiff: Welsh Office, published annually. Since July 1999, the Welsh Office has been known as the National Assembly for Wales.

Information and Statistics Division. *Scottish health statistics*. Edinburgh: ISD, published annually.

Department of Health and Social Services. *Hospital statistics*. Belfast: DHSSPS, published annually.

Department of Health and Social Services. *Community statistics*. Belfast: DHSSPS, published annually.

NHS staff

Sources of data

In each of the four countries of the UK, there are separate systems for collecting data for staff employed by the NHS: staff in training, staff employed in the private sector, and independent practitioners and contractors providing NHS services.

STAFF EMPLOYED BY THE NHS

The Department of Health's annual census of the medical, dental and non-medical workforce, PD(STAT), is the main source of data about all staff directly employed by the NHS in England. It counts staff in post on 30 September each year. This census includes staff working in health authorities and NHS trusts, including ambulance services, and staff directly employed by other NHS bodies such as postgraduate special health authorities, the Dental Practice Board, the Prescription Pricing Authority, the Health Development Agency, formerly known as the Health Education Authority, and the Public Health Laboratory Service.

Up to 1994, non-medical staff were classified according to their pay scale. With the introduction of local pay bargaining under the internal market, this became impossible and in 1995 a system of occupational codes was introduced. This caused a discontinuity, as staff who had been paid on managerial pay scales were reclassified according to their professional background, making trends over time difficult to monitor. Changes in higher training of doctors in the late 1990s affected the ways in which they were classified in statistics. The changes were introduced by specialty at different times, making it difficult to monitor trends in numbers of doctors in training.

In Wales, similar data about staff employed by health authorities and trusts, Health Solutions Wales and the Welsh Health Promotion Trust from 1996 onwards are collected through NHS personnel systems. Data for previous years were collected from the NHS payroll system. As in England, this change involved a move from pay scale to occupational codes.

The Information and Statistics Division, Scotland collects data about staff in post on 30 September through its Medical and Dental Census and by deriving national 'manpower' statistics from payroll. It still attempts to classify non-medical staff by pay scale, but points out that local pay bargaining makes this difficult and that the regrading of whole groups of staff through pay negotiations makes it difficult to interpret time trends.

NHS and personal social services staff employed in Northern Ireland are counted through the Personnel Information Management System.

Because many NHS staff work part time, staff are counted not only as numbers but also as 'whole-time equivalents'. This is the number of hours each person is contracted to work, expressed as a proportion of the full-time contract hours. This gives a better measure of the staff resources available, but is sensitive to changes in contract hours. When the contract hours of full-time nurses, midwives and health visitors were reduced from 40 to $37\frac{1}{2}$ in the early 1980s, this artificially inflated the numbers of whole-time equivalents. The reduction of the contract hours of doctors in training during the 1990s means a reduction, in terms of the hours worked at least, in the capacity of a whole-time equivalent doctor.

None of the data collection systems includes information about staff of private contractors who provide catering, cleaning, laundry or other services to NHS hospitals and trusts. This makes it difficult to interpret trends. For example, there has been an extensive decline in numbers of whole-time equivalent ancillary staff employed by the NHS since compulsory competitive tendering started from the mid-1980s onwards, but no data are collected about staff employed by private contractors who replaced them.

NURSES, MIDWIVES AND HEALTH VISITORS IN TRAINING

In the past, student nurses, midwives and health visitors were employed by the NHS and put in considerable numbers of hours' work. From 1989 onwards, training was progressively transferred to higher education institutions under 'Project 2000' and trainees became students and funded by bursaries. Statistics about these students are collected by the English National Board for Nursing, Midwifery and Health Visiting and its counterparts in Wales, Scotland and Northern Ireland.

INDEPENDENT CONTRACTORS PROVIDING SERVICES TO THE NHS

The General Medical Services database is a computerised register of all doctors who have a contract with a health authority in England and Wales to provide general medical services. It contains details of all general practitioners, with their age, sex and qualifications, details of the partnership, list size and whether certain allowances such as deprivation allowance are payable. Each year, health authorities use this census to update their records about numbers of practice staff, services offered by practices and achievement of targets for immunisations. Health authorities also collate information about numbers of community pharmacists and opticians who are contracted to supply services for their population. Information about dentists in general practice, as opposed to those employed by hospital or community trusts, is collated at a national level by the Dental Practice Board.

In Scotland, the Information and Statistics Division collects data about general practitioners in its General Medical Practitioner Database. The Dental Practice Division of the Common Services Agency collects similar data about general dental practitioners in Scotland. In Northern Ireland, the Central Services Agency compiles statistics about general medical practitioners and general dental practitioners, but they are not routinely published.

STAFF IN THE PRIVATE SECTOR

As part of the process of registering private hospitals and nursing homes, health authorities in England and Wales collect data on returns K036 and K037. These include the numbers of qualified and unqualified nursing staff and resident doctors employed. Data are collated centrally by the Department of Health and the National Assembly for Wales, but responsibility for doing so in England will pass to the new Care Standards Commission. In Scotland, the Information and Statistics Division collects data about qualified nurses employed in private nursing homes and hospitals subject to the Nursing Homes Registration (Scotland) Act of 1938. Apparently, no data are collected about staff working in the private sector in Northern Ireland.

These data do not cover the activities of doctors who work in these hospitals but are not employed by them, or the activities of the private sector outside these registered premises. Data are not collected about the work of dental practitioners practising outside the NHS or about care given privately by self-employed practitioners in a range of professions including home nursing, chiropody, physiotherapy and osteopathy.

Publications

Data for England are published in *Health and personal social services statistics for England*. Up to 1993, more detailed information about NHS staff was published every year in *NHS workforce in England*, otherwise known as the 'Blue book'. This is no longer published, but the information it contained is still collated and is available on request from the NHS Executive.

Four separate statistical bulletins, published annually, contain data about NHS staff and general practitioners. *Hospital, public health medicine and community health service medical and dental staff in England* contains tabulations of medical and dental staff by grade, sex and geographical distribution. Data about other directly employed staff are published in another statistical bulletin, *NHS hospital and community health services non-medical staff in England*. As well as data about NHS staff, there are some data about nurses in private hospitals and homes. Statistics about staff employed in private hospitals and nursing homes can be found in *Private hospitals, homes and clinics registered under section 23 of the Registered Homes Act 1984*, and national and regional summaries are published in the statistical bulletin of the same name.

Statistics for general medical practitioners in England and Wales contains data about the age, sex and status of general practitioners and the numbers of support staff, such as practice nurses or receptionists, that they employ, and fuller data are published in *General medical services statistics, England and Wales*. Finally, less detailed statistics about the number of pharmacies and opticians in contract with health authorities are published in bulletins on *General pharmaceutical services in England* and *Ophthalmic services statistics, England*.

There is no statistical bulletin relating to general dental services. Information about numbers of dentists in general practice in England and Wales and their geographical distribution is published in the *Annual report of the Dental Practice Board* and in its quarterly bulletins.

Data about staff employed by the NHS in Wales are published annually in *Health statistics, Wales* and summary data are published in *Health statistics Wales, quarterly statistics*.

The Information and Statistics Division, Scotland publishes a range of workforce statistics in *Scottish health statistics*. More detailed data can be found in its specialised publications, *Agency nursing staff*, *Ethnic group of staff directly employed by the NHS in Scotland*, *Medical manpower*, *General ophthalmic services* and *General practitioner and practice profile statistics*.

Hospital-based staff employed in Northern Ireland are tabulated by category and trust in *Hospital statistics*, while a similar tabulation of community-based health and personal social services staff appears in *Community statistics*.

Clinical activities in hospitals and the community

NHS hospitals

Statistics about activities and beds in NHS hospitals are derived both from aggregated 'returns', which are counts of numbers of events or activities, and from person-based datasets, based on data about in-patient and day case care given to individual people. These are collected using the minimum datasets shown in Table 8.1. Apart from data about admissions for in-patient or day case care, which are described later, only aggregated data are collected at a national level, but the person-based data are used increasingly at local level and are passed from trusts to health authorities. Publications based on aggregated returns are listed in Table 8.2.

The Performance Analysis Branch of the NHS Executive collects data about the average numbers of beds available daily in NHS hospitals in England on form KH03 and publishes them each year by trust and sector in the booklet *Bed availability and occupancy in England*. The form was revised in 1996–7 and extended to residential care wards and homes managed by the NHS. Counts of occupied bed days were added and ward categorisations were changed. The booklet includes time trends by trust and regional office area. Changes from directly managed units to trust status in the early 1990s and trust mergers in the late 1990s mean that those series are relatively short.

Table 8.1   Minimum datasets used for aggregated returns in England

Admitted patient care	Waiting list
Patient's GP, GP practice and referring GP	Patient's GP, GP practice and referring GP
Consultant	Consultant
Intended management	Decided to admit date
Health authority of residence	Priority
	Offered admission date
Out-patient care	Intended management
Patient's GP, GP practice and referring GP	Intended procedure
Attendance date and whether attended	Admission offer outcome
Clinic purpose	Duration of elective wait
Consultant	List removal date
Source of referral	List removal reason
Data request for referral received	
First attendance	**GP referral letter**
Outcome of attendance	Patient's GP, GP practice and referring GP
Operative procedure	Consultant
Priority type	Specialty
	Overseas visitor status
Accident and emergency	Date referral request received
Patient's GP, GP practice and referring GP	
Consultant	**Ward attenders**
Mode of arrival	Patient's GP and GP practice
Disposal	Attendance data
Investigation, diagnosis and treatment	Patient group
code	Intended clinical care intensity
Staff member	
Time of arrival, initial assessment,	
treatment, departure	

Activity data are published in two further booklets. *Ordinary admissions and day cases* contains counts of finished consultant episodes by trust derived from form KP70. *Outpatients and ward attenders* summarises data from form KH09, which counts attendances at out-patient clinics and accident and emergency departments, and form KH05, which counts people who attend wards for care without being admitted. Each of these contains data by trust and specialty, as well as 10-yearly trends for regional office areas.

Summaries of these aggregated activity data for England are published annually in the statistical bulletin *NHS hospital activity statistics, England* and in *Health and personal social services statistics for England.*

These publications also include data about use of hospital facilities for peo-ple with mental illness or learning disabilities. Use of NHS day care by men-tally ill and elderly people is shown in the publication *NHS day care facilities.* A statistical bulletin, *In-patients formally detained in hospital under the Mental Health Act 1983 and other legislation,* based on KP90, contains 5-year trends for England, while a longer publication with the same name contains more detailed regional statistics.

Data about the activities of diagnostic departments, including pathology, radiology, nuclear medicine and medical physics, collected on form KH12 are published in *Imaging and radiodiagnostics.* The blood transfusion service is now a separate authority, the National Blood Service. Statistics about its activ-ities are published in its annual report.

Table 8.2 Publications containing data from aggregate returns about facilities and activities undertaken in hospitals in England

Title	Data source	Coverage	Contents
NHS hospital activity statistics, Statistical bulletin	Körner returns, KH03, KH05, KH09 and KP70. Summary of finished consultant episodes from Hospital Episode Statistics. Prior to 1987: SH3, HIPE, HAA	Historical summaries England	Admissions, day cases, available beds, throughput, out-patient and ward attendances, accident and emergency attendances, average length of stay, selected operations, percentage discharged dead by sector: acute surgical, acute non-surgical, general and acute, maternity, mental illness, mental handicap and well babies
Ordinary admissions and day case admissions	Based on KP70	Historical summaries England/regions/provider units	Finished consultant episodes, ordinary and day case admissions by sector and speciality code
Out-patients and ward attenders.	Based on KH09, outpatient and accident and emergency activity, KH05, ward attenders Before1987: based on SH3	Historical summaries England/regions/provider units	Consultant out-patient clinic activity by sector and speciality code. A&E activity. Summary of ward attenders
Bed availability and occupancy, England	Based on KH03 which replaced SH3	Historical summaries England/regions/provider units	Beds by sector; separate tables for 24-hour wards, day wards and neonatal intensive care
Imaging and radiodiagnostics	KH12	1995/6 onwards England/regions	New examinations and tests in pathology, radiology, nuclear medicine and medical physics; includes microbiology from Public Health Laboratory Service; electrocardiogram and electroencephalogram data no longer collected centrally
NHS day care facilities England	KH13	Time trends England/regions/districts	Use of NHS day care facilities; total attendances, first attendances, re-attendances by patient group such as elderly, mentally ill

Health Solutions Wales collects similar data. Form QS1 is used to collect data about bed availability and use by people admitted as in-patients and day cases, together with numbers of attendances at out-patient and accident and emergency departments. Data are published by the National Assembly for Wales in the two volumes of *Hospital activity statistics*. The first volume covers bed use by in-patients and day cases and the second contains data about out-patients. Data are also published in *Health statistics Wales*, the *NHS Wales performance tables* and in *NHS Wales, quarterly statistics*. In addition, form KH14 is used to collect data about NHS day care. Activity data are also collected by district of residence.

Similar data collected in Scotland are published in *Scottish health statistics*. A more detailed publication, *Scottish hospital in-patient and day case statistics*, is under review at the time of writing. Data for Northern Ireland are published by trust and specialty in *Hospital statistics*.

Waiting lists

Waiting lists have had a high political profile under both Conservative and Labour governments, so considerable effort is invested in collecting data about them. This is despite the fact that only about half the admissions to NHS hospitals are from waiting lists. The numbers of publications on the subject and the frequency with which they are published increased considerably during the 1990s. After the Conservative government found it impossible to reduce the numbers on the lists, it concentrated on shortening waiting times. The Labour government, on the other hand, has pledged itself to reducing the numbers on the lists by 100 000 by the end of its first term of office.

In England, waiting list information is collected from health authorities about their residents who are waiting for treatment and from trusts about people who are waiting for the treatment that they provide. The data from the two sources differ by 2–3 per cent, as resident-based figures exclude people living outside England and privately funded patients waiting for NHS treatment. Resident-based data include residents waiting for treatment in other countries of the UK or abroad, as well as people waiting for NHS-funded treatment in private hospitals.

People's waiting time is counted from the time when the clinician decided to admit them to hospital. If they are offered a date but are unable to attend, their waiting time is reduced to zero and then counted from the time when they were offered treatment. This is known as self-deferral.[8]

At the time of writing, waiting list and time statistics are published in monthly press releases and quarterly bulletins, *Elective admissions and patients waiting*. Each bulletin is accompanied by a detailed booklet, which gives data for individual trusts. There were concerns that consultants may have kept waiting times short by delaying people's first out-patient appointment after being referred by a general practitioner. The Conservative government therefore introduced a further statistical return to monitor the time people waited for this first appointment. Data from this are published quarterly in a statistical bulletin, *Waiting times for first outpatient appointments in England*.

Waiting list data for Wales are also collected on both a provider and a resident basis. They are published in *Health statistics Wales*, the *NHS Wales performance tables* and *NHS Wales, quarterly statistics*.

In Scotland, waiting list data are compiled from a variety of sources, by both provider and health board of residence, but a different approach is used. If a person 'self-defers', they are removed from the 'true waiting list', which is used for monitoring waiting times, and placed on a 'deferred waiting list'. Data are collected in *Scottish health statistics*. A more detailed publication, *NHSiS patient treatment and waiting times statistics*, is currently under review.

In-patient, day case and out-patient waiting list data for Northern Ireland are published in *Hospital statistics*.

STATISTICS ABOUT PATIENTS ADMITTED TO HOSPITAL AND THEIR TREATMENT

As mentioned earlier, the limited data in the aggregated returns are complemented by fuller, person-based data.

Hospital Episode Statistics (HES) is a database of all episodes of care in NHS hospitals, including mental illness hospitals, in England. The Patient Episode Database Wales (PEDW) and the Hospital In-patients System in Northern Ireland work on similar principles. In Scotland, the 'core patient profile in Scottish hospitals' (COPPISH) system brings together the SMR1 records for in-patient admission, SMR2 records for maternity admission and the SMR11 records for newborn babies. Record linkage is much more developed in Scotland than in the other three countries.

The data items in the Hospital Episode Statistics are those in the admitted patient care minimum dataset shown in Table 8.3. Each Hospital Episode Statistics record contains personal details such as date of birth, administrative details, including the dates of admission and discharge, and clinical details, including the diagnosis and operative procedure. The patient's postcode is used to derive the region, county, health authority, local authority and electoral ward of residence. Up to 1994/5, diagnoses were coded according to the ninth revision of the *International classification of diseases*, and from 1995/6 onwards they have been coded using the tenth revision. Operative procedures are coded using the OPCS-4 operation code. This information has been used to derive a Healthcare Resource Group for each episode. Approximately 11 million records are added each year. The data items and the system are described much more fully in publications from the Department of Health[9,10] and elsewhere.[11]

Hospital Episode Statistics was designed to count episodes of care, known as finished consultant episodes, rather than numbers of admissions or numbers of individuals treated. Nevertheless, attempts have been made to overcome this restriction. Firstly, it is possible to ascertain whether a given episode began with admission or ended with discharge and to count the numbers of 'hospital spells'. From 1998 onwards, this has been increasingly used in preference to counting episodes. Secondly, from 1997/8 onwards, NHS numbers were included in Hospital Episode Statistics records, offering the potential to link successive episodes of care for the same person.

Additional items of data are collected on several specific categories of patients. One is women having babies. The additional data items in the 'maternity tail' are shown in Table 8.3 and Maternity Hospital Episode Statistics is discussed more fully in Chapter 3. Another category is long-term or detained patients in psychiatric units or hospitals. This applies to patients

Table 8.3 Hospital Episode Statistics dataset for in-patients 1997–8

Data about the contract	**Pregnancy and delivery**
Organisation code of provider	Birth date of mother
Site code of provider	First antenatal assessment date
Organisation code of purchaser or primary	Total previous pregnancies
care group	Length of gestation
General practitioner	Delivery place type (intended)
Referrer	Delivery place type (actual)
	Delivery place type (reason for change)
Patient	Labour/delivery onset method
Date of birth	Delivery method
Postcode of usual address	Status of person conducting delivery
NHS number	Anaesthetic given in labour/delivery
Sex, marital status	Anaesthetic given post-labour/delivery
Ethnic origin	Number of babies
Record type	Birth date of baby or babies
Carer support indicator	Sex of baby or babies
Intended management	Birth order
Local patient identifier	Live or stillbirth
Spell number	Birthweight
	Method of resuscitation
Provider spell	
Admission method	**Psychiatric census – detained or long**
Decided to admit date	**term**
Start date	Date detained
Duration of elective waiting time	Status of patient
Source of admission	Age at census
Category of patient	Duration of care to census date
	Legal status
Consultant episode	Mental category
Age at start of episode	Ward type
Episode number	Diagnosis on census date
Start of episode date	
End of episode date	**Augmented care**
Duration of episode	Start date
General Medical Council code of	Where patient came from
consultant	Location of care
Specialty function code	Whether planned
Specialty function code for shared care	Specialty of management
Patient diagnosis/diagnostic code	Duration of high dependency care
Patient operative procedure	Duration of intensive care
Operative procedure date	Number of augmented care periods in
Neonatal level of care	episode
	Number of organs supported
Data about discharge of patient	Care period number
Discharge date	Outcome
Discharge method	Disposal
Discharge destination	End date
Patient classification	

occupying NHS beds on 31 March and who are either formally detained under the Mental Health Act or had been in hospital for a year or more. The data items recorded are shown in Table 8.3. From October 1997 onwards, a third category, augmented care, was added. Thirteen additional items of data are collected for episodes including either high dependency or intensive care.

The quality and timeliness of the Hospital Episode Statistics data were poor at the start, but improved as the system got under way. In 1987–8, the first year of operation, coverage was only 88 per cent, with only 75 per cent of records coded for diagnosis. Coding of operative procedures was the most incomplete. By 1993–4, coverage was 98 per cent, with 96 per cent of records coded. The maternity, psychiatric census and augmented care records are much less complete, with a third of maternity data records being missing in the mid-1990s.[12]

In the late 1990s, considerable advances were made in the timeliness of the Hospital Episode Statistics. By 1998, annual data files were becoming available within a year, instead of taking nearly 2 years to compile, as had been the case previously. From the financial year 1998–9 onwards, Hospital Episode Statistics data have been produced on a quarterly basis.

During the early years of operation, access to the complete database was difficult. It was mainly used within the Department of Health to examine public expenditure on NHS, and to monitor activity levels, trends in specific conditions, and health care initiatives. In the mid-1990s, the Department of Health developed policies to enable it to be used more widely. The Hospital Episode Statistics system now has a more 'user friendly' front end and can be accessed by people in regional offices. In addition, the Department of Health has developed a protocol for its use, analysis and dissemination and a charging policy. Standard outputs include aggregated annual summary tables in paper 'reference volumes' containing data for England and regional office area of treatment and on a CD-ROM containing data for England, regional office area of treatment and health authority of residence. The paper publication is in three volumes and the CD-ROM has a similar structure:

Volume 1   Finished consultant episode statistics by diagnosis and operative procedure; injury/poisoning by external causes.

Volume 2   Finished consultant episodes: administrative tables.

Volume 3   Finished consultant episodes: waiting times.

Summary data are also published in *Health and personal social services statistics for England* and in the statistical bulletin *NHS hospital activity statistics, England*.

The Department of Health also provides advice about the dataset and tabulations for people working in the NHS or funded by grants from the Department of Health. If the Department of Health authorises access, then IBM Global Services, which is contracted to manage the database for the department, can process the data on a fee-paying basis. Most of the data are generally made available at the level of individual NHS trusts. In some more sensitive areas, such as sexually transmitted diseases, it may be possible to identify both individual patients and individual consultants. In these cases, data will be made available at trust level only by special request and subject to approval from the Security and Confidentiality Advisory Group.

A similar national system has been proposed for out-patient attendances, as this is becoming an increasingly important part of care. As this would involve some 35 million records each year, the size of the task is daunting and there are no definite plans as yet. As mentioned earlier, there are some locally collected datasets on out-patients, waiting lists, general practitioners' referral letters, accidents and emergency, and ward attenders, based on the datasets shown in Table 8.1.

In Wales, the Patient Episode Database Wales works on similar lines to the Hospital Episode Statistics, except that the augmented care recorded was not implemented in Wales. The 'maternity tail' is even more incomplete than in England and data from it are not published routinely.[13] The Patient Episode Database Wales data are collected by Health Solutions Wales on behalf of the National Assembly for Wales and data are published in *Health statistics Wales*. Further analyses are available from the Health Solutions Wales' information request service, details of which are given below.

The Regional Information Branch of the Department of Health, Social Services and Public Safety in Northern Ireland runs the Hospital Inpatients System, which is also similar to the Hospital Episode Statistics. As in the other countries, the maternity data are very incomplete and are not published. The augmented care record has not been implemented. Unlike the other countries, data from psychiatric hospitals and units are processed separately in the Mental Health Inpatients System. Data are published in *Hospital statistics* by programme of care and in a less formal publication, *Hospital statistics by specialty.* Data from the Mental Health Inpatients System are published separately in *Mental health standard analyses.* At the time of writing, these are about 4 years behind the other hospital data, but work is underway to clear this backlog.

Scotland has a different system of hospital statistics. The Scottish Hospital In-Patient Statistics developed from the 1960s onwards and is now run by the Information and Statistics Division of the Common Services Agency. An SMR1 record is generated for every in-patient stay in hospital other than in a maternity unit. A separate record, SMR2, is completed for every hospital admission to a maternity unit, while a SMR11 neonatal record is used for all hospital treatment given to the baby during its stay, including transfers from department to department. It can be linked to the SMR2 delivery record and these can also be linked with SMR1 records about any previous in-patient stays by the mother.[14]

The whole system was revised in the mid-1990s in preparation for the introduction of the tenth revision of the *International classification of diseases* in 1996, and is now known as Core Patient Profile Information in Scottish Hospitals (COPPISH). Data are published in *Scottish health statistics*. The changes made in April 1996, mean that 1996/7 was a transitional year. In many cases, data for 1997/8 are not compatible with those for previous years.

Private hospital care

USE OF NHS PAY BEDS

Data are collected in Hospital Episode Statistics about episodes of care in NHS pay beds and a table summarising these can be found in Volume 1 of the annual Hospital Episode Statistics publication. Analyses of trends in these data and comparisons with data from other sources found that some pay bed units appeared to have submitted no data to the Hospital Episode Statistics and that overall pay bed activity is under-represented in the system.[15,16] A brief summary of pay bed utilisation is published in *Health statistics Wales* and in *Hospital statistics* for Northern Ireland.

PRIVATE HOSPITALS, CLINICS AND HOMES

Data about private facilities are collected as part of the process of registration by health authorities under Section 23 of the Registered Homes Act 1984. Legislation before parliament in 2000 will transfer responsibility for registration to a new Care Standards Commission for England and to the National Assembly for Wales. These include both residential homes, which provide long-term nursing care primarily for elderly people, as well as private acute hospitals. Data about residential homes are described in detail in Chapter 9. Before 1993/4, only a crude distinction was made between nursing homes with operating theatres, which were assumed to be acute hospitals, and those without. These were assumed to be purely long-stay homes for elderly and disabled people. Information is collected on return KO36 about numbers of beds available and occupied, about nursing staff in post and whether there is a resident doctor. Data for England are published in a statistical bulletin, *Private hospitals, homes and clinics*, and further data are made available in electronic format.

Data for Wales are published in *Health statistics Wales*. In Scotland, data are collected on form ISD(S)34 from private nursing homes registered under the Nursing Homes Registration (Scotland) Act 1938 or the Mental Health Act 1960/1984. The data published in *Scottish health statistics* exclude those from private hospitals. From 1996/7, residents have been classified by care group. In 1997/8, about a third were classified as having dementia.

Much more detailed data, including financial data, are collected privately and published annually in *Laing's review of private healthcare*.[17] These publications are very expensive and can be found only in a few specialised libraries.

With two exceptions, no data are collected routinely about episodes of care given to individual private patients, nor are aggregated data collected routinely about the activities undertaken in these facilities, for example about the number of operations performed. The two exceptions to this are induced abortions, which must be notified to the Chief Medical Officers of England, Scotland and Wales, as described in Chapter 3, and in-patients formally detained in hospital under the Mental Health Act 1983 and other legislation, which must be notified using return KP90. These are published in the statistical bulletin mentioned earlier. It shows that very few people are formally detained in private hospitals.

The issues and problems connected with the lack of routine data about the private sector are discussed more fully below and in Chapter 9. Because of the lack of routine data, Sheffield University has done periodic surveys of the clinical activity in private hospitals. The results of three of these have been published to date and results of a fourth in 1997–98 are about to be published at the time of writing.[18–20] The General Household Survey collects data about whether people have private health insurance, whether they or their employers pay for it, and whether other family members are covered. In addition, data about spending on private health insurance and private health care are collected in the Family Expenditure Survey.

Diagnostic and therapeutic facilities and activities in hospitals and the community

Aggregated returns are used to collect data about areas of hospital activity not covered by Hospital Episode Statistics and about other services provided in hospital and the community. They include diagnostic and therapeutic facilities and activities and patient transport.

Paramedical staff and services based in either hospitals or the community

A number of returns are used to collect data about the activities of paramedical staff based primarily but not exclusively in hospitals. These include form KT23, used to collect data about chiropodists, KT24 for clinical psychologists, KT26 for occupational therapists, KT27 for physiotherapists and KT29 for speech therapists. The statistics about their activities are limited to the total number of 'face-to-face contacts' and the number of 'initial face-to-face contacts', with some breakdown by age and source of referral. The data are published informally in booklets, details of which are shown in Table 8.4.

Return KA34 collects data from the thirty-seven ambulance services in England, including numbers of patient journeys by priority of journey and population, response times for emergency calls and arrival times for urgent journeys. Data from this return are published in a statistical bulletin, *Ambulance services, England*. It includes time trends as well as details about performance against standards in the Patients' Charter.

Summary data are published in *Health and personal social services statistics for England*. Similar data for Wales, Scotland and Northern Ireland are published in *Health statistics Wales*, *Scottish health statistics*, and *Hospital statistics* for Northern Ireland.

Community nurses and midwives

This section discusses data available about NHS services provided in the community by nurses and midwives employed by hospital and community trusts.

Table 8.4 Statistical returns used to collect data about paramedical staff and services in England

Title	Data source	Coverage	Contents
Chiropody services: summary information from form KC23	KT23	Annual with summaries from 1988–9 onwards England/regions/provider units	Total face-to-face and initial face-to-face contacts; initial contacts by age
Clinical psychology services: summary information from form KC24	KT24	Annual with summaries from 1988–9 onwards England/regions/provider units	Total face-to-face and initial face-to-face contacts; initial contacts by age and source of referral
Occupational therapy services: summary information from form KT26	KT26	Annual with summaries from 1988–9 onwards England/regions/provider units	Total face-to-face and initial face-to-face contacts; initial contacts by age, sex, location and source of referral
Physiotherapy services: summary information from form KT27	KT27	Annual with summaries from 1988–9 onwards England/regions/provider units	Total face-to-face and initial face-to-face contacts; initial contacts by age, sex, and source of referral
Speech therapy services: summary information from form KT29	KT29	Annual with summaries from 1988–9 onwards England/regions/provider units	Total face-to-face and initial face-to-face contacts; initial contacts by age, sex, location and source of referral
Ambulance services, England: *Statistical Bulletin*	KA34	Annual with summaries from 1988–9 onwards England, Ambulance service areas	Covers 37 ambulance services in England; number of patient journeys by priority of journey and population; response times of emergency call and arrival times for urgent journeys

Data on local authority services are described in Chapter 9. Very few data are collected about the community care activities of general practitioners or the nurses or other staff they employ. Private sector activity is monitored only where services are contracted to the local authorities or the NHS.

All the data are collected through aggregated returns. Return KC54 collects data about maternity services and clinics provided by midwives and health visitors. Data are collected in terms of 'face-to-face contacts' and subdivided by whether they are antenatal or postnatal, domiciliary or at a clinic, and whether they involve midwives or health visitors. Other contacts by health visitors are monitored in return KC55, while data about district nurses are collected through return KC56. These are subdivided by age of client and location of contact, for example at home, in a general practitioner's surgery or in some other place. Similar data are collected about community psychiatric nurses on return KC57 and about community mental handicap nurses on return KC58. Return KC59 collects data about specialist nurses such as Macmillan nurses and stomatherapists.

The categories identified have changed as new specialties have developed in community nursing. The data in these returns are all very limited and are restricted largely to the numbers of initial and total face-to-face contacts for each group by age of clients, location of contact and the source of referral. The returns which they replaced contained much more detail. For example, up to the mid-1980s, data were collected about births attended by community midwives at home and in hospital.

For England, data from each return are published in the booklets described in Table 8.5. Summary data are published in *Health and personal social services statistics for England*. Similar data for Wales and Scotland are published in *Health statistics Wales, Scottish health statistics*, and some data are published in *Community statistics* for Northern Ireland. In Northern Ireland, community maternity services were specifically mentioned in the 1997–8 volume of *Community statistics* as an area for which no data are published as they are of poor quality and are being reviewed.

General medical, dental, optical and pharmaceutical services

Sources of statistics about the numbers of general practitioners, dentists, pharmacists and opticians who have a contract with a particular health authority to provide primary care services are discussed above. This section describes the statistics collected about the work done by these practitioners. The introduction of primary care groups in April 1999 is likely to change both the information collected about general practitioners and the information they require. In addition, primary care groups will themselves have information needs, but these are not yet defined at the time of writing. In the longer term, the information strategies envisage general practices holding an electronic health record for each patient with summaries of care received from other providers.[5–7] If successfully implemented, these would make general practice

Table 8.5 Staistical returns used to collect data about community nurses and midwives in England

Title	Data source	Coverage	Contents
Community maternity services: summary information	KC54	Annual with summaries from 1988–9 onwards England/regions/provider units	Maternity advice and support programmes carried out by midwives and health visitors either as domiciliary visits or in clinics run by midwives; total face-to-face and initial face-to-face contacts by programme, staff groups and location; antenatal and postnatal contacts by location and staff group
Profession advice and support programmes in the community: summary information	KC55	Annual with summaries from 1988–9 onwards England/regions/provider units	Face-to-face contacts with health visitors and other staff, first contacts by age
Patient care in the community, district nursing: summary information	KC56	Annual with summaries from 1988–9 onwards England/regions/provider units	District nurses, SGNs, enrolled nurses and unqualified nurses; face-to-face contacts by location; first contacts by age and sex
Patient care in the community, community psychiatric nursing; summary information	KC57	Annual with summaries from 1988–9 onwards England/regions/provider units	Face-to-face contacts by location; first contacts by age and sex
Patient care in the community, ommunity mental handicap nursing: summary information	KC58	Annual with summaries from 1988–9 onwards England/regions/provider units	Face-to-face contacts by location; first contacts by age and sex
Patient care in the community, specialist care nursing: summary information	KC59	Annual England/regions/provider units	Macmillan nurses, hospice nurses, Marie Curie nurses, stomatherapists, continence nurses, premature baby nurses, diabetes nurses and other nurses; face-to-face contacts by staff group providing care

systems a major source of person-based data. At the time of writing, it is unclear to what extent resources will be available to bring this about.

General practice

The main centralised source of information about general practice in England and Wales is the General Medical Services database, which was described earlier. This provides a limited amount of information about activities for which a reimbursement or 'item of service' fee is due. Therefore, data are collected about activities such as achievement of targets for immunisation and cervical cytology, and providing contraceptive advice and doing minor surgery. In addition, there are details of the numbers of support staff, such as nurses and receptionists, that practices employ. As mentioned earlier, few data are collected routinely about the clinical activities of these staff or the people who consult them. Activity information from the General Medical Services database, as well as demographic and professional information about general practitioners, is published in the statistical bulletin *Statistics for general medical practitioners in England and Wales*. More detailed data are published in *General medical service statistics.*

As general practitioners are the gatekeepers for other forms of care, their systems should, in theory, be a source of data about all the care an individual obtained from the NHS. This is the rationale behind the proposals for electronic health records. Two approaches have been used for deriving data from general practice records.

In the first of these, data about consultations with general practitioners were collected in a series of studies of *Morbidity statistics from general practice*. In the first three surveys, covering 1-year periods in 1955–6, 1970–1, and 1980–1, the general practitioners taking part undertook to keep an age/sex register of their patients and to supply certain details about each consultation.[1,21-4] In the fourth survey in 1991–2, the general practitioners included had to have certain types of computer systems, whose manufacturers wrote additional software for the survey.[25] Sixty practices in England and Wales with a total of about 500 000 patients took part.

Data were recorded about each episode of illness leading to one or more consultations within the survey year and about each consultation, irrespective of whether or not a prescription was issued. Items recorded included the date and place of consultation, the diagnosis, whether this was the first consultation in the current illness and whether the patient was referred elsewhere. In addition, every person registered with the practices was interviewed. This was to record socio-demographic data, including marital and cohabiting status, housing tenure, ethnic group, household composition and occupation and employment status.

Since participation involves a considerable amount of work, volunteer general practitioners had to be used instead of a random sample. This is thought to have led to certain biases, because of the nature of the volunteers, who were more likely to be research oriented and less likely to practise in inner cities than general practitioners as a whole. Nevertheless, the characteristics of the patients were found to be similar to those recorded in the 1991 census. Manual checks found that over 95 per cent of contacts with doctors and 93 per cent of diagnoses were recorded in the study, although referrals to out-patient departments were under-reported and some practices did not record consultations with practice nurses.

Many analyses of the data were published in *Morbidity statistics from general practice, Series MB5 no.3*[25] and on a CD-ROM. They have been used extensively for comparisons with local data and, in conjunction with data from the earlier surveys, to look at trends over time.

The second approach is to extract data directly from general practice systems. A number of projects were set up to extract data for epidemiological studies, as general practices became computerised during the 1980s. Some of the earliest projects were funded by pharmaceutical companies and were therefore biased towards data about prescriptions issued and linked to particular computer systems.

The best known of these is the General Practice Research Database, originally set up by VAMP Health Ltd and subsequently operated by the Office for National Statistics (ONS) and owned by the Department of Health. In April 1999, ownership was transferred to the Medicines Control Agency, with the ONS continuing to operate the database. In the mid-1990s, it covered over 2 million people registered with 288 practices in England, Scotland, Wales and Northern Ireland. By the end of the decade, it covered over 400 practices. It is used for special projects, many, but by no means all, related to prescribing. It also contains information about diagnoses, chronic conditions and whether a referral is made. Data from it are published by the ONS in *Key health statistics from general practice, Series MB6*.

The NHS Executive Information Management Group set up the 'MIQUEST' pilot project in 1997 to develop methods for extracting data from a variety of general practice computer systems. The health authorities taking part have used the techniques for a variety of purposes, including collecting health promotion data and supporting clinical audit.[26] The general practices involved used it to inform decisions on clinical priorities and commissioning. Although the results of the pilot have an important potential for meeting the information needs of primary care groups, the data it produced initially were mainly for local use. In addition, some regions and districts have projects collecting morbidity and other information about use of services from individual practices.

The approaches used in *Morbidity statistics from general practice* and in downloads from practice systems each has its strengths and limitations. Continuous downloading generates a live database, enabling individuals' diagnoses and outcomes to be monitored over time. On the other hand, the survey included socio-economic data about the patients, recorded all consultations and made comparisons with previous surveys. It also collected complete data about activity in each participating practice, including all consultations in each spell of illness. As data were collected with special software as part of a special study, they are likely to be more consistent with each other than data downloaded from operational systems in the absence of specific agreements about coding and recording.

The other source of data about general practice is the weekly returns service operated by the Royal College of General Practitioners Research Unit at the University of Birmingham. Volunteer practices submit information about their assessment and diagnoses of patients they have seen in the previous week. As described in Chapter 3, these contribute to the surveillance of communicable diseases by the Communicable Disease Surveillance Centre. The research unit also produces annual summaries and trends in disease, diagnosis and demand for health care services in *The weekly returns service: annual report*.

Between 1 April 1991 and 31 March 1999, when the general practice fundholding scheme was in operation, statistics were collected about the numbers of fundholders and the population covered by fundholding practices. These were published in *Health and personal social service statistics for England* and in the statistical bulletin, *Statistics for general medical practitioners in England and Wales*. Similar data were published in *Health statistics Wales* and *Scottish health statistics*.

Dentists

The Dental Practice Board is the main source of statistics about the activities of dentists in general practice in England and Wales. Its role is to process claims for payment by dentists who have contracts with health authorities. Data from these claims for payment are published in the *Annual report of the Dental Practice Board*, the *Digest of statistics* and quarterly bulletins. These reports contain information about the expenditure on dental care, the number of dentists, the number of adults and children registered with a dentist and the treatment undertaken. Some data items are analysed by region. There are no statistical bulletins on general dental practitioner services, but information from the Dental Practice Board is included in *Health and personal social services statistics for England* and *Health statistics Wales*. In Scotland, data are collected by the Common Services Agency's Dental Practice Division and published in *Scottish health statistics*. Data about dental practice in Northern Ireland are collected by the Central Services Agency, but are not routinely published.

Data about dentists employed in NHS hospitals or community dental services are collected through the census of NHS workforce. Numbers of staff are published in the statistical bulletin *Hospital, public health medicine and community health service medical and dental staff in England*. Data about the staff and activities of the hospital and community dental services are also published in *Health and personal social services statistics for England* and *Health statistics Wales*. Data about hospital dental services in Northern Ireland are published in *Hospital statistics*. In Scotland, data about dentists employed in the hospital and community health services are collected through the Information and Statistics Division's medical and dental manpower census. They are brought together with data from the Dental Practice Division in *Scottish health statistics*.

These data relate to the activities of dentists. To complement them, surveys are done to collect information about the dental health of the population and dental care received. The Office of Population Censuses and Surveys (OPCS) undertook separate surveys of adults' and children's dental health at 10-yearly intervals and these are now done by the ONS. The most recent survey of adult dental health was undertaken in 1998, and is described in Chapter 2. A dental survey accompanies the National Diet and Nutrition Survey. The General Household Survey asks people whether or not they have their natural teeth and whether they have recently made a visit to a dentist. These surveys are described more fully in Chapter 2. The British Association for the Study of Community Dentistry also conducts regular surveys and the results are published in the journal *Community dental health*. In Scotland, an Adult Dental Health Survey was done in 1993 and questions on dental health were included in the 1995 Scottish Health Survey, described in Chapter 2.

A growing proportion of dentistry is being carried out privately, although it is difficult to estimate how much. No data are available on the proportion of time a general dental practitioner spends on private work or on the activities undertaken. This makes it impossible to draw together a complete picture of dental care in any particular area. Data about the proportion of income families spend on private dental care and NHS dental charges are included in the Family Expenditure Survey, which is described in Chapter 2.

Prescriptions and pharmacies

All prescriptions dispensed in England by community pharmacists, appliance contractors, and dispensing doctors and prescriptions submitted by doctors for items they administer themselves are sent to the Prescription Pricing Authority, a special health authority. The information derived from these is made available to individual general practitioners, health authorities and the Department of Health in the form of prescription analysis and costs tables (PACT). These contain information about numbers and costs of items prescribed, subdivided by therapeutic group. Data are available electronically to health authorities and the Department of Health via a computer system known as EPACT. As the data are confidential, they are not made available more widely. Limited information is published in the Prescription Pricing Authority's annual report. Similar data for Wales are available from Prescription Pricing Services at the Welsh Health Service Common Services Agency, now known as Health Solutions Wales.

Information about prescriptions dispensed in England is also made available to the Department of Health through the prescription cost analysis (PCA) system. Unlike prescription analysis and cost tables, this also includes prescriptions written by dentists and those written outside England and dispensed in England. The prescription cost analysis system was introduced in January 1991. Prior to this, data were based on a one in twenty sample of prescriptions dispensed by community pharmacists and appliance contractors only, and was based on fees rather than items. This means that data from this system are not directly comparable with those currently collected.

Summary information about prescriptions dispensed over a 10-year period and more detailed information are available in the statistical bulletin *Statistics on prescriptions dispensed in the community, England.* As well as data about numbers and costs of prescriptions, the bulletin also includes data about prescriptions for groups of people exempt from charges. More detailed data about numbers and costs of prescriptions for individual preparations are published in *Prescription cost analysis.* For each item, the number of prescription items, the net ingredient cost and the class of preparation are given. For confidentiality reasons, preparations where less than fifty items were dispensed are excluded, but these are included in totals, unless the total itself relates to less than fifty items, in which case it is excluded.

Prescription data are potentially a very powerful tool for assessing clinical practice. On the other hand, the prescriptions are not linked to the characteristics of the people for whom they were prescribed or to other prescriptions they may have been given at the same time or on other occasions. Information about the number of pharmacies opening and closing and the special payments they receive is collected by health authorities and published in a 6-monthly statistical bulletin, *Community pharmacies in England and Wales,* and in an annual statistical bulletin, *General pharmaceutical services in England.* The annual publication contains further information from the Prescription Pricing Authority about prescriptions dispensed. Summary data are also published in *Health and personal social services statistics for England* and *Health statistics Wales.*

In Scotland, all prescriptions are sent to the Pharmacy Practice Division of the Common Services Agency. It produces statistics about the numbers of pharmacies, prescriptions dispensed and their cost. These are published in *Scottish health statistics* and include tables by health board and therapeutic classification. In Northern Ireland, prescriptions are sent to the Central Services Agency, which compiles statistics, but does not publish them routinely.

Ophthalmic services

Limited information about the range of ophthalmic services available and types of community opticians, based on data from health authorities is published in the statistical bulletin *Ophthalmic services statistics, England.* Summary data are also published in *Health and personal social services statistics for England* and *Health statistics Wales.* A survey is also undertaken of vouchers redeemed in Great Britain to ascertain the proportion which were for spectacles within the voucher value.

In Scotland, data about the numbers of ophthalmic opticians, ophthalmic medical practitioners, the sight tests given, the spectacles supplied and the costs to the exchequer of vouchers and free sight tests are published in *Scottish health statistics* and in a special briefing, *General ophthalmic services, Scotland.* In Northern Ireland, data are compiled by the Central Services Agency, but are not routinely published.

Health promotion and contraception

The NHS collects information about health promotion in terms of the performance of screening programmes, immunisation and vaccination rates, the activities of family planning and genitourinary medicine clinics and statistics about drug misuse. Some information about the involvement of general practitioners in health promotion activities is available from the National Survey of Morbidity in General Practice, the General Practice Research Database and the other projects which extract data from general practice systems. These contain information about consultation rates for health promotion purposes. Information on health-related behaviours is available from surveys. The General Household Survey and the Health Survey for England collect some information about these topics. Since 1995, the Health Education Authority has commissioned a series of annual Health Education Monitoring Surveys. These ask questions about attitudes to smoking, drinking, exercise, nutrition and sexual behaviour.

Immunisation programmes

Data about the uptake of immunisation in childhood are collected for the whole of the UK through the Coverage of Vaccination Evaluated Rapidly (COVER) system operated by the Communicable Disease Surveillance Centre. In addition, each of the countries has its own returns. In England, Wales and Northern Ireland, data are collected using return KC50. Wales collects additional data through Health Solutions Wales' child health system. Northern Ireland still uses return KC51, which was dropped in the other countries. In Scotland, a revised data collection form, ISD(S)13 Part 2, was introduced in April 1995. One reason for the change was to make the data more compatible with those collected through the Coverage of Vaccination Evaluated Rapidly system.

Data are published in *Health and personal social services statistics for England*, *Health statistics Wales*, *Scottish health statistics* and *Community statistics* for Northern Ireland. In England, more detailed information was published informally in booklets until 1997–8, when they were superseded by a statistical bulletin, *NHS immunisation statistics, England*. This contains time trends for England and gives the uptake by region and district for measles mumps rubella (MMR), tetanus, diphtheria, polio, pertussis and *Haemophilus influenzae* immunisation. Data about tuberculosis skin tests and BCG vaccinations are also included. In addition, data on performance of general practitioners in relation to targets for childhood immunisation are included in the statistical bulletin *Statistics for general medical practitioners in England and Wales*.

Screening programmes

CERVICAL CANCER SCREENING

Data about the uptake, coverage and test results from the computerised call and recall system for cervical cancer screening are collected through return KC53, while pathology laboratories complete return KC61. The latter summarises the results of all smears, whether they were taken as part of the screening programme or for some other reason, together with information about laboratory backlogs. From 1996–7 onwards, data from these two returns have been brought together in a statistical bulletin, *Cervical screening programme, England*. The Welsh Health Statistics and Analysis Unit has issued a similar publication, *Cancer screening programme, Wales*. These contain data by age and district. In Scotland, data are collected by ISD and are included in the *Annual report of the cervical screening programme*.

Data are also published in *Health and personal social services statistics for England*, *Health statistics Wales*, *Scottish health statistics* and *Community statistics* for Northern Ireland. Data on performance of general practitioners in relation to targets for cervical smears are included in the statistical bulletin *Statistics for general medical practitioners in England and Wales*.

BREAST CANCER SCREENING

Return KC62 is used to collect information from screening units about the operation and outcomes of their call and recall systems. Health authorities complete return KC63 about the population coverage of the programme. In England, the data are collected by the Department of Health and published in a statistical bulletin, *Breast cancer screening programme, England*. The number of cancers detected and the interval between detection and treatment are reported. This publication also contains information about women who were not screened as part of the programme but either referred themselves or were referred by their general practitioner. The publication also discusses the performance of the programme in relation to preset standards or targets. In Wales, the data are collated by 'Breast test Wales'. In Scotland, the Scottish Breast Screening Programme collects data on many aspects of each screening programme, including the number of films taken, radiation doses, and about cytology, pathology, surgery and radiotherapy. Data are also published in *Health and personal social services statistics for England*, *Health statistics Wales*, *Scottish health statistics* and *Community statistics* for Northern Ireland.

Contraception

Data about contraceptive advice and services provided by NHS family planning clinics are collected through return KT3. The data collected include numbers of clients of family planning clinics by age, sex and method of contraception. Data for England are published in a statistical bulletin, *NHS contraceptive services, England*. It shows increasing use of clinics by young people and declining use by people in the older age groups, who are more likely to seek contraceptive advice from general practitioners. The bulletin also discusses the limitations of data about services provided by general practitioners. These are based on item of service payments, and are therefore subdivided only into women registered for fitting of intrauterine devices and women registered for all other forms of contraception combined. Data are also published in *Health and personal social services statistics for England*, *Health statistics Wales* and *Scottish health statistics*. Data are collected in Northern Ireland, but not published because of their poor quality.

Data about the numbers of general practitioners providing contraceptive advice are published in the statistical bulletin *Statistics for general medical practitioners in England and Wales*. Data from general practice systems, including the General Practice Research Database, also contain some limited information about contraceptives prescribed. The prescribing statistics described earlier give an indication of the types of contraceptives prescribed, but not of the numbers of people or couples using them.

Because of the deficiencies in routinely collected data, surveys are essential to monitor trends in contraceptive use in the population. The General Household Survey has asked questions about use of contraception in 1983, 1986, 1989, 1991, 1993, 1995 and 1998 and will include such questions again in the future. Meanwhile, similar questions were asked in 1997 in the ONS' Omnibus Survey.[27] Data about legal abortion are described in Chapter 3.

Sexually transmitted diseases

The data collected and collated by the Communicable Disease Surveillance Centre and its counterparts in the other countries of the UK are described in Chapter 3.

Health-related behaviour

Many of the surveys described in Chapter 2 include general questions about health-related behaviour. In particular, these are included in the General Household Survey, the health surveys for England and Scotland and the Health and Lifestyle surveys.

The Health Education Monitoring Surveys were commissioned by the Health Education Authority and undertaken by ONS from 1995 onwards. The series aims to ascertain the health-related knowledge, attitudes and behaviour of adults between the ages of 16 and 74 in England. The survey focuses on health behaviours which are associated with the Health of Nation target areas, which are heart disease, cancer, mental illness, accidents, HIV / AIDS and sexual health. Interviewees are asked about their attempts to give up smoking, attitudes towards physical activity, knowledge about how to reduce the risks of skin cancer, sensible drinking levels and healthy diet. They are also asked about their alcohol consumption, participation in exercise, number of sexual partners and use of condoms. In 1996, questions were also asked about attitudes to drugs and about drug use. The sample size was around 4700 and attempts were made to make some questions comparable with other relevant surveys such as the Health Survey for England and the Health and Lifestyle Survey. The 1997 survey was a follow-up of the 1996 sample, and a new sample was selected in 1998 when associations between social inequalities and health were also investigated.

In addition, data about specific aspects of health-related behaviours are either collected specifically or collated from a number of different sources, These are summarised in what follows.

DRUG MISUSE

Information is collected by the drug misuse agencies about people with problem drug use who use their services either for the first time or for the first time after a break of 6 months or more. Selected personal details and information about the type of drugs used and the agency attended are forwarded to the relevant regional drug misuse database. Between 1 October 1992 and 31 March 1996, summaries of these data were forwarded to the Department of Health on form KO71. On 1 April 1996, the form was replaced by a system in which the regional databases forward anonymised individual electronic records. These include fuller information than the earlier form, including details of injecting and sharing equipment. The data are published 6 monthly by the Department of Health in a statistical bulletin, *Statistics from the regional drug misuse databases*. In Scotland, the Information and Statistics Division runs the Scottish Drugs Misuse Database, and data for Wales are collected by the Welsh Drug and Alcohol Unit. In Northern Ireland, the Department of Health and Social Services is considering whether to set up similar systems.

Up to March 1997, the Home Office operated an Addicts' Index. Under the 1973 regulations of the Misuse of Drugs Act 1971, general practitioners notified the Home Office of patients who were addicted to drugs. The Home Office published data derived from this source. The last publication from this system, the Home Office statistical bulletin *Statistics of drug addicts notified to the Home Office, United Kingdom, 1996* was published in October 1997.

In addition, a number of surveys have asked questions about drugs. Questions were asked in 1996 in the British Crime Survey.[28] The Health Education Authority undertook a survey in 1995.[29] As was mentioned above, questions were also asked in the 1996 Health Education Monitoring Survey.

SMOKING AND DRINKING

Although people using health services are often asked if they smoke or drink alcohol, data are not collected and compiled routinely by the NHS. The exception is the attempt to monitor the proportion of women who give up smoking before and during pregnancy. Few health authorities are able to supply the data at the time of writing, so these are not published.

On the other hand, information on smoking and drinking is collected in many surveys. These surveys (described in Chapter 2) include the health surveys, the General Household Survey, the Family Expenditure Survey, the ONS Omnibus Survey and the Health Education Monitoring Survey. In addition, ONS does special surveys about smoking and drinking among secondary school children, and information about smoking and drinking before and during pregnancy is collected in the 5-yearly infant feeding surveys. In Scotland, data about smoking at the start of pregnancy are collected through the SMR2 system. HM Customs and Excise collects information about numbers of cigarettes released for home consumption in the UK as a whole. This does not include duty free or smuggled cigarettes.

Data from these sources are brought together in an annual Department of Health statistical bulletin, *Statistics on smoking, England*. This includes trends in smoking prevalence by age and sex, cigarette consumption, smoking-related behaviour, tar and nicotine yields and the costs of smoking, together with estimates made by the Health Education Authority of premature deaths attributable to smoking. As well as being reported along with the results of individual surveys, summary data about smoking and drinking are published in *Health and personal social services statistics for England, Health statistics Wales* and *Scottish health statistics*.

DIET

The National Diet and Nutrition Survey programme (described in Chapter 6) is the major source of information about what adults and children eat. Data about attitudes towards healthy diets can be found in the Health Education Monitoring Survey. The diet of babies is monitored in 5-yearly Infant Feeding Surveys.

EXERCISE, SPORTS AND LEISURE ACTIVITIES

These have been regular topics in the General Household Survey and are now covered in the Health Education Monitoring Survey. Statistics about how people travel to work are compiled from census data and published in the volume on *Workplace and transport to work*. Data are also collected in the Labour Force Survey. A report, *Cycling in Britain*,[30] compiled by the Department of the Environment includes statistics from many different sources on characteristics of cyclists, cycling to work and accidents.

ACCIDENTS

Statistics about fires, road accidents, violent deaths and injuries, accidents at home and sports and leisure accidents are collected in a number of ways. Data about accidents at work are described in Chapter 6, and those about transport accidents are described in Chapter 7. Accidents can lead to deaths, data about which are described in Chapter 3, or use of hospitals as in-patients or out-patients, data about which are described earlier in this chapter. The Home Office collects data about accidents recorded by the police.

Public expenditure on health care

The main publications providing information on the finances of the NHS fall into the following categories:

1. 'Command papers' prepared for the parliamentary authorisation and scrutiny of public expenditure by the Department of Health, known as 'departmental reports', by the House of Commons Health Committee, known as 'public expenditure memoranda', and by HM Treasury, for example the Supply estimates.

2. ONS economic publications, in particular *the National accounts* and *Financial statistics.*

3. The accounts of Health Authorities and NHS trusts, in particular the *NHS England summarised accounts,* and other documents prepared for financial and performance management purposes by the NHS Executive, such as the 'Scottish costs book' and Health Authority revenue cash limits exposition book.

These publications are produced for different purposes and frequently use different conventions in recording and presenting data, leading to inconsistencies between figures given in different publications, which can, on occasion, be irreconcilable. Moreover, recording and presentation are subject to changes in practice, leading to inconsistencies between years. This is particularly true of information prepared for parliament by the Department of Health, and reconciliation of figures produced using different conventions is generally not taken back further than 6 years. Finally, the fundamental reorganisation of the finances of the NHS resulting from the 1990 NHS Community Care Act led to major breaks in time series. The 1990 reforms also led to the creation of flows of funding internal to the health service from NHS trusts to the Department of Health. These are not always adequately distinguished from flows of funding from the health service to the general economy via wages and payments for goods and services.

NHS expenditure at a national level

DEPARTMENTAL REPORTS AND OTHER COMMAND PAPERS

In March of each year, government departments produce annual reports in which they set out their expenditure plans, along with selected statistics about the activities of the department and the activities and services funded from its budget. These are usually referred to as 'departmental reports'.

As mentioned earlier, the Department of Health is responsible for the NHS in England. It also has overall responsibility for personal social services. Before July 1999, the Welsh Office and the Scottish Office had similar responsibilities, but on devolution these passed to the National Assembly for Wales and the Scottish Executive. When the Northern Ireland Assembly came into operation, health and social services became the responsibility of the Department of Health, Social Services and Public Safety, a single department within the Northern Ireland Office. On devolution, a new executive agency will take over its responsibilities and those of the four health and social services boards.

Reports prepared for presentation to the Westminster parliament are referred to as 'command papers'. The establishment of devolved government in Scotland, Wales and Northern Ireland will mean that information will in future have to be presented to the representative assemblies for those countries. It is unclear what information will continue to be presented to the Westminster parliament. Except in Scotland, the devolved assemblies have no tax-raising powers, but they will be able to vary health expenditure within the total budget determined by the UK parliament at Westminster. This means that decisions on aggregate NHS expenditure and resource allocation within the countries will no longer be confined to the Westminster parliament. Moreover, the assemblies may develop their own ways of reporting and monitoring expenditure. Westminster 'command papers' may therefore become less useful as a source of NHS financial information for the UK as a whole, although they will remain an important source of information for England.

The financial information presented in departmental reports is geared towards parliamentary scrutiny of expenditure plans, and includes spending for recent years along with projections for the following 3 or 4 years. The Department of Health 'departmental report' *The government's expenditure plans* is supplemented in the late summer by an annual publication of the House of Commons Health Committee, *Public expenditure on health and personal social services*, more commonly known as the 'public expenditure memorandum'. This consists of a memorandum produced by the Department of Health in response to a questionnaire from the Health Committee on various aspects of expenditure and policy. It provides much information which is not included in the 'departmental report'. The exact form of the questions changes from year to year, but broadly similar questions are asked each year about aggregate spending and the application of funds.

Because departmental reports are geared to parliamentary scrutiny of public expenditure, the financial information they present is based on the annual cash plans of departments concerned. The same overall format is used in the presentation of the cash plans of all four countries. Expenditure is presented for two main programmes, hospital and community health services and family health services. Together, these accounted for 96 per cent of health service expenditure in England in 1998/9. Other programmes presented in the cash plans vary from one country to another. The Department of Health's cash plans include the department's own expenditure on personal social services, but not local authority expenditure, and health service expenditure is totalled separately. This is not possible in Northern Ireland, where all expenditure on personal social services is combined with that on hospital and community health services. In Scotland, social work services were not the responsibility of the Scottish Office Department of Health and they are now split between two different departments of the Scottish Executive. It remains to be seen whether the proposed unification of family health services and hospital and community health services budgets in the hands of primary care groups will demand changes in the way expenditure is voted and reported.

The command papers also include tables setting out the cash plans in a different format according to 'area of expenditure'. Although these tables are derived from the cash plans, they depart from them in the way expenditure is scored to different programmes, leading to the potential for confusion. The Department of Health's report includes a table entitled 'NHS, England – by area of expenditure' and the House of Commons Health Committee's annual report on *Public expenditure on health and personal social services* includes a similar table. One of the most important differences is that, in the expenditure tables, cash-limited family health service budgets, which are held by health authorities, are included in spending on hospital and community health services. Another major difference is in the treatment of capital expenditure: in the cash plans, capital investment by NHS trusts is scored to current expenditure, whereas in the expenditure tables it is scored to capital. The notes to the published cash plan and expenditure tables generally allow figures to be reconciled.

The cash plan tables and their derivatives do not show the sources of the cash to be spent. Historically, there have been only two sources of NHS funding, general taxation and national insurance contributions, and charges made by NHS bodies for services to individuals or private sector organisations. Disposals of capital assets, such as land and buildings, release cash to the service, but are not an additional source of funding. This is not recognised in cash plan tables. The House of Commons Health Committee's report makes some attempt to account for sources of revenue, by including lines for 'charges and receipts' in the expenditure table, but this can lead to confusion: charges are a source of funding, whereas disposals are not.

Internal flows of funding can be identified by reconciling the cash plans with the parliamentary authorisation of expenditure. This takes two forms. Expenditure is either voted as 'supply grants' from the Consolidated Fund, the government's account at the Bank of England, or as 'appropriations in aid'. The latter represent funds which individual departments receive directly. Spending of these has to be authorised explicitly; otherwise, the funds have to be surrendered to the Consolidated Fund. The Department of Health's report includes an annex detailing the 'appropriations in aid' which contribute to expenditure for the current year. Since 1992, these have included flows of funds from NHS trusts to the Department of Health. These flows, described as capital refunds, are clearly not a source of funding for the system as whole, as they are themselves funded out of NHS revenue. To assess the real level of tax-funded expenditure on the health service, it is therefore important to check plans against the *Supply estimates*, published annually by HM Treasury, and the *Appropriation accounts*, published annually by the Comptroller and Auditor General.

NATIONAL ACCOUNTS

The *National accounts*, generally referred to as 'The Blue Book', is the main annual publication by the ONS giving information on public expenditure. Before 1984 it was called *National income and expenditure*, and before 1996 it was published by the Central Statistical Office. The national accounts present expenditure on health care as part of the economic activity of the government. International comparability is important, as is the construction of relatively extended time series. Neither of these is characteristic of the departmental reports.

ONS compiles the accounts by collecting data directly from departments on a quarterly basis. The data on expenditure do not align precisely with those provided for parliamentary scrutiny in the departmental reports. A Treasury publication, *Public expenditure statistical analysis*, gives a reconciliation between the national accounts and cash plans.

The *National accounts* have included series about NHS expenditure from 1948 onwards. The level of detail increased with changes to the presentation of government expenditure in 1955. From 1955 to 1977, the most complete data were presented in the combined accounts of central and local government. In 1977, this was renamed 'general government expenditure'. Central government expenditure was and continues to be dealt with separately in the central government current account. Expenditure is analysed in terms of 'final consumption expenditure' and 'gross domestic fixed capital formation', in other words, as current and capital. Current expenditure is divided between 'labour costs' and 'other'.

There are two important breaks in the series, both resulting from efforts in the 1970s to bring the UK's national accounts into line with methods proposed by international institutions. In 1977, a new classification of government expenditure by function, the United Nations Classification of Functions of Government (COFOG), was introduced. This led to changes in what was categorised as health expenditure, and it was not possible to reclassify pre-1977 data to take account of this. Data were not published using the United Nations Classification until 1984.[31]

The second break occurred in 1991, but was to some extent a consequence of changes made in 1977. In 1964, a new heading of 'public sector' was introduced. It included the accounts for public corporations such as nationalised industries as well as those of central and local government. In order to bring the accounts into conformity with the Organisation for Economic Co-operation and Development's system of national accounts, the concept of a public sector was dropped in 1977, effectively reverting to the pre-1964 position. The accounts of central and local government were combined and labelled 'general government expenditure' and public corporations were given a separate reading. The change had no effect on health service expenditure data at the time, but from 1991 onwards, NHS trusts were established as public corporations. This means that certain aspects of the economic activity of NHS trusts – in particular, capital expenditure – fall outside the category of 'general government expenditure'. Instead, they are consigned to the public corporations heading. Data on capital are collected by a survey of NHS trusts, but as one of the conditions of the voluntary agreement between the ONS and the trusts, the data can only be used to produce accounts for the public corporations sector as a whole; even aggregated data on the NHS trust sector cannot be released.

Financial information from health authorities and NHS trusts

The *NHS summarised accounts* for England, Scotland and Wales have been produced by the Office of the Comptroller and Auditor General since the foundation of the service. They represent the audited accounts of NHS bodies in the respective countries, prepared for the attention of the Public Accounts Committee of the House of Commons. As with other sources of financial information on the health service, they changed dramatically with the 1990 Act, under which NHS bodies were obliged to draw up their accounts on a commercial basis. As of the year 2000, the accounts for the NHS in Scotland and Wales will be produced by the Auditor Generals of those countries for the attention of their own representative assemblies.

Because the accounts are prepared on a commercial basis, they need to be treated with caution. For example, NHS bodies are obliged to account for future medical negligence claims as liabilities on their balance sheets, but are only funded for claims as and when they have to be met; this can lead to deficits on their accounts which have no economic significance. The general point here is that information derived from the financial performance management system, of which the accounts form part, does not necessarily say much about the economic condition of the service as a whole. On the other hand, the 'summarised accounts' give a clearer account of capital investment in the service than other publications.

NHS trusts' financial returns are intended to provide the Executive with data on hospital and community health services' net expenditure by programme and specialty and gross expenditure by staff, commodity and service groupings. Only Scotland produces a publication making extensive use of this material, *Scottish health service costs*, generally referred to as the 'Scottish costs book', produced by the Information and Statisctics Division, Scotland.

Information on expenditure by programme is published for England in the House of Commons Health Committee's *Public expenditure on health and personal social services* under the heading 'Programme budget'. Until 1998, this was based on returns from providers, but due to the expansion of NHS purchasing of care in the private sector, purchaser returns are now used. The rationale for this change is given in the 1998 edition.

Key official publications

Department of Health. *Departmental report: the government's expenditure plans.* London: TSO, published annually.

Scottish Office. *Departmental report: the government's expenditure plans.* London: TSO, published annually up to 1999.

Welsh Office. *Departmental report: the government's expenditure plans.* London: TSO, published annually up to 1999.

Northern Ireland Office. *Departmental report: the government's expenditure plans.* London: TSO, published annually.

House of Commons Health Committee. *Public expenditure on health and personal social services.* London: TSO, published annually.

HM Treasury. *Supply estimates: main estimates.* London: TSO, published annually.

Office for National Statistics. *National accounts.* London: TSO, published annually.

Comptroller and Auditor General. *Appropriation accounts.* London: TSO, published annually.

HM Treasury. *Public expenditure statistical analysis.* London: TSO, published annually.

Comptroller and Auditor General. NHS (England) summarised accounts. London: TSO, published annually.

Information and Statistics Division. *Scottish health service costs.* Edinburgh: ISD, published annually.

Other publications containing data about NHS expenditure

In addition to the detailed publications described above, some more general publications contain some data about NHS expenditure. The *Annual abstract of statistics* contains time series of NHS spending in each of the four countries of the UK. *Social trends* contains summarised data about NHS spending. Tables of data about expenditure on the NHS in each country are included in *Health and personal social services statistics for England*, *Health statistics Wales* and *Scottish health statistics*. Although these are not sufficiently detailed for people wanting to scrutinise NHS spending in depth, they give a general idea of how NHS funds are spent.

Monitoring NHS performance

We have shown in this chapter that a considerable amount of information is recorded about the resources, the activities and the finances of the NHS. To what extent are these used to monitor the performance of the services and is this possible with the data available?

One approach is to monitor complaints. In the 1990s, under the Patients' Charter, all the countries of the UK established systems for collecting and publishing data about patients' complaints about the care they receive. Although this can point to problem areas, it will always be unclear to what extent complaints may relate to relationships between staff and patients and to what extent they relate to quality of clinical care. In England, data collected on returns KO41(A), relating to the hospital and community health services, and KO41(B), relating to family health services, are published in *Handling complaints: monitoring the NHS complaints procedures*. Similar data are collected in Wales and published in an additional table on the free diskette issued to purchasers of *Health statistics Wales*. Satisfaction with services is monitored in the Welsh Health Survey. In Scotland, data are published in an Information and Statistics Division publication, *NHS complaints in Scotland*, and in *Scottish health statistics*. In Northern Ireland, the Central Services Agency monitors complaints made to the health and social services boards.

Although they have a much longer history, dating back to the nineteenth century, current statistical approaches started in the early 1980s, when the government started to collect 'performance indicators' in many public funded services. In the NHS in England, the first set of 'performance indicators', later known as 'health service indicators', was compiled. In general, they were expressed as rates, derived by dividing activity and resource data by an appropriate population denominator, so that comparisons could be made between districts. The way these and other indicators developed into the current high level performance framework[34] and clinical indicators is described in Chapter 3. Development is inevitably constrained by the extent and quality of the data available to construct them.

As we have seen in this chapter, three of the four countries of the UK rely on a system designed in the 1980s for administrative rather than clinical purposes. The system was designed for a system which was hierarchical and focused on care in hospital under the NHS. It therefore collects very few data from non-NHS providers and relatively few from general practitioners. No person-based data are collected routinely about care in general practice, the community or out-patient departments. With the increasing shift to care outside hospital, this lack of data is becoming an increasingly serious problem.

Monitoring community care

During the 1990s, a number of policy initiatives attempted to shift the balance of resources from secondary to primary care. In particular, one aim of general practitioner fundholding, introduced under the NHS and Community Care Act 1990, was to empower general practitioners to obtain more cost-effective secondary and community health care services for their patients. This same aim lies behind the creation of primary care groups in April 1999.

The 1990 Act also brought about changes to the way social care was allocated to individuals and to the responsibilities of different sectors. Local authorities replaced the NHS in taking the lead in organising care for elderly people. In the same way that fundholding gave general practitioners responsibility for purchasing secondary and community services, local authority care managers were given the task of purchasing social care. In addition, local authorities were encouraged to purchase services and residential care from the independent sector rather than providing it themselves.

Monitoring and planning community care have always been seen as problematic, with many difficulties involved in collaboration between the agencies involved and in joint planning. The internal market compounded these problems by further fragmenting the services and increasing the numbers of agencies involved. Five different types of organisations – hospital trusts, community trusts, general practitioner fundholders, local authorities and the private sector – were involved in providing care. District health authorities, fundholding general practitioners, and local authorities were all involved in purchasing care for client groups whose needs could not be clearly spilt between these agencies. Although fundholding was abolished in April 1999, two types of commissioning authorities – primary care groups and local authorities – remained.

Despite these major changes in entitlements to and organisation of care, it is very difficult to build up a complete picture of community care using only data available routinely. Little information is available to support the joint planning of services or to ascertain the impact of the changes on clients. Information is lacking in three areas. There is inadequate information about problems relating to interfaces between organisations, about the activities of community and primary care staff, and about the needs of the population.

INTERFACE PROBLEMS

Local authorities and health authorities do not necessarily have common geographical boundaries or use common definitions. As shown in Chapter 9, this leads to difficulties in comparing information from the two different systems. Moreover, general practices are based only loosely on geographical areas, so primary care groups do not cover geographically defined populations. Because the practice lists are not geographically based, problems will arise in using the census, birth and death statistics and any other data which are based on electoral wards. In addition, the many changes which have taken place make it almost impossible to monitor trends over time for local areas.

The artificial nature of the clear boundaries between health and social care drawn in the NHS and Community Care Act 1990 have been recognised.[5] For elderly and mentally ill people, in particular, the line between the two cannot be drawn precisely, because needs fluctuate. The boundaries between health and social care are locally negotiable, but health services are free at the point of delivery, whereas local authority care is means tested. There is no information about where particular social services departments and health authorities draw that line and therefore no information about geographical inequities. It may be that clients in some parts of the country are paying for services they would be receiving as a free entitlement elsewhere. Although plans for an electronic health record assume that it will contain records of social care as well as health care, it is unclear how the many conceptual and practical problems will be overcome or whether it will be possible to derive statistics from them.

DATA FOR ASSESSING NEEDS

The limited data from general practice described earlier do not cover all practices and do not measure the need for social care. It is not easy to monitor people's destination on discharge from hospital. Data can still be obtained from the Hospital Episode Statistics, but considerable skill and time are required to produce comparative information. Even then, they would not monitor the needs of people who had not been admitted to hospital. Both the Körner returns described in this chapter and the local authority returns described in Chapter 9 were devised primarily to provide information to enable local management to monitor activity rather than to measure the need for social care.

This could potentially be derived from the assessment process for individual social care which is undertaken by local authorities, but little information is collected about the process at a national level. There are no national data about the numbers of referrals, the numbers of assessments carried out, referral times, the numbers, content and cost of client care packages, how these packages are funded, or about their clients. No attempt is made to use the system to monitor unmet need and there are no means by which one authority can compare its assessment process with another. Such comparative information would be particularly valuable for local authorities in developing their own plans for community care.

DEFICIENCIES IN ACTIVITY DATA

NHS data are acknowledged to be inadequate for monitoring community care. In the past, data definitions have relied on who has provided a service and where it has been provided. This may have some relevance to hospital care, but for community services it can mean that indicators give a very incomplete picture. The need for either a functional or client-based approach to indicator definition will become increasingly pressing for all health care services.

At one time, there were plans to implement a new community minimum dataset in England by April 1993, but this did not happen. Subsequent plans were to implement it partially by April 1997. It would have included information about the core objectives of the care in terms of whether it was meant to cure, maintain or rehabilitate, and a description of the care programme. A dependency indicator, which would have been a measure of need, was dropped as it was said to require further development.

After the change of government, the community dataset was reviewed again, as part of the preparations for the information strategy. *Information for health* concluded that the minimum dataset proposed in 1995 was too contract oriented to meet the needs of local commissioning or the national performance framework.[5,32] While acknowledging the value of some of the work which had been done on mental health and maternity datasets, it concluded that 'the case to abandon the development of a single episodic minimum dataset for community services is strong'.[5] It also questioned the advisability of spending staff time on completing Körner returns, given the limited value of the resulting data.

Unfortunately, however, the alternatives proposed were disappointingly vague. *Information for health* recommended that primary care systems should be improved and that they should be integrated with community care systems. In addition, it restated the principle that information for secondary data flows should be derived from those captured in operational clinical systems, and that the means should be developed to extract data from them automatically. These are all very laudable aims, but they were stated to be 'clearly a medium to long term development agenda'.[5] All that is proposed for the short term is 'simple interim measures for benchmarking the relative value for money of local primary and community services.' In other words, data about community care have yet again dropped to the bottom of the queue.

Meanwhile, the lack of information about activities in and needs for community and social care means that resources cannot be allocated according to need, and gross inequities may occur. This has serious implications as increasing emphasis is placed on primary and community care.

What hope do the information strategies offer?

In proposing integrated person-based records, the information strategies offer the potential for record linkage and an enhanced ability to measure outcome. A number of key questions need to be asked, however. The first, and most crucial, is whether adequate resources will be made available to implement them, as considerable redevelopment will be needed, especially of primary care systems. The next, given the focus in the documents on assembling data for individual patient care, is whether it will actually be possible to derive statistical information from them. While the principle of deriving data from operational clinical systems is laudable, it also needs to be shown to work in practice.

An equally important question is what data items will actually be derived from these systems and collected locally and nationally? Will our national statistics be limited to a relatively small number of clinical indicators and an even smaller number of high level performance indicators? If so, the picture will be even more limited than it is at present. The Steering Group on Health Services Information focused its attention on the data items to be collected and gave little thought about how they were to be collected or analysed. In contrast to this, the information strategies talk more about how systems will operate, but say very little about what data might be needed for different purposes, how the items will be identified and how they will be derived.

The decision to put the development of data about community and primary care at the bottom of the queue is unfortunate, but perhaps not surprising. Although the documents talk about the needs of general practitioners as commissioners of care, the main thrust of the discussion is about the process of booking individual patients into hospital and obtaining reports about the care provided to individuals. Although the need for good aggregated data about hospital, community and primary care is stressed, this is mainly at a conceptual level, and more information is needed about how this can be translated into reality.

Contact addresses and web sites

Department of Health
Statistical bulletins and most other
publications are available from:
Department of Health
PO Box 777
London SE1 6XH
Telephone: 0541 555 455
Fax: 01623 724524
Web site: http://www.doh.gov.uk/

Branch SD2, Hospital and community
health services statistics
Skipton House
80 London Road
London SE1 6LW
Telephone:
Hospital in-patient activity
                        020 7972 5529
Maternity statistics   020 7972 5533
General dental and community health
statistics   020 7972 5392
General pharmacy services
                        020 7972 5504
General ophthalmic services
                        020 7972 5507
Prescription analysis   020 7972 5515

Quarry House
Quarry Hill
Leeds LS2 7UE
Telephone:
NHS medical staff statistics
                        0113 254 5881
NHS non-medical staff statistics
                        0113 254 5891
Finance statistics   0113 254 5389
Waiting lists   0113 254 5555
Hospital activity   0113 254 5522
NHS expenditure   0113 254 5356
Finance statistics   0113 254 5389

National Assembly for Wales, formerly
the Welsh Office, Health statistics,
Telephone: 029 20 825080

Statistical publications:
Publications Unit
Statistical Directorate 5
National Assembly for Wales
Cathay's Park
Cardiff CF10 3NQ
Email: Statswales@gtnet.gov.uk

Information and Statistics Division,
Common Services Agency for the NHS
in Scotland
Trinity Park House
South Trinity Road
Edinburgh EH5 3SQ
Telephone: 0131 552 6255
Web site: http: //www.show.scot.
nhs.uk/isd/index.htm

Department of Health, Social Services
and Public Safety
Regional Information Branch
Annexe 2
Castle Buildings
Stormont
Belfast BT4 3UD
Telephone: 028 90 522800
Web site: http://www.dhssni.gov.uk/
hpss/statistics/index.html

Central Services Agency
27 Adelaide Street
Belfast BT2 8FH
Telephone: 028 90 324431

HM Treasury publications in print are all
placed on the internet.
Web site: http: //www.hm-treasury.gov.
uk/pub/html/pip/main.html

References

1. General Register Office. *Morbidity statistics from general practice, 1955–56.* Studies on Medical and Population Subjects No. 14. London: HMSO, 1958.
2. Rayner D. *Review of the government statistical services: report to the Prime Minister.* London: Central Statistical Office, 1980.
3. Steering Group on Health Services Information. *First report to the Secretary of State.* London: HMSO, 1982.
4. Steering Group on Health Services Information. *Supplement to the first and fourth reports to the Secretary of State.* London: HMSO, 1985.
5. Department of Health, NHS Executive. *Information for health.* Leeds: NHS Executive, 1998.
6. National Information Management and Technology Board. *Strategic programme for modernising information management and technology in the NHS in Scotland.* Edinburgh: Scottish Office, 1998.
7. Welsh Office. *Better information, better health: information management and technology for health care and health improvement in Wales. A strategic framework 1998 to 2005.* Cardiff: Welsh Office, 1998.
8. Radical Statistics Health Group. NHS 'indicators of success': what do they tell us? *British Medical Journal* 1995; **305**: 1045–50.
9. Department of Health. *HES: the book.* London: Department of Health, published annually.
10. Department of Health. *How HES data is processed.* London: Department of Health, published annually.
11. Price S. Hospital episode statistics. In: Leadbeter D, Rigby M eds. *Harnessing official statistics.* Abingdon: Radcliffe Medical Press. In press.
12. Department of Health. NHS maternity statistics, England: 1989–90 to 1994–95. *Statistical Bulletin* 1997; **28**: 1–44.
13. Welsh Office. *Maternity aspects of child health in Wales,* third report. Cardiff: WHSCSA, 1998.
14. Kendrick S, Clarke J. The Scottish record linkage system. *Health Bulletin* 1993; **51**(2): 72–9.
15. Williams B. Utilisation of National Health Service hospitals in England by private patients, 1989–95. *Health Trends* 1997; **29**: 21–5.
16. Williams BT, Pearson J. Private patients in NHS hospitals: comparison of two sources of information. *Journal of Public Health Medicine* 1999; **21**(1): 70–3.
17. Laing W. *Laing's review of private healthcare.* London: Laing and Buisson, published annually.
18. Williams BT, Nicholl JP, Thomas KJ, Knowelden J. Analysis of the work of independent acute hospitals in England and Wales, 1981. *British Medical Journal* 1984; **289**(6442): 446–8.
19. Nicholl JP, Beeby NR, Williams BT. Role of the private sector in elective surgery in England and Wales, 1986. *British Medical Journal* 1989; **298**(6668): 243–7.
20. Williams BT, Nicholl JP. Patient characteristics and clinical caseload of short stay independent hospitals in England and Wales, 1992–3. *British Medical Journal* 1994; **308**(6945): 1699–701.
21. Royal College of General Practitioners, Office of Population Censuses and Surveys, and Department of Health and Social Security. *Morbidity statistics from general practice, 1971–72: second national study.* Studies on Medical and Population Subjects No. 36. London: HMSO, 1979.

22. Royal College of General Practitioners, Office of Population Censuses and Surveys, and Department of Health and Social Security. *Morbidity statistics from general practice, 1970–1971: socio-economic analyses.* Studies on Medical and Population Subjects No. 46. London: HMSO, 1982.

23. Royal College of General Practitioners, Office of Population Censuses and Surveys, and Department of Health and Social Security. *Morbidity statistics from general practice, 1981–82: third national study.* Series MB5 No. 1. London: HMSO, 1986.

24. Royal College of General Practitioners, Office of Population Censuses and Surveys, and Department of Health. *Morbidity statistics from general practice, 1981–82: third morbidity study: socio-economic analyses.* Series MB5 No. 2. London: HMSO, 1990.

25. Royal College of General Practitioners, Office of Population Censuses and Surveys, and Department of Health. *Morbidity statistics from general practice: fourth national study, 1991–1992.* Series MB5 No. 3. London: HMSO, 1995.

26. Department of Health, NHS Executive. *Collection of data from general practice: overview.* Leeds: NHS Executive, 1996.

27. Dodd T, Freeth S. *Contraception and sexual health, 1997.* Series OS11. London: Office for National Statistics, 1999.

28. *Drug misuse declared in 1996: latest results from the British Crime Survey.* Home Office Research Study 172. London: Home Office Information and Publications Group, 1997.

29. *Drug use in England. Results of the 1995 National Drugs Campaign Survey.* London: Health Education Authority, 1997.

30. Department of the Environment. *Cycling in Britain.* London: TSO, 1996.

31. Doggett EA. *National accounts: concepts, sources and methods.* Office for National Statistics. London: TSO, 1998, Annex 2, 497–501.

32. NHS Executive. *A national framework for assessing performance – consultation document.* Leeds: NHS Executive, 1997.

Social services

STATISTICS CHASING THE POLICY TAIL

Nick Miller and Robin Darton

Introduction

Personal social services statistics

Residential and nursing homes for elderly people

Introduction

Social care statistics, like policies for social care provision, were in a continual state of change during the 1980s and 1990s. The changes were driven by two conflicting agendas. The Department of the Environment efficiency scrutiny[1] attempted to reduce the burden of information collection on local authorities, while attempts by central government to increase the oversight of the activities of social services departments required more information from them. There is also a third agenda, the change in the role of social services departments from providers of care to commissioners of services. This has resulted in large-scale, ongoing privatisation of service provision.

The collection and publication of information on social care provision vary from one constituent part of the United Kingdom to another. This chapter concentrates on the collection of data for England. Data collected and published about services in Wales, Scotland and Northern Ireland are described briefly.

The first section of this chapter gives an overview of current social services statistics for all client groups, and then goes on to discuss the problem of using the statistics for monitoring the performance of social services departments. In any area, the local social services department is just one of a number of agencies which commission or provide social care. Comparisons between social services departments are complicated by the inability to measure the contribution of these other agencies, in particular the National Health Service (NHS). The second section reviews the statistics on the provision of residential and nursing home care. In the last two decades, there has been a substantial growth of independent, especially private sector, provision of residential and nursing home care,[2] but it has proved extremely difficult to chart this expansion through the official datasets on residential and nursing homes.[3] The expansion was financed to a large extent from the social security budget, which increased from £10 million in 1979 to £1390 million in 1990, and to an estimated

£2.4 billion in 1992–3.[4] Information collected on social security payments is completely separate from that collected about spending by local authorities on provision of services.

The information presented in this chapter concentrates on activity. Financial information relating to expenditure and income is collected by the Department of the Environment, Transport and the Regions (DETR) for each financial year, using the RO3 series of forms. Parallel to the information collected by government departments are the annual collections of personal social services statistics by the Institute of Public Finance Limited for the Chartered Institute of Public Finance and Accountancy (CIPFA). These include information about estimated and actual expenditure, income and provision for each local authority in England and Wales and, from 1994–5, Scotland. Two volumes are published annually, *Personal social services statistics estimates*[5] and *Personal social services statistics actuals*.[6] The statistics are predominately financial, but the publications also contain some limited information on provision of services. Although the majority of local authorities complete the Chartered Institute of Public Finance and Accountancy returns, a number either do not complete the returns or are unable to provide all the information requested. In recent years, complete non-response has principally affected the statistics for metropolitan districts.

Beginning with 1987/8, the Department of Health has published indicators of social services provision in the publication *Key indicators of local authority social services*.[7] The indicators are presented for each local authority, groups of local authorities and England as a whole. They include financial information submitted to the Department of the Environment, Transport and the Regions and information derived from Chartered Institute of Public Finance and Accountancy data. Since 1997, the key indicators have been released in an electronic format,[8] which enables comparisons to be made over time. Following the introduction of the Citizen's Charter, the Audit Commission has collected information annually to monitor the performance of local authorities against the Citizen's Charter standards.[9] These performance indicators are also available in electronic format.

The annual Department of Health publication entitled *Health and personal social services statistics for England* contains an overview of the information collected about social services provision. The volume of information was reduced substantially from the 1997 edition onwards, following a complete revision of its content and format.[10] Details of the sources of information and the statistical returns from local authorities and health authorities to the Department of Health on personal social services, including nursing homes, are contained in the *Personal social services statistical information directory*.[11]

Personal social services statistics

Local authority social services departments, like the NHS, provide services from the cradle to the grave. Although the sector has grown significantly since 1993, compared to the NHS it is still small. In 1999, there were 151 English social services departments. Their overall estimated annual expenditure in 1996/7 was over £9 billion gross, compared with NHS gross expenditure of nearly £35 billion in the same year.[10] In September 1997, social services departments in England directly employed 229 000 whole-time-equivalent staff, while the NHS employed 758 000.[10] Unlike services provided by or through the NHS, services provided by social services departments are not 'free at the point of delivery' and service users may be charged depending on their income and savings.

Most social services departments now organise their services around 'client groups'. Adult client group 'specialisms' often include older people, adults with severe learning disabilities, adults with mental health problems and adults with physical and sensory disabilities. Adult subspecialisms may include services related to people with HIV/AIDS or substance abuse problems. Services for children and their families may have subspecialisms relating to children with disabilities, youth justice, child protection, child and adolescent mental health, and support for families with pre-school children.

Defining the core purposes of social services departments is difficult, given the enormous range of their 'activity', and personal social services statistics have been under continuous revision since the mid-1990s. This section describes the current data collected by social services departments and published by the Department of Health for adults, children and families, including changes currently being implemented or proposed.

What statistics are available on personal social services?

Unlike the NHS, social services departments are subject to control and scrutiny, not only from central government but also from locally elected councillors. Information on activity, staffing and expenditure is a critical part of this accountability. Most social services departments collect data regularly at locality level for internal management purposes. Data collection includes workload measures such as referrals and caseloads, activity data such as levels of provision of services, and waiting lists. Local authorities usually have their own 'performance' indicators including some comparison with targets, such as whether complaints are responded to in a given time period. They will also collect separate financial and staffing data. While there is overlap between internal management information and the Department of Health's statistical returns, data definitions are not standardised. Each department decides what is collected, how it is reported and how the information is used.

The Department of Health requires social services departments to submit a series of annual returns about their activities. The returns can be divided into two groups. Returns for 1998/9 relating to services for adults are shown in Table 9.1 and returns for the same year relating to services for children and families are shown in Table 9.2.

Table 9.1 Social services departments returns to the Department of Health, adults 1998/9

Return (return reference)	Topic	Coverage	Units reported
Local authority-supported residents in residential and nursing care (SR1)[13]	Adults funded in residential/nursing home care at 31 March and new admissions in previous 12 months (permanent/short term)	Numbers funded by social services departments at 31 March	Numbers for each social services department in four different client groups
Day centre provision for adults (DC3)[12]	Numbers of day care centres in a social services department's area; numbers of places per week; adults provided with care	Sample week in September annually	Numbers for each social services department in four different client groups and a 'mixed' client group
Home help and home care (HH1)[12]	Hours of home care provided to residents of a social services department's area funded by the social services department; number of clients to whom provided; matrix of hours and visits	Sample week in September annually	Includes children; double counting of recipients who had services from more than one provider should be eliminated
Meals services (MS1)[12]	Meals provided to adult clients through day care centres, lunch clubs, meals on wheels schemes, frozen meals schemes	Sample week in September annually	Numbers of meals and recipients by age group
Registered homes for adults returns (forms A/B/C) (formerly returns RAC5 and RAU1)[13]	Numbers of homes and residential and nursing places at 31 March; number of admissions in year and discharges in year; reason for discharge; day care provision in homes	At 31 March	Unit return on each home including small homes with fewer than 4 places

Registers of disabled people: blind/partially sighted (SSDA 902)[32]*	Numbers of people known to the social services departments at 31 March who are registered as blind/partially sighted; also those registered as having a visual handicap with other disabilities	Every third year only at 31 March	Summary return from each social services department by age group; includes children
Registers of disabled people: deaf/hard of hearing (SSDA 910)[34]*	Numbers of people known to the social services departments at 31 March who are registered as deaf or hard of hearing	Every third year only at 31 March	Summary return from each social services department by age group; includes children
Registers of disabled people: physical handicap (SSDA 911)[33]*	Numbers of people known to the social services departments at 31 March who are registered as having a physical disability	Every third year only at 31 March	Summary return from each social services department by age group; includes children
Mental Health Act Guardianship (SSDA 703)[86]	All subject to guardianship in a year	Annual	Unit return for each person subject to guardianship in year: section of Mental Health Act, reason for guardianship, age and gender
Expenditure (return RO3 to the Department of the Environment, Transport and the Regions)*	Expenditure by principal areas of activity of social services departments for financial year	Annual	Expenditure and income for some 6 activity areas for each of 5 adult client groups
Staffing (SSDS001): ADSS/Local Government Management Board Workforce surveys[17,18]	SSDS001 covers all staff in post within social services departments as at 30 September	Annually at 30 September	Numbers full time and part time and whole-time equivalent in post in each of approx. 40 different staff groups

* Information also relates to social services departments' involvement with children and their families – see text.

Table 9.2 Social services departments returns to the Department of Health – children and families

Return	Topic	Coverage	Units reported
Children 'looked after' by social services departments in a year (CLA100: SSDA903)[21]	Children/young people under 18 looked after for 1 or more nights by social service departments: includes those in residential care and fostering.	Annually at 31 March, excluding those placed for respite care under short-term agreements	Returns from each social services department. Aggregated numbers per local authority and unit return on 1/3 sample of all children looked after in year
Secure units (SSDA 912)[24]	Places in secure units; number in secure units	Annually at 31 March	1 return per secure unit
Children's residential establishments (CH1)[25]	Gazetteer	At 31 March Returns now triennial from each social services department	Each home registered within social services department area
Child protection (CPR1)[22]	Children on child protection registers at 31 March, and those added to and removed from registers; number looked after at 31 March and their placements; number subject to initial child protection conferences in year	Annually at 31 March	Returns from each social services department
Criminal Supervision Orders (SSDA 906)[23]	Number of young people on supervision orders to social services departments at year end/started in year	Annually at 31 March	Returns from each social services department

Day care provision for under 8s (was SSDA 503, now via Department for Education and Employment)	Number of nurseries, playgroups, childminders, holiday schemes, after-school clubs; family centres; number of registered places; number of children placed and funded by social services department	Annually at 31 March	Returns from each social services department
Families with children receiving home care support through the social services departments (HH1)[12]*	Hours of home care provided to residents of a social services department area funded by the social services department; numbers of clients provided in sample week; matrix of hours and visits	Numbers receiving support in sample week in September	Annual return for social services departments for a sample week in September
Registers of those with disabilities (see text): blind/partially sighted, deaf/hard of hearing, physical handicap[32-4]*	Numbers of people known to the social services departments at 31 March who are registered	Every third year only at 31 March	Summary return from each social services department; includes children
Personal social services expenditure (Return RO3 to DETR)*	Expenditure (gross and net) by principal areas of activity of social services departments for financial year	Annual returns	Activity areas by client group; central management costs redistributed
Staffing (SSDS001): ADSS/Local Government Management Board Workforce surveys[17,18]*	SSDS001 covers all staff in post within social services departments at 30 September	Staff in post on 30 September	Numbers full-time and part-time and whole-time-equivalent staff in post in each of approximately 12 different staff groups

*Information also relates to social services departments involvement with adults. See text.

ADULT CARE RETURNS: CHANGES IN THE LATE 1990S AND PRIORITIES FOR FURTHER DEVELOPMENT

Most of the data from the annual returns are published in two detailed annual publications, one covering domiciliary and day care[12] and the other residential care.[13] Two statistical bulletins cover similar areas, but their titles and content change from year to year.[14,15]

Following the Department of the Environment, Transport and the Regions Efficiency Scrutiny in 1996/7,[1,16] the level of detail in many returns was reduced. As a result, many datasets now have discontinuities and lack comparability with previous years. For example, in 1998, the return for adult day care (DC3) collected data on attenders in a sample week, while the total number of attendances was collected previously. In addition, social services funded day care in residential and nursing homes was included for the first time. As this cannot be separately identified, the data are not comparable with those for previous years. The annual expenditure return to the Department of the Environment, Transport and the Regions (RO3) was also 'slimmed down' from 1998/9 onwards and revised. Data about staffing, including qualifications, vacancies, turnover and staffing ratios, collected by the Local Government Management Board are also under review. In 1998, the Local Government Management Board undertook two major surveys to 'map' the workforce providing residential and day care in independent agencies and their perceived training needs.[17,18]

As well as revising the returns, the Department of Health introduced a new system of data collection for adults. This attempts to link demand for services and assessment of individual need with the care actually provided. The complex series of twelve forms, known as the 'Referrals, assessments and packages of care' returns, is being fully implemented in April 2000.[19] These returns cover three broad areas: first, referrals to social services departments and how departments responded to them; second, assessments and subsequent reviews by social service staff, including those of informal carers; and third, clients provided with 'packages of care' or services.

Much of this information was already collated by social service departments using local definitions. Definitions have now been standardised, so that comparable data are collected in every authority. Returns will be aggregated for each authority, but could also be disaggregated by social services departments to different geographical levels, including, for example, NHS primary care groups.

The Department of Health has indicated that it is proposing to develop the referrals, assessment and packages of care returns further to cover time lapsed between referral, completion of assessments and subsequent delivery of services. It is assessing use of the new data for estimating unit costs of activities and service packages.

CHILDREN'S RETURNS: CHANGES IN THE LATE 1990S AND PRIORITIES FOR DEVELOPMENT

The data from the returns about services for children (shown in Table 9.2), appear in six separate annual publications. These relate to children's day care,[20] children 'looked after' by local authorities,[21] child protection registers,[22] supervision orders,[23] children accommodated in secure units[24] and children's homes.[25]

In the late 1990s, the returns for children were slimmed down. In 1997/8, the annual return on each child 'looked after' (SSDA 903) was reduced to a sample of a third and there are plans to prune this further.[26] Departments were strongly encouraged to record the circumstances of 'looked after' children in considerable detail, using 'Looked after children' forms[27] introduced in 1996. Data from these, if retrievable from computer systems, can significantly add to the information available about this group.

Returns in use up to 1999 covered only about 20 per cent of children receiving services from or through social services departments at any one time. From 1999/2000 onwards, a new return, the *Children in need* dataset,[28] is being completed about all individual children supported by social services departments in a sample week. Social services departments' staff categorise each child or young person worked with, and record time spent in the week with each client. The Department of Health aims to relate this to costs, services and social work time so that authorities can be 'bench-marked' and compared. From 1999/2000 onwards, social services departments have to provide the Department of Health with a series of outcome indicators for children they 'look after' continuously for more than a year.[29] These indicators focus on educational attainment, further education, offending, employment and health. Health indicators include conceptions under the age of 16, attendances at accident and emergency departments in the year, routine immunisations, and failure to visit a dentist in the year. For children aged under 5, they include developmental reviews, the presence of ongoing health conditions or disability, and the proportion who have received 'adequate' treatment for these conditions.

The 'referrals, assessments and packages of care' proposals for adult care are being developed to include data collection about levels of referral and social services department responses. At the time of writing, there are no proposals to collect similar data for children, nor is it proposed to collect other relevant information, such as the impact of the criteria which social services departments use to screen referrals.

Priority needs to be given to linking data on individual children with data about the families in which they live. The circumstances of children living in three different types of household are of particular interest. First, there is a strong relationship between the activity of social services departments and family poverty. Data on income support recipients at a level below that of the local social services department office or local authority are difficult to obtain, although in 1998 the Benefits Agency released data on recipients at ward level for August 1996.[30] Few social services departments record or analyse information focusing on levels of family income, and none of the government's development proposals addresses this. Social services departments have powers to assist families with children in poverty under the 1989 Children Act, but little is known about the use made of these powers, apart from occasional local analyses.

Secondly, the majority of children 'looked after' away from their own homes by social services departments are placed in foster homes, either on a permanent basis or for relief care. In 1996/7, there were 34 000 children in foster care in England, with a further 6300 placed on one or more occasions during 1996/7 for relief care. No data are collected centrally on the availability of foster homes, the quality of foster care, including training and qualifications, or about the levels of 'difficulty' of the children placed.

Third, there is concern over children living in households where adults have mental health problems or learning difficulties, or where the child is a carer. No official statistics are collected about this at the time of writing.

Children with disabilities are also a group which has been neglected, but is now receiving attention under the *Quality protects* proposals.[31] Little information is currently collected centrally on this group. Children with disabilities can be registered on the different local authority disability registers listed in Table 9.2. Data from these are collected nationally every 3 years by the Department of Health,[32-4] but children with disabilities are particularly likely to be under-reported. Social services departments have a statutory responsibility under the Children Act 1989 to hold a 'register' of children with disabilities, in collaboration with education departments and the NHS. Information from these registers is not collated centrally. Sources of data about people with disabilities are described more fully in Chapter 4.

Key problems in measuring the performance of personal social services

The changes in community care for adults introduced in April 1993 and the Department of the Environment, Transport and the Regions Efficiency Scrutiny reviews[1,16] led to significant change in data collection. Although data collection is now more closely focused on monitoring policy, there are still fundamental problems in using personal social services statistics to assess the performance of individual departments or to compare departments in different local authorities.

MONITORING THE POLICY GOALS OF SOCIAL SERVICES

Both the Social Services Inspectorate and the Audit Commission are increasingly using centrally collected statistics to monitor the work of social services departments. Despite this, it is questionable whether these data can provide adequate information about whether social services departments achieve the four policy goals of efficiency, responsiveness, effectiveness and equity set out by the Audit Commission.[35]

The statistics provide some clues about efficiency, but reliance on 'unit costs' as a measure of efficiency is problematic. Social services departments vary significantly in the way they report their expenditure to the Department of the Environment, Transport and the Regions on the main financial return, RO3. Responsiveness is difficult to assess at a national level. Official datasets do not currently allow much examination of the extent of innovation and flexibility of 'packages of care', or of the extent to which they are integrated with health care. The Department of Health has funded a major academic programme reviewing research on outcomes of social care. This may make it possible to assess the effectiveness of care given to individuals. Without this, social services departments and other related agencies will not be able to move towards 'evidence-based practice'.

COMPARING LIKE WITH LIKE

The statistics currently collected appear to be better for assessing *equity*, as many of the activity, expenditure and staffing data are 'standardised' by being expressed as rates per 1000 relevant population. Closer scrutiny reveals that these comparisons are shaky.

First, there has been little investment in developing standard definitions, and social services departments vary in the way they record their activities. The Department of Health annual statistical returns on personal social services department activity, services and staffing include a series of definitions. The Chartered Institute of Public Finance and Accountancy has produced a series of comprehensive definitions for accounts and, by inference, for most core services of social services departments.[36] Despite this, analysis of the data returned too often highlights the wide variation in local interpretation of these 'national' definitions. Moreover, for some important measures such as referrals, caseloads, workloads and reviews, there are no national definitions. Each authority will currently use its own, reflecting local recording practice and software design. Critical issues are left to each social services department to resolve, include defining who becomes a 'client' and how they should be categorised. This includes deciding who should be defined as having a learning disability or being 'elderly mentally ill'. The 'referrals, assessments and packages of care' proposals will move social services departments towards clearer standardisation. Even so, it remains to be seen how far all the variety of initial processes whereby a client makes contact with a social services department can reliably be measured to a common defined standard.

Second, there is little information about 'need' for social care within the general population. In its absence, 'need' is often equated with demands that have been met or services that have been provided. This is influenced by many confounding factors, in particular how the services are configured. For example, how can rates of home care provision per 1000 people aged 65 and over be compared in authorities with broadly comparable populations of older people? Apparent variations can arise if one of the authorities has historically funded more residential care for its population, or provides 'meals on wheels' more extensively, while another makes more use of home care services to meet needs for meals. One authority may define 'need' more strictly than another by applying tighter eligibility criteria for its services. On the other hand, an authority with higher charges for its home care services reduces 'expressed' need.

Third, there is little information about the characteristics of service users. In particular, standard measures of the 'dependency' of service users are urgently required. The NHS is increasingly moving towards standardised measures of 'casemix', such as the Health of the Nation Outcomes Scoring system. In contrast to this, in mental health, social services departments are still choosing or making up their own measures at a local level. This limits the scope for comparisons between social services departments and between NHS agencies and social services departments. At the time of writing, no data are collected on the ethnic origin of people referred or those receiving or providing services. The Social Services Inspectorate has been seeking information on the topic for a number of years, but progress in collecting and using the data in policy analysis is still very patchy.[37,38] The Department of Health is reviewing the possibility of adding indicators of ethnicity such as ethnic group, first language or religion to data collected about children 'looked after'. Ethnic group is also included in the 'referrals, assessments and packages of care' dataset.

The final problem is that social care may be provided by many agencies other than social services departments. Local authority education and housing departments, the NHS and private or voluntary agencies may all provide forms of social care. Some information on the contribution of the private sector in providing residential and nursing home care is available, either from limited data collected by the Department of Health[13] (which is described more fully in the next section) or from the more comprehensive data collected by independent analysts.[39–41] Little is known of the extent to which people pay privately for domiciliary care from the independent sector. Without this, assessing the impact of change in personal social services and also NHS commissioning is difficult. It also makes any comprehensive analysis of provision and its relation to 'need' virtually impossible.

COLLABORATION BETWEEN THE NHS AND SOCIAL SERVICES

Obstacles to sharing data between the NHS and social services include differences in geographical boundaries, differences in definitions and confidentiality constraints. Boundary problems may be resolved, as social services departments postcode all their client records. The problems of confidentiality posed when health practitioners provide information for recording by social services departments were highlighted in the Caldicott report on patient-identifiable information.[42,43]

Attempts to develop common definitions to enable assessment of the contributions of the NHS, social services departments and private and voluntary providers have a very long history. Many attempts have been made to define a common minimum dataset for mental health, but it can seem like an ever-receding mirage. If NHS and social services departments shared mainframe systems data, it would be advantageous to both agencies, but there are both technical problems and issues of responsibility for shared data. In 1998, a report on the feasibility of using common 'headings' in shared communications between the NHS and social services departments was submitted to the NHS Executive Clinical Systems Group. [44]

The move towards more coherent interagency working on issues like community safety and social exclusion will provide an impetus to resolve these problems. For organisations supposedly committed to 'seamless care' with other agencies, there has been a singular lack of success in breaking out of a 'single-agency' perspective. 'Joined up' problems need not only 'joined up' solutions but 'joined up' data collection and data analysis.

THE ROLE OF CENTRAL GOVERNMENT

Central government direction is important in overcoming these problems. Whereas the NHS has had a strategy for information for some years, there was no formal national strategy for personal social services information until 1997.[45] A new 'performance management framework' has been developed and the first data were published by the Department of Health in 1999.[46] A wider collaborative statement involving all the key stakeholders was proposed by the Local Government Management Board.

Increased central government direction will undoubtedly compromise the historical 'autonomy' of local authorities. There is also a danger that the innovative work of social services departments will not be visible in the statistics. Important service developments, like ordinary housing with care and support or voluntary agencies working with families at risk, may never feature in annual returns to central government or in 'performance management frameworks'.

Measures of performance and outcomes look set to play an increasingly important part, both in local management and in monitoring policy changes. An indication of possible future central demand for information may be seen in targeted funding programmes such as the Mental Illness Specific Grant, special funding for AIDS/HIV, 'challenge funds' and special funding for 'winter pressures'. In these, there have been requirements for reporting not only levels of expenditure but also achievements, such as activity measures.

The more sophisticated data required by these strategies and by the trend towards targeted funding will overburden many social services departments unless they invest more realistically in both information systems and information staff. As with the NHS, social services departments have found it difficult to collect data directly from practitioners. There have been moves to provide practitioners with more user-friendly and flexible information systems, but these are costly. Social services departments have not been provided with the level of resources promised to the NHS in its new information strategy.[47] This means that resources for information within social services departments will compete directly with those for service developments.

Personal social services: some indicators of progress and pointers for the future

To conclude more positively, recent developments from the Department of Health have focused on slimming down existing national personal social services data collections.[1,16,45] Those which remain should form a more usable set of information.

In the late 1990s, the Department of Health moved to gather new information going beyond collections of activity data, relating data on services to expenditure and staffing data. The 'referrals, assessments and packages of care' proposals for adults aim to give a fuller picture of social services departments' activities in response to local people seeking help. Data on children 'looked after' will provide new outcome measures for care of such children. The *Children in need* initiative aims to offer a more meaningful overview of social services departments' activity with the children with whom they are working. The Citizen's Charter Performance Indicators started to explore users' views of quality of services. A framework for performance management for the personal social services should assist in clarifying the information requirements which are needed to support the large number of seemingly discrete policy initiatives.[48]

The Department of Health Statistics Branch responsible for personal social services statistics has speeded up the processing of returns and started to use sophisticated graphical analysis systems more widely, for example in the Key Indicator Graphical System.[8]

There is clear evidence of increasing dialogue between 'players' who have information to hand. This is happening at all levels. At the time of writing, discussions are taking place between the Department of Health, social services departments and the Information Management Groups of the Association of Directors of Social Services and the NHS, and health authority staff are talking to local social services information managers. With the coming of primary care groups, Health Improvement Programmes and Joint Investment Programmes, this dialogue will be taken down another 'level' and become more focused. Other agencies, such as education, housing and justice agencies, will come into the arena at an appropriate time. Increasing work locally on shared datasets[49,50] may provide good models for more focused official data collection by government. In the future, the proposed Care Standards Commission will be responsible for collecting data about the services it regulates.

Within the next decade, considerable further progress should have been made and many of the deficiencies in the official statistics discussed in this chapter will have at long last been resolved. This will be of great benefit to service users and policy makers and will reduce stress levels of information workers in social services departments and the NHS.

Residential and nursing homes for elderly people

Overview

This section is mainly concerned with data about provision of residential and nursing home care for elderly people. The systems for collecting information cover services for several adult client groups, including, in some cases, services for children. Information about these other client groups is therefore included, where appropriate. Since the terminology used for different client groups has changed over time, it has sometimes been necessary to use the terminology current at the time. Thus, people with physical disabilities are also referred to as younger physically handicapped people, and people with learning disabilities are also referred to as mentally handicapped people.

Independent residential care and nursing homes in England and Wales are regulated under the Registered Homes Act 1984.[51] This will be superseded by the proposals in the Care Standards Bill. Local authorities are responsible for registering and inspecting private and voluntary residential care homes, while health authorities are responsible for the registration and inspection of private and voluntary nursing homes. Since 1991, local authorities have become responsible for providing an 'arm's length' inspection of their own homes.[52] Nearly all of the residents in local authority homes are financially supported by a local authority. In 1993, following the 1990 National Health Service and Community Care Act,[53] local authorities also became responsible for assessing and financing publicly funded residents in independent residential care and nursing homes. By May 1997, 46 per cent of residents in independent homes for elderly and physically handicapped people were supported by a local authority.[54] Residents who had been admitted prior to April 1993 had preserved rights to the previous system of income support payments. In May 1997, 22 per cent of residents in independent homes for elderly and physically handicapped people were funded by income support, 28 per cent were self-funded and 4 per cent were funded by the NHS.[54] Homes with fewer than four places were not required to register with the local authority until April 1993.[55] Homes constituted by an Act of Parliament or incorporated by Royal Charter and Christian Science nursing homes are exempt from registration, although the current government has indicated its intention to remove the exemptions.[56] In Scotland, separate Acts of Parliament regulate residential and nursing homes.

Residential care homes are distinguished from nursing homes in the 1984 Act as being those providing board and personal care only, whereas nursing homes are those intended to accommodate patients requiring constant or frequent daily nursing care. In order to enable homes to provide personal care and nursing care within the same premises, the 1984 Act included a provision for the dual registration of homes as both residential and nursing homes.

In each country of the UK, separate information about residential and nursing homes is collected from local and health authorities. The Care Standards Bill and similar legislation in Scotland and possibly in Northern Ireland is changing this. Since there are geographical differences between health authorities and local authorities, their overall level of provision of residential and nursing home care has to be estimated. In addition, it is difficult to monitor the changes over time for individual authorities because of the reorganisation of local government from 1996, and the many changes made to health authorities since 1991.

Currently, the Department of Health publishes a detailed annual volume of statistics on residential and nursing home care for adults in England, the RA series, plus an annual statistical bulletin providing summary information and more detailed commentary. The annual volume of statistics contains time series information tabulated for England as a whole and information for the particular year tabulated by local authority or health authority. It also includes descriptions of the methodology used for collecting information and speci-men copies of the return forms. The first edition of the annual volume related to 1995 and the first edition of the statistical bulletin related to 1993. Informa-tion on nursing homes was collected from district health authorities and pub-lished separately until 1997, when statistics on nursing homes were also included in the RA volume and the associated statistical bulletin. As a con-sequence of the changes in coverage, the titles of the two publications have varied from year to year. The volumes for 1997 and 1998 in the RA series were entitled *Community care statistics. Residential personal social services for adults. Detailed statistics on residential and nursing care homes and local authority supported residents, England.*[57,58] The companion statistical bulletins were entitled *Community care statistics. Residential personal social services for adults, England.*[59,60]

The Department of Health combined the system of data collection for resi-dential care for elderly people and people with physical or sensory disabilities with that for residential care for people with learning disabilities or mental ill-ness in 1987. Despite this, two separate series of statistics were published until 1995. Two annual volumes were published for residential homes for elderly people and people with physical or sensory disabilities. One was called *Resi-dential accommodation for elderly people and people with physical and/or sensory dis-abilities: all residents in local authority, voluntary and private homes* (reference number RA/2) and the other was called *Residential accommodation for elderly people and people with physical and/or sensory disabilities: local authority supported residents* (reference number RA/1). Prior to 1987, information on residential accommodation for people with mental illness or learning disabilities was published in a single volume (reference number A/F 11). From 1987, it was published in two volumes: *Residential accommodation for mentally ill people and people with learning disabilities: number of local authority, voluntary and private homes and places* (reference number A/F 11A) and *Residential accommodation for people with mental illness and people with learning disabilities: local authority sup-ported residents* (reference number A/F 11B). The volume containing informa-tion on the number of homes and places was discontinued after the publication of the 1991 issue.[61] In addition to the annual RA/2 volumes, the Department of Health has also published historical volumes of statistics for 6-year periods (reference number RA/2(H)), beginning with the period 1981–6. The latest of these historical volumes relates to the period 1989–94.[62]

Until 1996, information on nursing homes in England was tabulated by district health authority in a publication entitled *Private hospitals, homes and clinics registered under Section 23 of the Registered Homes Act 1984*. In 1996, the format was changed to a statistical bulletin, with the same title, and detailed district health authority information was available only in spreadsheet for-mat. In 1997, statistics on nursing homes were also included in the RA volume and the associated statistical bulletin. The RA volume and the statistical bulletin for 1998 were expanded to cover nursing homes in more detail, the information being collected on a new form introduced in that year.

The annual Department of Health publication entitled *Health and personal social services statistics for England* contains summaries of the information collected about residential homes for England as a whole, presented in the form of time series. As noted earlier, the volume of information was reduced substantially from 1997 onwards.[10] This and subsequent editions contain information only on the number of local authority-supported residents in residential and nursing home care. As in earlier years, they include the number of beds in residential and nursing homes for people with learning disabilities and mental illness.

Residential homes in England

THE DATA COLLECTION SYSTEM

The current system of the collection of data about residential homes was introduced in 1997, following the efficiency scrutiny undertaken by the Department of the Environment.[1] Despite this, the system is based on the gazetteer systems introduced in 1981. The gazetteer systems introduced the principle of 'change reporting', in which a central computerised register of all homes in each local authority was established by the Department of Health and Social Security, and each year lists of homes were sent to local authorities for checking.

Prior to 1981, separate returns were used for homes for elderly people and younger physically handicapped people, homes for mentally handicapped people and homes for mentally ill people, and information was collected about all residents. These were replaced in 1981 by separate gazetteers and associated return forms for the different types of home. Information was collected on homes and places and on residents supported by local authorities for each client group; information about all residents was collected only for homes for elderly people and younger physically handicapped people. In 1987, following the Registered Homes Act 1984, a single system was introduced and the separate return forms were replaced by a new return which included staffed local authority homes and registered private and voluntary homes for all client groups. The new return also collected information about residents, but the separate returns used to collect information about the number of residents supported by the local authority in residential accommodation were retained. A number of changes were made in 1989 to reduce the amount of information collected. In 1994, following the introduction of the community care arrangements in 1993 under the 1990 National Health Service and Community Care Act, the forms were redesigned again, and a single return was introduced to collect information about the number of residents supported by the authority.

CAPACITY OF THE RESIDENTIAL CARE HOME SECTOR

Between 1981 and 1986, information on homes for elderly people and younger physically handicapped people, and on the number of places in these homes, was collected on a set of three forms (RA5A, RA5B and RA5C). For homes for mentally handicapped and mentally ill people, separate forms were used for local authority homes (RA9A and RA13A), including staffed and unstaffed homes, and for private and voluntary homes (RA9B and RA13B). Homes with fewer than four places, which were not required to register, were not included, but homes exempt from registration for other reasons were included. Following the introduction of dual registration in 1984, information was collected on the number of residential and nursing care places in dual registered private and voluntary homes.

The reliability of the statistics for homes for mentally handicapped or mentally ill people declined between 1981 and 1983, although it appeared to improve from 1984 onward.[63] There were continuing problems arising from different interpretations by local authorities of the types of home that should be included, and from apparent under-reporting of the numbers of private and voluntary homes.[61,63] Some authorities were including group homes or half-way homes and others were excluding them. The new return introduced in 1987 (RAC5) was expected to overcome some of the problems,[64] although the collection of information about the number of places for each client group was discontinued when the form was shortened in 1989. The RAC5 return covered all homes, with the exception of local authority unstaffed homes for mentally handicapped and mentally ill people, which were still covered by the RA9A and RA13A returns. In 1994, the RAC5 return was redesigned as a single form, and an additional return (RAC5(S)) was introduced to collect more limited information on registered homes with fewer than four places. In addition, the separate returns for unstaffed local authority homes were replaced by a single return (RAU1).

One of the main reasons for introducing the computerised register was to mitigate the effects of non-response from private and voluntary homes by enabling the Department of Health and Social Security to impute information for the current year. Non-response was greater for private and voluntary homes than for local authority homes. Two local authorities did not submit any returns for residential homes for elderly people and younger physically handicapped people for several years following the introduction of the gazetteer system. Gaps in submissions continued to occur following the introduction of the new return in 1987. The use of data for previous years meant that the size of the growing private sector would be underestimated for non-responding or partially responding authorities, and hence in the national figures.

The introduction of the RAC5 form in 1987 resulted in a change in the way homes for elderly people and younger physically handicapped people were classified in Department of Health and Social Security and Department of Health publications. Prior to 1987, these homes were classified as homes for elderly people, homes for younger physically handicapped people, or homes for mixed client groups. Until 1985, the groups were based on the proportion of residents aged 65 or over. In 1985 and 1986, homes were classified according to the recorded client groups. From 1987 to 1993, up to three client groups could be recorded on form RAC5, but this was then reduced to two from 1994. Homes catering for more than one client group were classified according to the largest client group, and information was not published on the degree to which homes catered for more than one client group. Homes classified as for elderly people included those catering primarily for elderly mentally infirm or elderly disabled people, but excluded homes for elderly people with learning disabilities. In the statistics of residential care for people with learning disabilities or mental illness, homes were classified in three groups: homes for children with learning disabilities, homes for adults with learning disabilities, and homes for adults with mental illness.

The report of the efficiency scrutiny conducted by the Department of the Environment in 1996 recommended that the RAC5 form and the separate return on local authority-supported residents should be restructured into a shorter, single annual return. It also recommended that local authority inspectorates should assist in data collection.[1] In the review which followed the efficiency scrutiny report, the Department of Health indicated that more detailed information was required than the original report envisaged.[65] In 1997, the RAC5 and RAC5(S) forms were replaced with a new return (RA). In 1998, the RUA1 return on unstaffed local authority homes was discontinued, and the return on local authority-supported residents was retained in a shorter form, as described below. The RA return consisted of three forms. Form A was an aggregate local authority return designed to collect information on the number of homes and places. It did so separately for staffed residential care homes and dual registered homes, by type of home and client group. Form B collected information on the type of home, its category of registration and capacity, the number of residents by age group and type of stay, and information on resident turnover. Form B was designed to be completed at the time the home was inspected and separate information was collected from homes with fewer than four places. Form C was designed to obtain some specific information on local authority-supported residents aged under 65. This represents a substantial shift in the method of data collection, and the Department of Health has reported that the response to form B has been poor.[58] In relation to this, the Social Services Inspectorate has reported that local authority inspection units often failed to achieve the required number of inspections.[52,66]

Since its introduction in 1984, dual registration has become increasingly important. Although separate information for dual registered homes was presented in the annual volumes of statistics for 1985 and 1986, no further information was published until 1995, when approximately 18 per cent of the places in residential and dual registered homes were in dual registered homes.[54] Aggregated figures for England as a whole were published for 1995,[67] but detailed information was not published by local authority until 1997.[57] By this time, 29 per cent of places in residential and dual registered homes were in dual registered homes.[54] Separate information on residential and nursing places in dual registered homes was published in the statistical volume for 1997, but in 1998, this information was shown only for residential places. In the 1997 publication, detailed information on private and voluntary residential homes by local authority, which previously had been shown separately for the two types of home, was combined. The distinction between private and voluntary homes is important, because the voluntary sector includes local authority homes which have been transferred to independent trusts.

CHARACTERISTICS OF RESIDENTS

Between 1981 and 1986, information was collected about all residents in homes for elderly people and younger physically handicapped people on forms RA2, RA3 and RA4. Data about residents supported by local authorities was collected on form RA1. Information was collected on local authority-supported residents only in homes for mentally handicapped people and mentally ill people (forms RA6 and RA10). The RAC5 return introduced in 1987 replaced the separate returns for the different client groups, and collected information about homes and residents for all homes except local authority unstaffed homes for mentally handicapped and mentally ill people. The separate forms for information on local authority-supported residents (RA1, RA6 and RA10) were retained. For 1987 and 1988, the RAC5 return collected information about individual residents. This information was used by the Department of Health to prepare a special report on the age, sex and length of stay characteristics of residents at 31 March 1988.[68] In 1989, the RAC5 return was redesigned 'to reduce the burden of form-filling', and aggregated information on the number of residents subdivided by age and type of stay was collected instead of information about individuals. Problems of missing data remained greatest for private and voluntary homes, although gaps in submissions by local authorities continued to occur following the introduction of the new return in 1987. For some homes, information was not supplied for residents. As a result, either the information published on places and residents would refer to different years, or the information on residents would be missing. The RAC5(S) return introduced in 1994 included the number of residents by age group (under 65, and 65 or over).

In 1997, the RAC5 and RAC5(S) returns were replaced by the new RA return. The collection cycle for form B of the return, relating to residents, had not been completed when the 1997 volume of statistics was being prepared, so it contained only estimated numbers of residents for England as a whole, based on the returns received.[57] The 1997 publication indicated that a special publication giving more detailed information on residents would be produced. As noted above, the 1998 publication reported that the response to form B was poor and, as for 1997, the 1998 volume contained only a table of estimated numbers of residents for England as a whole.[58] For 1997, information on the estimated number of residents was shown separately for private and voluntary residential homes, but for 1998 the information was shown for the two types of home combined. Comparisons with the figures obtained in 1996 suggest that there may be problems with the reliability of the new system. The estimated number of residents reported in private and voluntary residential homes in 1998 was 2.9 per cent lower than the number shown in the 1996 publication,[69] whereas the number of places in these homes increased by 7.4 per cent between 1996 and 1998.[58]

Although information about residents in homes for people with a 'mental handicap' or a mental illness was collected on the RAC5 return from 1987, the published statistics were not amended until 1995. Until 1995, only information on local authority-supported residents, obtained from separate returns, was

included in the published tabulations. For 1993 and 1994, the statistical bulletins included the number of residents by client group for England as a whole
and the total number of residents, for all client groups combined, by local
authority.[70,71]

From 1981 to 1993, information about residents supported by local authorities
was collected on separate returns for the different types of home, as described
above. In 1994, the separate returns were replaced by a single return. The new
return (SR1) classified homes according to five primary functions: elderly people, people with physical disabilities, people with learning disabilities, people
with mental illness, and alcohol/drug misusers and others or as unstaffed local
authority homes. It also classified homes by the type of care provided, residential care or nursing care. Information was collected on the number of supported residents by age group and type of stay, but not sex. Supported
residents in homes for elderly mentally infirm people were reclassified as people with mental illness, although the classification of homes on the RAC5 form
was not amended. The SR1 return also collected information on the number of
supported residents in dual registered homes. As for the previous returns, all
residents receiving some contribution from a local authority to their fees were
included on the SR1 return, but no information was collected on the distribution of levels of financial support.

Until 1993, information on supported residents was tabulated by age group
for the three categories of home defined by the separate forms. The same
grouping of homes was used for the corresponding statistics for 1994, although
residents in homes for elderly mentally infirm people were included in the
tables for people with mental illness, and children with learning difficulties
were not included in the tables for people with learning difficulties. The published statistics for 1994 contained fewer tables than in previous years, and the
tables for homes for people with mental illness or learning disabilities did not
separate residents by age group, except in the summary for England. On the
other hand, they did contain separate tables for individuals supported in nursing homes. From 1995 onwards, information on supported residents was tabulated by the revised classification of homes in the published statistics.[67]

In 1998, a shorter version of the SR1 form was introduced, although its
coverage was extended to include information on the number of local authority-
supported residents in unstaffed local authority and independent residential
homes. The age bands for each client group were reduced to two categories –
18 to 64, and 65 or over – and the separate classification of placements within
and outside the authority was dropped. Individuals were classified according
to client group rather than to the type of home to which they were admitted,
with elderly people being classified according to the main reason for the provision of care. More detailed information on age group and information on
placements outside the authority and in unstaffed homes was obtained for
each authority as a whole. The change in the method of classifying individuals means that the information presented in the 1998 volume of statistics[58]
cannot be compared directly with information published for previous years.

An important consequence of the changes to the SR1 form is that the lack
of information about age structure will preclude any estimation of likely

length of stay, and hence the financial commitment of local authorities. Individuals admitted to care due to age and infirmity, and who are typically in their late seventies or older, cannot be distinguished from younger elderly people. The latter are more likely to have been admitted due to physical disability, learning disability or mental health problems. This is likely to be particularly important for elderly mentally infirm people. Furthermore, the requirement to classify elderly people according to the main reason for provision of care may lead to differences in interpretation between local authorities, despite the availability of a 'not allocated' category.

With the exception of residents supported by local authorities, the Department of Health does not collect information about the source of finance of residents. The Department of Social Security produces a quarterly publication containing aggregate information on the number of residents receiving income support, including those with preserved rights to the previous system, entitled *Income support statistics quarterly enquiry*. This covers Great Britain and the most recent issue relates to November 1998.[72]

UTILISATION

When the RAC5 return was introduced for all homes in 1987, it included a section on the number of admissions to local authority homes. Information about admissions was collected for all homes in the revised RAC5 form introduced in 1994 and this information was published in the RA/2 volume for 1994. A report on admissions to residential care for all client groups from the 1994 RAC5 return was also published.[73] From 1997, information on the number of admissions and discharges has been collected on the RA form, as part of the inspection visit. From 1994, the return SR1 collected information on the number of short-stay admissions of supported residents. The collection of information on supported residents placed in permanent care during the year did not begin until the revisions to the SR1 form in 1998. No information is collected on the source of admission, for example whether from hospital or the community, or the destination on discharge.

STAFFING

Information on staffing for registered homes, including those exempt from registration, was collected on the RAC5 return in 1987 and 1988, but was not published. This information was discontinued when the form was shortened in 1989, and no further information has been collected. Information on staffing in local authority homes in England, which now constitute a minority of homes, is included in the annual collection of information on the staff of social services departments in post at 30 September on form SSDS 001. Prior to 1996, this information was published in a Department of Health publication entitled *Staff of local authority social services departments* (reference number S/F 1). In 1996, the format was changed to a statistical bulletin entitled *Personal social services staff of social services departments*, the most recent issue of which relates to 1998.[74]

Nursing homes in England

Information on registered nursing homes is collected annually by health authorities for the Department of Health. Between 1982 and 1986, information was collected on form SBH 212, and between 1987 and 1997 the equivalent information was collected on form KO36. For 1998 onwards, a new return was introduced, form RH(N), which was intended to bring the collection of information on nursing homes and residential care homes closer together. The returns include private hospitals and clinics, as well as nursing homes. In contrast to residential homes, the information collected does not distinguish between private and voluntary establishments, nor is it clear whether nursing homes exempt from registration are included.

The information collected prior to the financial year 1993–4 included the category of registration, the number of registered beds classified by intended use, whether a resident medical practitioner was employed and the number of full-time and part-time nursing staff, by grade. The information on the intended use of beds was designed to correspond to NHS ward use. The classification included broad patient groups and whether the intended occupants were children, elderly long-stay or other patients. Initially, long-stay was defined as 3 months and over,[75] but was later redefined to refer to an intended stay of over a year.[76] From 1985, information on dual registered establishments was collected and, for these homes, only beds registered as nursing beds were recorded on the return form.

Until 1993–4, the returns did not distinguish nursing homes from private hospitals and clinics. It was possible to estimate the number of nursing homes from the total number of establishments minus the number with operating theatres, and the total number of beds in nursing homes from the information published about individual institutions with operating theatres. The annual publications did not contain sufficient information to determine the number of beds in nursing homes for different types of patient. The growth in independent sector hospital and nursing home beds during the 1980s was dominated by the growth in beds recorded as for elderly patients.[2] The size of the market catering for elderly people may have been underestimated by the recording of beds in homes catering exclusively for elderly people as for 'general specialties', rather than for long-stay elderly patients.[77] There were large inconsistencies in the information collected on nursing home beds for elderly people for 1982 and 1984. It was estimated that over 18 per cent of district health authorities with beds for elderly people had submitted incorrect original returns to the Department of Health and Social Security.[78]

In 1993–4, form KO36 was amended to separate nursing homes from private hospitals and clinics and to collect information on the number of occupied beds by patient group and age group. The intended use categories and patient groups were also amended to correspond to the client groupings used by local authority social services departments and, with the exception of maternity and terminal care, to the income support payment categories for nursing homes. Although information on the number of beds for terminal care was included on the KO36 form prior to 1993–4, and constituted an income support payment category, it was deleted from the form for 1993–4.

The RH(N) form, introduced in 1998, is in three parts. Form A collects parallel information on the aggregate numbers of homes and places for dual registered homes and all nursing homes. It has a more detailed list of intended use categories, including a hospice category. It also collects information on the number of residential places in dual registered homes. The same groupings of patient type were used as in the previous returns, although the elderly category no longer refered to elderly long-stay. Form B collects information on the facilities provided by the home and the number of occupied beds by patient type in five age groups – under 18, 18–64, 65–74, 75–84, and over 85. Form S collects information about qualified and unqualified permanent and agency nursing and care staff. Forms B and S were designed to be collected by Registration and Inspection Units.

From 1985 to 1995, information on nursing homes was tabulated by district health authority in a publication entitled *Private hospitals, homes and clinics registered under Section 23 of the Registered Homes Act 1984*. Prior to 1985, the information was published only for England as a whole and for each regional health authority. From 1993–4 onwards, separate information was presented for nursing homes and for hospitals and clinics.[79,80] In addition, the published statistics included regional summaries of provision relative to population and time series of numbers of beds, and details of individual establishments with operating theatres. In 1996, the format of the publication was changed to a statistical bulletin.[81] This contained summary information for each health authority, while detailed information for each health authority was available only in spreadsheet format.

The statistical bulletin on residential care for 1996 included some limited information on nursing home provision.[82] Both the statistical bulletin and the annual volume of statistics on residential personal social services for 1997 contained information on nursing home provision, tabulated by local authority, and summary information for 1993 to 1997.[57,59] The figures given in these publications for nursing homes for the years prior to 1997 appear to have been obtained from the nursing home statistics by subtracting the number of dual registered homes from the total number of nursing homes. The numbers of dual registered homes obtained from the statistics on residential care homes were lower than the numbers obtained from the statistics on nursing homes, and the lower figures are given in the statistics on residential personal social services. Thus, for the years prior to 1997, the total number of nursing homes, including dual registered homes, derived from these statistics is less than the total number shown in the statistics on nursing homes. Following the introduction of the RH(N) form in 1998, the information collected on nursing homes was published in the statistical bulletin and the annual statistical volume on residential personal social services,[58,60] tabulated by health authority.

The descriptions of the collection of data in the annual publications indicate that the process relied on information supplied by the establishments and that the information was not independently verified, although missing or inconsistent information was followed up and information imputed to make the returns as complete as possible. For the financial year 1993–4 onwards, some of the information collected was recorded during routine inspection visits, thus reducing the reliance on information supplied by the establishments themselves.

Residential and nursing homes in Wales, Scotland and Northern Ireland

The Welsh Office, now known as the National Assembly for Wales, has also employed gazetteer systems to collect information on residential homes, and has used the same form as in England to collect information on nursing homes. Information on residential accommodation in Scotland is collected annually by the Scottish Executive Social Work Statistics Group, and information about nursing homes is collected by the Information and Statistics Division of the National Health Service in Scotland, using different return forms. In Northern Ireland, information is collected by the Department of Health, Social Services and Public Safety.

Prior to 1996, health boards corresponded to regions in Scotland and health authorities corresponded to local authorities in Wales. Following local government reorganisation in 1996, the five new health authorities in Wales corresponded to groups of the twenty-two new unitary local authorities, but health boards in Scotland did not correspond exactly to groups of the new local authorities.[83]

Of all the countries in the UK, Scotland collects the most comprehensive data for residential homes. Data are collected on the characteristics of residential homes and staffing, the age and length of stay of residents and their funding source. For residential homes for elderly people, data are also collected on the disabilities of residents. Data collected in Wales broadly follow those collected in England. In Northern Ireland, information is collected about numbers of residential homes and places for each client group and the overall numbers of nursing homes and beds. For publicly owned residential accommodation, data are collected about numbers of residents. Data are also collected about people receiving publicly funded packages of care.

Prior to 1995, the Welsh Office published annual volumes of statistics containing detailed information on residential homes by local authority and summaries of the information collected about residential homes for Wales as a whole in the publication *Health and personal social services statistics for Wales*. Until 1994, detailed statistics on residential homes for elderly people and people with physical disabilities were published in *Residential accommodation for elderly people and people with physical or visual disabilities*, while information on residential homes for people with a mental illness or learning disabilities was published separately in *Activities of social services departments*. In 1994, the publication on residential care homes was expanded to include information on homes for people with a mental illness or learning disabilities and their residents. This publication also included information on small homes, catering for fewer than four residents, and on nursing homes and their residents, and was renamed *Residential care homes and nursing homes in Wales: 1994.*[84] Prior to 1994, information on nursing homes was published by health authority in *Health and personal social services statistics for Wales*, beginning with the 1989 edition.[85] Information on the number of beds for each category of patient was shown separately for nursing homes and private hospitals, unlike the information published on nursing homes in England. In addition, summary information was shown for nursing homes and private hospitals separately for the previous 5 years.

Since 1994, the Welsh Office has revised its publications, and has replaced *Health and personal social services statistics for Wales* with separate publications on health statistics and personal social services statistics. The first edition of *Health statistics Wales* was the 1996 edition,[86] published in 1997, but the first edition of *Social services statistics Wales* did not emerge until 1999.[87] In addition, an annual *Digest of Welsh local area statistics* was introduced in 1997.[88] The *Digest of Welsh local area statistics* includes some of the information on residential and nursing homes now available in fuller detail in *Social services statistics Wales*. The tables in *Health statistics Wales* and some more detailed tables are also available in spreadsheet format.

The publication *Social services statistics Wales 1999* includes separate tables on residential care homes for each client group for the new unitary authorities. The information published includes the number of homes, places and residents, and the number of local authority-supported residents, but information for private and voluntary homes has been combined, and information for small homes has been excluded. More detailed information is shown for homes for elderly people, including the number of residents by age and sex. This publication also includes time series of data for homes for each client group for Wales as a whole and information on the staffing of local authority social services departments.

The series of statistics on nursing homes previously published in *Health and personal social services statistics for Wales* has been continued in *Health statistics Wales*. The 1996 edition shows information for the pre-1996 health authorities, and subsequent editions show information for the five new health authorities.[89,90] Numbers of nursing homes, places and residents, and the number of residents by age and source of funding, each tabulated by local authority, are included in *Social services statistics Wales 1999*.

For Scotland, the most comprehensive publications about residential and nursing homes were produced by the Scottish Office as statistical bulletins and are now known as information notes. In 1990, separate statistical bulletins on residential accommodation and home and day care services were replaced with a bulletin covering community services generally. The community care bulletins have included information on sheltered housing, NHS hospital beds and nursing homes from the first issue.[91] Information on residential accommodation for elderly people, people with physical disabilities, people with learning disabilities and people with mental health problems is shown separately in the statistical bulletins by local authority or, prior to 1997, by region. Data for private and voluntary homes are shown separately for 1985 or 1986 onwards. The exception is for residential homes for people with physical disabilities, for which detailed information by sector has been published only for 1995 onwards.

The statistics of residential accommodation for Scotland cover a wider range of information than those for England and Wales. They include home size and staffing, ages, turnover, length of stay and source of financial support of residents. For homes for elderly people, they include information on the number of residents with different disabilities. A separate series of statistical bulletins covers staff of Scottish social work departments.[92] The bulletins on community care services show the number of nursing homes catering for elderly people by local authority or region, and the numbers of places in these homes, as well as the total number of beds in nursing homes and private hospitals for 1987 onwards. In the bulletin for 1997, the time series information is shown only for nursing homes.[93] These publications are being restructured as information notes following devolution.

Information on nursing homes in Scotland has also been published annually from 1987, by health board, in *Scottish health statistics*, produced by the Information and Statistics Division of the National Health Service in Scotland.[94] Prior to 1994, the number of homes and beds was published for nursing homes and private hospitals combined. From 1994, the information was published separately, private hospitals being defined as providing acute surgical services. The number of residents in different categories in nursing homes and private hospitals, including elderly long-stay residents, was also published from 1994 onwards. Following local government reorganisation in 1996, health boards and local authorities no longer had common geographical boundaries, but the information on nursing homes has been tabulated for both local authority areas and health boards from 1997. *Scottish health statistics* also includes information on the number of qualified nursing staff in nursing homes and private hospitals. Prior to 1997, it included the total number of staff in these establishments.

Information about nursing homes in Northern Ireland is collected by the registration and inspection units of health and social services boards, and information about residential care is collected centrally by the Department of Health, Social Services and Public Safety. *Community statistics* contains data on the numbers of residential and nursing homes and their beds. Information about the numbers of people receiving 'packages of care', in other words publicly funded, is shown separately for private and voluntary residential and nursing homes and for statutory residential homes.

Unofficial sources of information on residential and nursing homes

The main unofficial publications on residential and nursing home care are those produced by Laing and Buisson. These contain summaries of statistics drawn from official sources, information collected in their own surveys, and extensive commentary on developments in the independent sector. Their current principal annual publications relating to residential and nursing home care are *Laing's healthcare market review*,[95] formerly *Laing's review of private healthcare*, and *Care of elderly people: market survey*.[54] They also produce a monthly newsletter, *Community care market news*. These publications include more information than the official publications on such topics as the owner-ship of independent residential and nursing home care, the proportion of homes in each sector owned by major providers, the quality of provision, for example the provision of single rooms and en suite facilities, and fees charged. Regional information on fees, together with indicators of demand and supply, is shown in the *Market survey*. These publications are not easily accessible because of the high price, for example the cost of the 1998 edition of *Market survey* is £360.[54]

An electronic database of residential and nursing homes is available from Laing and Buisson on CD-ROM. Another commercial database is the *A–Z Care Homes Guide data-on-disk* database, which includes local authority homes. The addresses from which these databases can be obtained are given below.

Conclusions

The information which would provide a comprehensive picture of the care home sector can be grouped into five different categories: the capacity of the sector, the characteristics of homes, the characteristics of residents, the utilisa-tion of homes and the quality of the care they provide. Although some infor-mation is available for each of these categories, the construction of an overall picture is severely limited by three factors: differences between the informa-tion available on residential and nursing homes, changes over time in the information collected and variations between the different constituent parts of the United Kingdom.

Information has been collected about the number of residential homes and places in England for all client groups over the period from 1981. Information about the number of nursing homes and the number of nursing home beds in England has been collected since 1982, but was not collected separately from private hospitals and clinics until 1993–94. Before that date, the number of nursing homes and nursing home beds had to be estimated. Information on homes in England with dual registration was not published until 1995. Infor-mation about residential and nursing homes is collected separately from local authorities and health authorities and, with the exception of 1997, has been published separately for each type of authority. Thus, although the overall level of residential and nursing home provision can be derived from the data, only approximate estimates can be made at a local level.

An important characteristic of homes is ownership. This information has been collected for residential homes throughout the period from 1981. Although the information has been collected separately for dual registered private and voluntary homes, it is not shown separately in the publications. For nursing homes, the information collected does not distinguish between private and voluntary establishments. These limitations have severely ham-pered the examination of trends in private and voluntary provision.

Information on the number of residents in different age groups in residen-tial care homes for elderly people and for people with physical disabilities has been collected in England throughout the period from 1981. Information about all residents in homes for people with learning disabilities or mental illness has been collected only since an integrated return form was introduced in 1987. Similar information is available for Scotland and Wales, but the information collected on residents in Northern Ireland is limited to those in statutory residential care. Information about the number of occupied beds in nursing homes is collected by age group in England and Wales and by category of resident in Scotland. Other information about the characteristics of residents is very sparse. Scotland is the only country which collects information about the disabilities of residents, but this is collected only for elderly people in residential care. All countries of the UK collect information about publicly funded residents, but information about the source of financial support is only collected for residents of residential homes in Scotland and nursing homes in Wales.

Information has been collected on the number of admissions to residential homes in England since 1994, and from 1997 information has been collected on the number of discharges. Information is collected on turnover in residential homes in Scotland, and includes the destination on discharge. No information is collected on turnover for nursing homes, and no information is currently collected on the source of admission to either residential or nursing homes anywhere in the UK.

Staffing is the only information collected which relates to the quality of care. Information on staffing is collected for local authority residential homes in England and Wales, but it is collected for all residential homes in Scotland. Information on staffing is collected for nursing homes in England and Scotland, but has not been included in the most recent publications for England.

The collection of administrative statistics on residential and nursing homes is linked to the registration and inspection systems. An alternative would be to use the payment systems for residents, but as the financial support of residents is shared between local authorities, the Department of Social Security and private individuals, and, to a limited extent, the NHS, it would be difficult to collect information through this route. The systems of data collection introduced in England in 1993–94 for nursing homes and in 1997 for residential homes made more use of the inspection process. The system introduced for residential homes was intended to focus more on the needs of residents and less on the services provided.[65] Despite this, the information collected about residents has been reduced and problems of response have occurred. The work of the Social Services Inspectorate[52,66] suggests that such problems of response should have been foreseen.

In its efficiency scrutiny, the Department of the Environment recommended that an annual sample survey of homes should be undertaken to complement the collection of administrative statistics.[1] The Department of Health reported that local authorities tended to be unenthusiastic about the use of sampling.[65] Unless some form of more detailed sample survey is used to compensate for the reduction in the amount of information collected, the data available will not be sufficient to provide crucial information on residential and nursing home care and its recipients. The current government's emphasis on national standards[56] is likely to require information on provision as well as on residents. A strategy of collecting basic census information about all homes, complemented by more detailed sample information, would provide much more useful information than the fragmented system that exists at present. Under the proposals in the Care Standards Bill, a National Care Standards Commission will be responsible for collecting information on the availability of care home provision and the quality of care for England, but it is as yet unclear how it will approach this task.

Key official publications

Overviews

Department of Health. *Health and personal social services statistics for England.* London: TSO, published annually.

Department of Health. *Key indicators.* Published on CD-Rom twice yearly. (Available from DH Statistics Division 3C, telephone: 020 972 5602.)

The National Health Service in Scotland Information and Statistics Division. *Scottish health statistics.* Edinburgh: ISD Publications, published annually.

Scottish Executive. Series of annual statistical bulletins on community care and children, available from the Scottish Executive, Edinburgh.

National Assembly for Wales. *Digest of Welsh local area statistics.* Cardiff: National Assembly for Wales, published annually.

National Assembly for Wales. *Health statistics Wales.* Cardiff: National Assembly for Wales, published annually.

National Assembly for Wales. *Social services statistics Wales.* Cardiff: National Assembly for Wales, published annually.

Department of Health, Social Services and Public Safety. *Community statistics.* Belfast: Department of Health, Social Services and Public Safety, published annually.

Performance indicators

Department of Health. *Key indicators graphical system.* From DH Key Indicator team. User licence other than to social services departments and DH, £20.

Audit Commission. *Local authority performance indicators.* London: Audit Commission, published annually.

Residential and nursing homes

Department of Health. Community care statistics. Residential personal social services for adults, England. *Statistical Bulletin.* London: Department of Health, published annually.

Department of Health. *Community care statistics. Residential personal social services for adults. Detailed statistics on residential and nursing care homes and local authority supported residents, England.* Series RA. London: Department of Health, published annually.

Scottish Executive. Community care, Scotland. *Statistical bulletin.* Edinburgh: Scottish Executive, published annually.

Contact addresses and web sites

Department of Health
DH Statistics Division
Room 452C
Skipton House
80 London Road
London SE1 6LH
Telephone: 020 7972 5582
http://www.doh.gov.uk

Key Indicators Team
Room 452C
Skipton House
80 London Road
London SE1 6LH
Telephone: 020 7972 5571

National Assembly for Wales
Cathays Park
Cardiff CF10 3NQ
Telephone: 029 20 825041

Department of Health, Social Services
and Public Safety
HQ Annexe 2/3
Castle Buildings
Stormont BT4 3HD
Telephone: 028 90 520500

Scottish Executive Health Department
Community Care Statistics
James Craig Walk
Edinburgh EH1 3BA
Telephone: 0131 244 3777

Scottish Executive Children's Social
Work Statistics
1B Victoria Quay

Edinburgh EH6 6QQ
Telephone: 0131 244 3745/3607
http://www.scotland.gov.uk

Audit Commission
1 Vincent Square
London SW1P 2PN
http://www.audit-commission. gov.uk

Chartered Institute of Public Finance
and Accountancy (CIPFA)
3 Robert Adam Street
London WC2N 6BH

Association of Directors of Social
Services Information Management
Group
Chair: Tony Hunter
East Riding of Yorkshire Social Services
Department
County Hall
Cross Street
Beverley HU17 9BN

Social Services Research Group
http://www.ssrg.demon.co.uk

Laing and Buisson
38 Georgiana Street
London NW1 0EB

A–Z Care Homes Guide
PO Box 7677
Hungerford 1
Berks RG17 0FX

References

1. Department of the Environment. *Lifting the burden: less data, better understanding. An efficiency scrutiny on information flows between central and local government.* London: Department of the Environment, November 1996.
2. Darton RA, Wright KG. Changes in the provision of long-stay care, 1970–1990. *Health and Social Care in the Community* 1993; **1**(1): 11–25.

3. Macfarlane A, Pollock A. Statistics and the privatisation of NHS and social services. In: Dorling D, Simpson S, eds. *Statistics in society.* London: Arnold, 1999, pp. 252–61.

4. House of Commons Health Committee. *Community care: funding from April 1993.* Third Report, Session 1992–3, HC309–I. London: HMSO, 1993.

5. Chartered Institute of Public Finance and Accountancy. *Personal social services statistics estimates.* London: Chartered Institute of Public Finance and Accountancy, published annually.

6. Chartered Institute of Public Finance and Accountancy. *Personal social services statistics actuals.* London: Chartered Institute of Public Finance and Accountancy, published annually.

7. Department of Health. *Key indicators of local authority social services, 1987/1988.* London: Department of Health, July 1990.

8. Department of Health. *Key indicators 1997 graphical system.* London: Department of Health, 1997.

9. Audit Commission. *Local authority performance indicators 1997/98. Services for people with special needs in England.* London: Audit Commission, 1999.

10. Department of Health. *Health and personal social services statistics for England*, 1997 edition. London: The Stationery Office, 1998.

11. Department of Health. *Personal social services statistical information directory.* London: Department of Health, August 1996.

12. Department of Health. *Community care statistics: day and domiciliary personal social services for adults.* Series HMD. London: Department of Health, published annually.

13. Department of Health. *Community care statistics: residential personal social services for adults. Detailed statistics on residential and nursing care homes and local authority supported residents, England 1997.* London: Department of Health, 1998.

14. Department of Health. *Community care statistics. Personal social services day and domiciliary services for adults, England. Statistical Bulletin.* London: Department of Health, published annually.

15. Department of Health. *Community care statistics. Residential personal social services for adults, England. Statistical Bulletin.* London: Department of Health, published annually.

16. Department of Health. *A review of personal social services statistics.* London: Department of Health, 1997.

17. Local Government Management Board. *Survey of independent sector residential and nursing homes – staffing and training needs.* London: LGMB, 1998.

18. Local Government Management Board. *Survey of independent sector day care – staffing and training needs.* London: LGMB, 1998.

19. Department of Health. *Referrals, assessments and packages of care proposals* (papers for briefing on 15.9.98). London: Department of Health, 1998.

20. Department of Health. *Children's day care facilities* (A/F 6)(to 31.3.97 only). London: Department of Health, published annually.

21. Department of Health. *Children 'looked after' by local authorities* (A/F 12). London: Department of Health, published annually.

22. Department of Health. *Children and young people on child protection registers* (A/F 13). London: Department of Health, published annually.

23. Department of Health. *Supervision orders* (A/F 16). London: Department of Health, published annually.

24. Department of Health. *Children accommodated in secure units* (A/F 21). London: Department of Health, published annually.

25. Department of Health. *Children's homes* (A/F 22). London: Department of Health, published annually.

26. Department of Health. *Proposals to revise SSDA 903* – consultation paper. London: Department of Health, 1998.
27. Department of Health. *'Looked after' children forms.* London: Department of Health, 1996.
28. Department of Health. *Children in need study newsletter* (from DH Statistics Branch). London: Department of Health, 1998.
29. Department of Health. *Proposals for outcome indicators for LAC.* London: Department of Health, 1998.
30. Local Government Management Board. *Recipients of income support in English wards at August 1996 supplied by the Benefits Agency.* London: LGMB, 1998.
31. Department of Health. *Quality protects.* London: TSO, 1998.
32. Department of Health. *Registered blind and partially sighted people* (A/F 7). London: Department of Health, published triennially.
33. Department of Health. *Registers of people with physical disabilities* (A/F19). London: Department of Health, published triennially.
34. Department of Health. *People registered as deaf or hard of hearing* (A/F 20). London: Department of Health, published triennially.
35. Boyne G. Comparing the performance of local authorities: an evaluation of the Audit Commission indicators. *Local Government Studies* 1997; Winter: 17–43.
36. Chartered Institute of Public Finance and Accounting. *Accounting for social services in Great Britain.* London: CIPFA, 1993.
37. Commission for Racial Equality. *Racial equality means equality: a standard for racial equality in local government.* London: CRE, 1993.
38. Commission for Racial Equality. *Race, culture and community care: an agenda for action.* London: CRE, 1997.
39. Laing and Buisson. *Laing's review of private health care.* London: Laing and Buisson, 1998.
40. Laing and Buisson. *Community care market news.* London: Laing and Buisson, decennial 1998.
41. Laing and Buisson. *Care of elderly people: market survey.* London: Laing and Buisson, 1998.
42. NHS Executive. *The Caldicott Committee: report on the review of patient-identifiable information.* Leeds: NHSE, 1997.
43. NHS Executive. *The role and responsibilities of Caldicott guardians and access controls for the NHS Strategic Tracing Service.* Leeds: NHSE, 1998.
44. Glastonbury B, Spackman B, Gilbert D. *Testing headings for clinical communication – report on an analysis to test the feasibility of using headings in shared communication with SSDs.* London: Department of Health, 1998.
45. Department of Health. *Personal social services information strategy statement – 1998/9–2000/1.* London: Department of Health, 1997.
46. Department of Health. *Social services performance in 1998/99.* London: Department of Health, 1999.
47. NHS Executive. *Information for health.* Leeds: NHSE, 1998.
48. Audit Commission. *Getting the best from social services. Learning the lessons from joint reviews.* London: Audit Commission, 1998.
49. Department for Education and Employment. *Local audits of child care need and provision (circular 31.7.98).* London: DfEE, 1998.
50. Home Office. *Youth justice teams.* London: TSO, 1998.
51. Registered Homes Act 1984. c. 23. London: HMSO, 1984.
52. Department of Health Social Services Inspectorate. *Social services department*

inspection units: the first eighteen months. Report of an inspection of the work of inspection units in ten local authorities. London: HMSO, 1993.

53. National Health Service and Community Care Act 1990. London: HMSO, 1990.

54. Laing and Buisson. *Care of elderly people: market survey 1998,* 11th edition. London: Laing and Buisson, 1998.

55. Department of Health. *Registered Homes Act 1984. Registered Homes (Amendment) Act 1991 and Commencement Order 1992; Residential Care Homes (Amendment) (No.2) Regulations 1992.* LAC(92)10. London: Department of Health, 1992.

56. Department of Health. *Modernising social services. Promoting independence, improving protection, raising standards.* Cm 4169. London: TSO, 1998.

57. Department of Health. *Community care statistics. Residential personal social services for adults. Detailed statistics on residential and nursing care homes and local authority supported residents, England 1997.* RA/97. London: Department of Health, 1998.

58. Department of Health. *Community care statistics. Residential personal social services for adults. Detailed statistics on residential and nursing care homes and local authority supported residents, England 1998.* RA/98. London: Department of Health, 1999.

59. Department of Health. Community care statistics 1997. Residential personal social services for adults, England. *Statistical Bulletin,* 1997/26. London: Department of Health, December 1997.

60. Department of Health. Community care statistics 1998. Residential personal social services for adults, England. *Statistical Bulletin,* 1998/37. London: Department of Health, December 1998.

61. Department of Health. *Residential accommodation for mentally ill people and people with learning disabilities: number of local authority, voluntary and private homes and places at 31 March 1991. England.* A/F 91/11A. London: Department of Health.

62. Department of Health. *Residential accommodation for elderly people and people with physical and/or sensory disabilities: all residents in local authority, voluntary and private homes. Year ending 31 March 1989 to year ending 31 March 1994. England.* RA/89–94/2(H). London: Department of Health, 1995.

63. Department of Health and Social Security. *Homes and hostels for the mentally ill and the mentally handicapped, at 31 March 1985. England.* A/F 85/11. London: Department of Health and Social Security.

64. Department of Health. *Residential accommodation for mentally ill and mentally handicapped people: number of local authority, voluntary and private homes and places at 31 March 1987. England.* A/F 87/11A. London: Department of Health.

65. Department of Health. *A review of personal social services statistics.* London: Department of Health, August 1997.

66. Department of Health Social Services Inspectorate. *Almost half. Social services department inspection units – fourth overview 1996.* London: Department of Health, September 1996.

67. Department of Health. *Residential accommodation: detailed statistics on residential care homes and local authority supported residents, England 1995.* RA/95. London: Department of Health, 1996.

68. Department of Health. *Survey of age, sex and length of stay characteristics of residents of homes for elderly people and younger people who are physically handicapped in England at 31st March 1988.* London: Department of Health.

69. Department of Health. *Residential accommodation: detailed statistics on residential care homes and local authority supported residents, England 1996.* RA/96. London: Department of Health, 1997.

70. Department of Health. Personal social services: residential accommodation in

England 1993. *Statistical Bulletin*, 1994/2. London: Department of Health, March 1994.

71. Department of Health. Personal social services: residential accommodation in England 1994. *Statistical Bulletin*, 1994/13. London: Department of Health, November 1994.

72. Department of Social Security Analytical Services Division. *Income support statistics quarterly enquiry, November 1999*. Newcastle upon Tyne: Department of Social Security, 2000.

73. Department of Health. *Residential accommodation for all client groups: admissions to local authority, voluntary and private homes, 1994. England.* London: Department of Health, 1995.

74. Department of Health. Personal social services staff of social services departments at 30 September 1998. England. *Statistical Bulletin*, 1999/8. London: Department of Health, March 1999.

75. Department of Health and Social Security. *Independent sector hospitals, nursing homes and clinics in England. A national and regional analysis of information recorded on form SBH 212 about institutions registered with English district health authorities under the Nursing Homes Act 1975 on 31 December 1982.* London: Department of Health and Social Security.

76. Department of Health. *Private hospitals, homes and clinics registered under Section 23 of the Registered Homes Act 1984. England – Position at 31 March 1992.* London: Department of Health, 1993.

77. Laing and Buisson. *Laing's review of private healthcare 1988/89 and directory of independent hospitals, nursing and residential homes and related services. Volume 2. Long-term health and social care.* London: Laing and Buisson, 1988.

78. Larder D, Day P, Klein R. *Institutional care for the elderly: the geographical distribution of the public/private mix in England.* Bath Social Policy Papers No. 10. Bath: Centre for the Analysis of Social Policy, University of Bath, 1986.

79. Department of Health. *Private hospitals, homes and clinics registered under Section 23 of the Registered Homes Act 1984. Volume 1 – England, regional health authorities and regional office areas. Financial year 1993–94.* London: Department of Health, 1995.

80. Department of Health. *Private hospitals, homes and clinics registered under Section 23 of the Registered Homes Act 1984, Volume 2 – District Health Authority Summaries. Financial Year 1993–94.* London: Department of Health, 1995.

81. Department of Health. *Private hospitals, homes and clinics registered under Section 23 of the Registered Homes Act 1984, England, 1996. Statistical Bulletin*, 1997/5. London: Department of Health, March 1997.

82. Department of Health. *Residential accommodation statistics 1996. Personal social services: residential care homes and supported residents, England. Statistical Bulletin*, 1996/25. London: Department of Health, December 1996.

83. Jackson G, Lewis C. Local government reorganisation in Scotland and Wales. *Population Trends* 1996; **83**: 43–51.

84. Welsh Office. *Residential care homes and nursing homes in Wales: 1994.* Cardiff: Welsh Office, 1995.

85. Welsh Office. *Health and personal social services statistics for Wales.* No. 16, 1989. Cardiff: Welsh Office, 1990.

86. Welsh Office. *Health statistics Wales 1996.* Cardiff: Welsh Office, 1997.

87. Welsh Office. *Social services statistics Wales 1999.* Cardiff: Welsh Office, 1999.

88. Welsh Office. *Digest of Welsh local area statistics 1997.* Cardiff: Welsh Office, 1997.

89. Welsh Office. *Health statistics Wales 1997.* Cardiff: Welsh Office, 1998.

90. Welsh Office. *Health statistics Wales 1998.* Cardiff: Welsh Office, 1999.

91. Scottish Office. *Community care bulletin 1989–90. Statistical Bulletin*, No. CMC1/1991. Edinburgh: Scottish Office, December 1991.
92. Scottish Office. *Staff of Scottish social work departments, 1997. Statistical Bulletin*, No. SWK/S/1998/20. Edinburgh: Scottish Office, August 1998.
93. Scottish Office. *Community care, Scotland 1997. Statistical Bulletin*, No. SWK/CMC/1998/8. Edinburgh: Scottish Office, November 1998.
94. The National Health Service in Scotland Information and Statistics Division. *Scottish health statistics*. Edinburgh: ISD Publications, published annually.
95. Laing and Buisson. *Laing's healthcare market review 1998–99*. London: Laing and Buisson, 1998.
96. Department of Health. *Social services: achievement and challenge*. Cm 3588. London: TSO, 1997.

Acronyms

ADSS	Association of Directors of Social Services
AHC	after housing costs
ARIC	Atmospheric Research and Information Centre
BHC	before housing costs
CDR	Communicable Disease Report
CDSC	Communicable Disease Surveillance Centre
CEMD	Confidential Enquiry into Maternal Deaths
CESDI	Confidential Enquiry into Stillbirths and Deaths in Infancy
CHCS	child health computing system
CiN	children in need
CIPFA	Chartered Institute of Public Finance and Accountancy
CISH	Confidential Enquiry into Suicide and Homicide by People with Mental Illness
CJD	Creutzfeldt Jacob Disease
CLS	Centre for Longitudinal Studies
CO(NI)	Census Office (Northern Ireland)
COMEAP	Committee on the Medical Effects of Air Pollutants
COPPISH	Core Patient Profile Information in Scottish Hospitals
CRI	Chemical Release Inventory
DCO	death certificate only
DETR	Department of the Environment, Transport and The Regions
DfEE	Department for Education and Employment
DH	Department of Health
DSS	Department of Social Security
EHCS	English House Condition Survey
EL	executive letter
EPIC	European Prospective Investigation into Cancer and Nutrition
FES	Family Expenditure Survey
FHS	family health services
FRS	Family Resources Survey
GDP	gross domestic product
GHS	General Household Survey
GP	general practitioner
GRO	general register office
GRO(S)	General Register Office for Scotland
GUM	genitourinary medicine
HBAI	households below average income
HCS	housing and construction statistics
HES	hospital episode statistics
HMSO	Her Majesty's Stationery Office
HSE	Health and Safety Executive
ICD	International Classification of Diseases
ICIDH	International Classification of Impairments, Disabilities and Handicaps
IIAC	Industrial Injuries Advisory Council
IIS	Industrial Injuries Scheme
ILO	International Labour Organisation

IPC	integrated pollution control
IPPC	integrated pollution prevention control
IS	income support
ISD	Information and Statistics Division of the Common Services Agency for the NHS in Scotland
JSA	Job Seekers Allowance
JUVOS	Joint Unemployment and Vacancies Operating System
LATS	London area travel survey
LFS	Labour Force Survey
LGMB	Local Government Management Board
LIF	low income families
LS	Longitudinal Study
MAFF	Ministry of Agriculture, Fisheries and Food
MIMAS	Manchester Information and Associated Services
MOSA	Medical Officers of Schools Association
MRC	Medical Research Council
NAQS	National Air Quality Strategy
NDNS	national diet and nutrition surveys
NFS	National Food Survey
NHS	National Health Service
NHSE	National Health Service Executive
NHSiS	National Health Service in Scotland
NI	Northern Ireland
NIC	National Insurance contribution
NISRA	Northern Ireland Statistics and Research Agency
NOMIS	National Online Manpower Information System
NTS	National Travel Survey
ONS	Office for National Statistics
OPCS	Office of Population Censuses and Surveys
PAHs	polyaromatic hydrocarbons
PHLS	Public Health Laboratory Service
PM	particulate matter
PSS	personal social services
RCGP	Royal College of General Practitioners
RG	registrar general
RHA	regional health authority
RIDDOR	Reporting of Injuries, Disease and Dangerous Occurrences
RSC	Royal Society of Chemistry
SARs	samples of anonymised records
SB	supplementary benefit
SCIEH	Scottish Centre for Infection and Environmental Health
SEC	socio-economic class
SEG	socio-economic group
SEH	Survey of English Housing
SMR	standardised mortality ratio
SSD	social services department
STD	sexually transmitted disease
TB	tuberculosis
TRI	toxics release inventory
TSO	The Stationery Office
TTWA	travel to work area
WHO	World Health Organisation
WiE	workforce in employment
WRS	weekly return service

Index